Contemporary Occupational Health Psychology

Contemporary Occupational Health Psychology

Global Perspectives on Research and Practice, Volume 1

Edited by Jonathan Houdmont
and Stavroula Leka

⊛WILEY-BLACKWELL

A John Wiley & Sons, Ltd., Publication

Registered Office
John Wiley & Sons Ltd, The Atrium, Southern Gate, Chichester, West Sussex, PO19 8SQ, UK

Editorial Offices
The Atrium, Southern Gate, Chichester, West Sussex, PO19 8SQ, UK
9600 Garsington Road, Oxford, OX4 2DQ, UK
350 Main Street, Malden, MA 02148-5020, USA

For details of our global editorial offices, for customer services, and for information about how to apply for permission to reuse the copyright material in this book please see our website at www.wiley.com/wiley-blackwell.

Library of Congress Cataloging-in-Publication Data

Contemporary occupational health psychology / edited by Jonathan Houdmont and Stavroula Leka.
  v. ; cm.
  Includes bibliographical references and index.
  Contents: v 1. Global perspectives on research and practice.
  ISBN 978-0-470-68265-4 (hardcover : alk. paper)
  1. Job stress. 2. Psychology, Industrial. 3. Clinical health psychology. I. Houdmont, Jonathan. II. Leka, Stavroula.
  HF5548.85.C654 2010
  158.7–dc22

                                                                    2010003196

A catalogue record for this book is available from the British Library.

Set in 10.5/13pt Minion by SPi Publisher Services, Pondicherry, India
Printed in the UK

1 2010

To those whose progress through the ranks of the occupational health psychology research group at the Institute of Work, Health, & Organisations preceded mine: thank you for the introduction to the discipline, friendship, and support.

Jonathan

To all those who strive to make work what it should be: meaningful and inspiring.

Stavroula

Contents

About the Editors

Jonathan Houdmont
jonathan.houdmont@nottingham.ac.uk

Stavroula Leka
stavroula.leka@nottingham.ac.uk

Institute of Work, Health and Organisations, University of Nottingham, International House, Jubilee Campus, Wollaton Road, Nottingham, NG8 1BB, U.K.

Jonathan Houdmont BSc PGCE MSc PhD is a Lecturer in Occupational Health Psychology in the Institute of Work, Health, and Organisations at the University of Nottingham (U.K.). He earned his BSc in Psychology at the University of Leeds, postgraduate certificate in further and adult education (PGCE) at the University of Keele, followed by an MSc and PhD in occupational health psychology at the University of Nottingham. He is director of the Institute's Masters in Workplace Health. His current research interests focus on legal and policy issues in occupational health, specifically in relation to work-related stress, and the discipline of occupational health psychology with particular emphasis on education and training. He is the author of several journal papers, edited books, chapters, and commissioned reports on these topics. Jonathan is Executive Officer of the European Academy of Occupational Health Psychology. He has been the Academy's conference coordinator, having led the delivery of international conferences in Berlin (2003), Oporto (2004), Dublin (2006), and Valencia (2008). He is coeditor of *Occupational Health Psychology*, also published by Wiley-Blackwell. Further information about Jonathan and his work can be found at www.nottingham.ac.uk/iwho/people/

Stavroula Leka BA MSc PhD PGCHE CPsychol FRSPH is Associate Professor in Occupational Health Psychology in the Institute of Work, Health, and Organisations at the University of Nottingham (U. K.). She is director of the Institute's Masters in Occupational Health Psychology. Stavroula is a Chartered Psychologist, a Member of the British Psychological Society, the International Commission on Occupational Health, the European Association of Work & Organizational Psychology, and the European Academy of Occupational Health Psychology, and a Fellow of the Royal Society for the Promotion of Public Health. She studied psychology at the American College of Greece, followed by postgraduate studies in occupational health psychology at the Institute. Stavroula is Director of the Institute's World Health Organization Programme. She is a member of the Planning Committee of the WHO Network of Collaborating Centres in Occupational Health and Director of its programme of work on "Practical Approaches to Identify and Reduce Occupational Risks." She is Chair of the Education Forum of the European Academy of Occupational Health Psychology and secretary of the scientific committee Work Organization & Psychosocial Factors of the International Commission on Occupational Health. Stavroula's main research interests are the translation of occupational health and safety knowledge and policy into practice and psychosocial risk management. Her research is well published and she has been keynote speaker at a number of international conferences. She is coeditor of *Occupational Health Psychology*, also published by Wiley-Blackwell. Further information about Stavroula and her work can be found at www.nottingham.ac.uk/iwho/people/

Contributors

Carl Åborg

carl.aborg@ki.se
Karolinska Institute, Sweden

Yael Bacharach

yaelbacharach@nyc.rr.com
Cornell University, USA

Arnold B. Bakker

bakker@fsw.eur.nl
Erasmus University Rotterdam, The Netherlands

Peter Bamberger

peterb@tx.technion.ac.il
Technion: Israel Institute of Technology, Israel

Peggy Bernin

peggy@bernin.se
Stockholm University, Sweden

Michal Biron

m.biron@uvt.nl
Tilburg University, The Netherlands

Frank W. Bond

f.bond@gold.ac.uk
Goldsmiths, University of London, United Kingdom

Benjamin Brooks

b.brooks@amc.edu.au
Australian Maritime College, University of
Tasmania, Australia

Christine Busch

cbusch@uni-hamburg.de
University of Hamburg, Germany

Sara Casenave

casenave@ull.es
University of La Laguna, Spain

Karl Bang Christensen

k.christensen@biostat.ku.dk
University of Copenhagen, Denmark

Evangelia Demerouti   *e.demerouti@uu.nl*
                           Utrecht University, The Netherlands

Dolores Díaz-Cabrera   *mddiaz@ull.es*
                           University of La Laguna, Spain

Maureen F. Dollard   *maureen.dollard@unisa.edu.au*
                           University of South Australia

Antje Ducki   *ducki@beuth-hochschule.de*
                           University of Applied Sciences, Berlin, Germany

Paul E. Flaxman   *Paul.Flaxman.1@city.ac.uk*
                           City University, London, U.K.

Maya Golan   *mgolan@tx.technion.ac.il*
                           Technion: Israel Institute of Technology, Israel

Leslie B. Hammer   *hammerl@pdx.edu*
                           Portland State University, USA

Estefanía Hernández-Fernaud *efernaud@ull.es*
                           University of La Laguna, Spain

Aditya Jain   *aditya.jain@nottingham.ac.uk*
                           University of Nottingham, U.K.

Maria Karanika-Murray   *maria.karanika-murray@ntu.ac.uk*
                           Nottingham Trent University, U.K.

Robert A. Karasek   *robert_karasek@uml.edu*
                           University of Massachusetts Lowell, USA

Michiel A.J. Kompier   *m.kompier@psych.ru.nl*
                           Radboud University Nijmegen, The Netherlands

Stavroula Leka   *Stavroula.leka@nottingham.ac.uk*
                           University of Nottingham, U.K.

Karina Nielsen   *kmn@nrcwe.dk*
                           National Research Centre for the Working Environment, Denmark

Anna Nyberg   *anna.nyberg@ki.se*
                           Stockholm University and Karolinska Institute, Sweden

Gabriel Oxenstierna   *gabriel.oxenstierna@stressforskning.su.se*
                           Stockholm University, Sweden

Jane Parent   *parentj@merrimack.edu*
                           Merrimack College, USA

Tahira Probst

probst@vancouver.wsu.edu
Washington State University Vancouver, USA

Yeray Ramos-Sapena

yramos@ull.es
University of La Laguna, Spain

Raymond Randall

rjr15@leicester.ac.uk
University of Leicester, U.K.

Julia Romanowska

julia@romanowska.com
Stockholm University, Sweden

Susanne Roscher

susanne.roscher@vbg.de
Verwaltungs-Berufsgenossenschaft, Germany

Wilmar B. Schaufeli

w.schaufeli@uu.nl
Utrecht University, The Netherlands

Arie Shirom

ashirom@post.tau.ac.il
Tel-Aviv University, Israel

Robert R. Sinclair

rsincla@clemson.edu
Clemson University, USA

Lindsay E. Sears

lesears@clemson.edu
Clemson University, USA

Henning Staar

henning.staar@uni-hamburg.de
University of Hamburg, Germany

Alice Staniford

alistaniford@hotmail.com
PKF Organisation Development, Australia

Toon W. Taris

t.taris@uu.nl
Radboud University Nijmegen and Utrecht
University, The Netherlands

Noreen Tehrani

ntehrani@btinternet.com
Child Exploitation and Online Protection
Centre, U.K.

Töres Theorell

tores.theorell@ki.se
Stockholm University and Karolinska Institute, Sweden

Machteld van den Heuvel

m.vandenHeuvel@uu.nl
Utrecht University, The Netherlands

Ingrid van der Wal

ivanderwal@abvakabo.nl
Radboud University Nijmegen, The Netherlands

Marc van Veldhoven

m.j.p.m.vanveldhoven@uvt.nl
Tilburg University, The Netherlands

Hugo Westerlund

hugo.westerlund@stressforskning.su.se
Stockholm University, Sweden

Richard J. Wiseman

richard.wiseman@unisa.edu.au
University of South Australia

Mark Zajack

mzajack@clemson.edu
Clemson University, USA

Kristi L. Zimmerman

kzimmerm@pdx.edu
Portland State University, USA

Gerard Zwetsloot

gerard.zwetsloot@tno.nl
TNO Work and Employment, The Netherlands

Preface

Welcome to the first volume of *Contemporary occupational health psychology: Global perspectives on research and practice*. This groundbreaking biennial series is published by Wiley-Blackwell on behalf of the European Academy of Occupational Health Psychology and the Society for Occupational Health Psychology. We would like to use this foreword to introduce the series and share with you its aspirations.

Contemporary occupational health psychology has the following goals:

1. To publish authoritative, "stand-alone," reviews in the field of occupational health psychology.
2. To publish new empirical research, where it is appropriate to do so, to enable contributors to advance the field in ways that are not typically possible within the confines of the traditional journal article. This applies particularly to developments in professional practice, education, and training.
3. To attract contributions from an international constituency of experts which, in time, become citation classics.
4. To include topics of contemporary relevance to the interests and activities of occupational health psychology researchers, practitioners, educators, and students.

As such, each chapter:

1. contains a comprehensive state-of-the-art review of the literature in a topic area.
2. where appropriate, reports on new empirical data generated by the author.
3. places an emphasis on the organizational application of theory and evidence with a view towards bridging the science/practitioner divide.
4. is written in an accessible style.

In sum, the series aspires to nothing less than to emerge as *the* major reference work of choice for those with an active interest in occupational health psychology.

To achieve these goals the editors are assisted by an Advisory Board. As the series develops, this distinguished group of individuals will play a pivotal role in ensuring that it lives up to expectations and publishes contributions of the highest quality and contemporary relevance. The Advisory Board comprises:

Tom Cox	University of Nottingham, U.K.
Michiel Kompier	Radboud University Nijmegen, the Netherlands
Tage Kristensen	Task-Consult, Denmark
Jose Maria Peiro	University of Valencia, Spain
Steve Sauter	National Institute for Occupational Safety and Health, USA
Lois Tetrick	George Mason University, USA
Töres Theorell	Karolinska Institute, Sweden

As it grows, the series will address a wide range of contemporary topics that concern the application of psychological principles and practices to occupational health challenges and opportunities. Contributions are evaluated on the following criteria:

1. contemporary relevance of the topic to the activities of researchers, educators, practitioners, and students
2. appropriateness and strength of the literature review
3. conceptual strength
4. strength of methodology and data analysis (where a contribution contains new empirical data)
5. quality of writing
6. implications for professional practice.

The focus on topics that are of contemporary relevance ensures that the series remains a useful guide to developments in the field of occupational health psychology. Authors interested in contributing to the series should contact the first editor at jonathan.houdmont@nottingham.ac.uk to discuss ideas. We intend to commission approximately 15 chapters for publication in the second volume that will be launched at the 2012 conference of the European Academy of Occupational Health Psychology. We look forward to reviewing your excellent work.

Finally, a few words of thanks. We would like to express our deep gratitude to Darren Reed, Commissioning Editor for Psychology Books at Wiley-Blackwell, who, from the start, has demonstrated nothing but enthusiasm and support for our desire to take occupational health psychology to a wide audience. Thanks are also due to the European Academy of Occupational Health Psychology and the Society for Occupational Health Psychology; without the endorsement of these representative bodies this project would not have come into being. We are also grateful to Tom Cox, Director of the Institute of Work, Health & Organisations at the University of Nottingham. When presented with the idea for this series Tom immediately perceived value in the endeavor, and has supported us unrelentingly in its gestation.

Jonathan Houdmont and Stavroula Leka

1

A Multilevel Model of Economic Stress and Employee Well-Being

Robert R. Sinclair, Lindsay E. Sears, and Mark Zajack
Clemson University, USA

Tahira Probst
Washington State University Vancouver, USA

We write this chapter in the midst of a global economic crisis; international markets and financial systems have been disrupted and many companies have struggled, not always with successful outcomes. For example, a recent U.S. Bureau of Labor Statistics report (Bureau of Labor Statistics, 2009c) indicated that in the first quarter of 2009, 3,489 mass layoff events resulted in some 550,000 workers being separated from their jobs for at least 31 days, the most since the BLS began tracking these numbers in 1996. Many other workers now hold positions that are below their desired level of pay, responsibility, or hours of work; still others have given up searching for employment. As of May 2009, the U.S. labor force included 2.2 million marginally attached[1] workers, a 177% increase from the previous year, and 9.1 million workers in involuntary part-time positions, an increase of 4.4 million between December 2007 and May 2009. Including such underemployed, marginally attached, and discouraged workers yields a May 2009 unemployment rate of 16.4% for the United States (BLS, 2009a).

Of course, such trends are not limited to the United States; the International Labour Organization (ILO, 2009) predicted that 2009 would be the worst year for global job creation since it began keeping records in 1991. As many as 1.5 to 1.6 billion workers are in vulnerable employment worldwide, or up to 52.8 percent of the global workforce (ibid.). These workers are less likely to earn an adequate income, more likely to experience labor rights violations, and less able to protect themselves from abuse (ILO, 2009; U.K. Department of Trade and Industry, 2006). The financial crisis also has placed additional downward pressure on wages and the ILO estimates that between 38% and 45% of the world's workforce would meet the definition of "working poor" (i.e., people who earn less than US$2 per day) by the end of 2009. Worse, as many as 200 million workers, mostly in developing countries, could be pushed into extreme poverty (US$1.25, or less, per day). The downward trends of 2008–2009 seem unlikely to be permanent and, even as we write, there are some initial signs of economic recovery. However, international markets seem unlikely to reach the peaks of 2007 any time soon, and many important economic actors, such as banks and auto companies, seem likely to struggle well into the future.

Occupational Health Psychology (OHP) researchers have long recognized the threat of job insecurity, unemployment, and under-employment to employee well-being. Other important economic stress concerns have received less attention, such as workers' current financial status (including both household income and debt), their worries about financial issues, and, particularly in the United States, the large share of medical care costs borne by workers. One important challenge for researchers is that economic stressors result from interactions between multiple systems operating at different levels of analysis. Therefore, the central purpose of this chapter is to develop a multilevel model that describes the relationship between economic stress and well-being. We will extend a model of economic stress proposed by Probst (2005a), distinguishing individual, organizational, and macroeconomic antecedents of employees' economic stress. We also suggest several moderators of the effects of these antecedents and propose a multilevel framework for conceptualizing economic stress interventions.

Defining Economic Stress

Probst (2005a) drew from prior work by Voydanoff (1990) to offer a general definition of economic stress as "aspects of economic life that are potential stressors for employees and their families and consists of both objective and subjective components reflecting the employment and income dimensions of the worker-earner role" (p. 268). Probst distinguished employment-related and income-related stressors, both of which may be further divided into objective and subjective stressors. Thus, unemployment (i.e., actual loss of one's job) is an objective employment stressor whereas job insecurity is a subjective employment stressor. Similarly, economic deprivation concerns the objective inability to meet current financial needs whereas economic strain concerns the perceived inadequacy of one's income. A sizable body of literature indicates that employment stressors are associated with poor job attitudes and performance, lower physical and mental health, higher turnover intentions (e.g., Cheng & Chan, 2008; Feldman, 1996; Hanisch, 1999; McKee-Ryan, Song, Wanberg, & Kinicki, 2005; Sverke, Hellgren, & Näswell, 2002) and even a higher risk of death by suicide and homicide (Stuckler, Basu, Suhrcke, Coutts, & McKee, 2009). In contrast, the income-related stress literature is more fragmented and includes fewer studies directly related to OHP.

Sears' (2008) review of the income-related stress literature highlights the many ways researchers have measured objective income stressors, including total household income (e.g., Sinclair & Martin, 2006), financial resources (e.g., Conger et al., 1990), debt-to-asset ratios (e.g., Simons, Lorenz, Conger, & Wu, 1992), and composite measures of financial need based on demographic variables such as marital status and family size (e.g., Brett, Cron, & Slocum, 1995; Doran, Stone, Brief, & George, 1991; Shaw & Gupta, 2001). Sears also distinguished the affective and cognitive

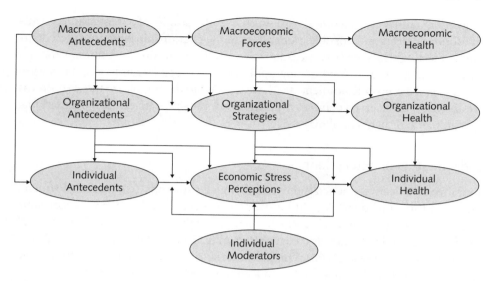

Figure 1.1   A Multilevel Model of Economic Stress

components of subjective income stressors. She defined *financial strain* as an affective construct consisting of negative emotional reactions related to one's current financial status. In contrast, she described *perceived income adequacy* (PIA) as a cognitive construct consisting of evaluations of one's current and expected future ability to afford basic living needs (PIA-needs), and the ability to afford current and future lifestyle desires (PIA-wants). This wide range of measurement options highlights the need for further attention to the connections between economic stress constructs, a point we return to later.

Figure 1.1. portrays a multilevel model of economic stressors that integrates macroeconomic processes, organizational policies and practices, and individual psychological processes. This model serves as a heuristic device highlighting the idea that individuals' economic stress perceptions are embedded in personal, organizational, and macroeconomic contexts. Each level of analysis shares the common theme of intervening processes linking antecedents to outcomes, albeit with considerably different variables at each level.

The Individual Level

Our central focus is on the individual level of analysis. Probst (2005a) discussed several individual outcomes of economic stress, including lower physical and psychological health, higher family/friendship strain and marital distress, poor job attitudes, more work withdrawal, and less workplace safety. Our model assumes that subjective economic stress mediates the relationship between personal economic antecedents and these outcomes. We discuss several examples of potential antecedents of economic stress and possible moderators of the relationship between antecedents and subjective stress, or between subjective stress and health outcomes. Although some research has examined demographic variables such as gender (e.g., Jacobson et al., 1996; Mauno & Kinnunen, 2002), we decided to de-emphasize those studies as we assume that observed demographic differences are indicative of some underlying psychological or behavioral difference.

Individual-level antecedents

Employees' objective financial and employment situations (e.g., unemployment, household income, debt) should be strongly associated with subjective economic stress (e.g., McKee-Ryan et al., 2005; So-hyun & Grable, 2004) as should individual differences in saving tendencies (e.g., Anderson & Nevitte, 2006), or debt accumulation (e.g., Norvilitis et al., 2006). This literature suggests the need for attention to the role of financial knowledge, skills, and abilities (KSAs) in economic stress (e.g., Howlett, Kees, & Kemp, 2008). As knowledge of sound financial principles and strategies increases, people should be less likely to make bad financial decisions. Thus, they should have better objective financial situations and, as a result, lower subjective financial stress. Consistent with this idea, consumer science literature has demonstrated positive effects for financial education programs (Fox, Bartholomae, & Lee, 2005). Although such programs cannot completely overcome the effects of severe income deprivation or extended unemployment, they can help employees make the best of bad situations.

Personality traits also may contribute to economic stress by making employees more vulnerable to subjective economic stress either through their more negative appraisals of the environment or their own ability to manage the environment. Research has examined three clusters of these traits: traits affecting the anxiety people experience in relation to stressors, such as neuroticism (Tivendell, & Bourbonnais, 2000), and tolerance for ambiguity (Adkins, Werbel, & Farh, 2001); traits reflecting employees' sense of control over their financial situation, such as locus of control (van Hooft & Crossley, 2008); and traits concerning employees' general sense of their self-worth, such as self-esteem (Lee, Bobko, & Chen, 2006; Mauno & Kinnunen, 2002; Pearlin, Lieberman, Menaghan, & Mullan, 1981). All of these traits reflect vulnerability to psychosocial threat, and most either directly or implicitly fit with research on core-self evaluations (CSE, cf. Judge & Bono, 2001). CSE research posits that people have general tendencies to appraise themselves and their environments positively or negatively and to feel in control of and capable of responding to environmental demands. Thus, low CSE should be associated with higher subjective financial stress. Consistent with this idea, Judge, Hurst, and Simon (2009) found that higher CSE was associated with lower financial strain, both directly and indirectly through a positive relationship between CSE and income. Thus, we would encourage economic stress researchers to examine CSE in future research.

Individual-level moderators

Relationships between economic stress and outcomes may depend on several individual factors, although research on any particular factor is limited and sometimes yields inconsistent conclusions. For example, some studies show that the relationship between financial stress and outcomes may not differ across gender (e.g., Elliot, 2001). However others report both age and gender interactions, such that the negative effects of job insecurity may be strongest for older workers in general (Finegold, Mohrman, & Spreitzer, 2002) and older women in particular (Rugulies, Aust, Burr, & Bültmann, 2008). Other research has found that personality traits moderate the relationship between economic stress and outcomes. Most of this research fits the CSE framework described above, including the moderating effects of self-efficacy (Adebayo, 2006), control (Creed & Bartrum, 2008), and control-focused coping (Wadsworth & Santiago, 2008). Finally, social support appears to protect people from the negative mental health outcomes of economic stress (Crosier, Butterworth, & Rodgers, 2007; Ferraro & Su, 1999). Supervisor and coworker support also appear to buffer negative effects of job insecurity (Lim, 1997), and interpersonal conflict exacerbates the negative effects of financial stress (Skinner, Zautra, & Reich, 2004). Research in each of these areas suggests promising findings, but there remains a definite need for more empirical studies.

The Organizational Level

The organizational level concerns the policies and practices organizations use to respond to changing competitive conditions and environmental constraints. Organizational theorists have described the strategies organizations use to adapt to their environments and defined several effectiveness criteria, including stakeholder satisfaction, goal accomplishment, market share, and long-term survival (Daft, 1995). The American Psychological Association has also developed a *Psychologically Healthy Workplace Award* program (www.phwa.org) which includes criteria such as work–life balance, workplace safety, and employee development, involvement, and recognition. Organizational variables may influence employees through several pathways, including (1) effects on individual economic antecedents, (2) direct influences on subjective economic stress, (3) moderating relationships between individual-level antecedents, responses, and outcomes, or (4) influences on individual-level moderators. Some of these pathways have been studied extensively, and others not at all.

Organization-level antecedents

Many organizational characteristics may influence economic stress. For example, research shows higher job security for people working in state-owned firms in China (Gong & Chang, 2008) and public sector employees in Finland (Mauno & Kinnunen,

2002), compared with employees in nonstate-owned and private sector organizations, respectively. An organization's financial status is perhaps its most important characteristic, as it influences organizational policies and practices likely to affect employees' economic stress.

Improving financial performance boils down two basic strategies: increasing revenue and reducing costs. Worker pay and benefits account for a large share of operating expenses, leading companies to cut costs through workforce reductions or downsizing (Said, Le Louarn, & Tremblay, 2007) and related strategies, such as mergers. Such practices create considerable stress for employees (Ashford, Lee, & Bobko, 1989; Probst, 2002; Reisel et al., 2003; Sverke et al., 2002) as they redefine the work environment (Ahuja & Katila, 2001), increase role stressors (Jimmieson, Terry, & Callan 2004) and reduce employee commitment (e.g., Brotheridge, 2003; Dackert, Jackson, Brenner, & Johansson, 2003). These human costs are particularly unfortunate given that reorganization does not always achieve its intended goals (Cascio, 2002; Said, 2007). Even when downsizing yields gains in profitability, the gains may be short-lived (McKinley, Sanchez, & Schick, 1995) and often harm a firm's reputation (Love & Kraatz, 2009).

Organization-level moderators

Organizational-level moderators influence the individual-level relationship between antecedents and subjective stressors or between stressors and outcomes. For example, income-related stressors might have stronger effects on well-being for workers in a declining industry because the stress caused by income deprivation might be exacerbated by their limited future prospects. Two examples of organization-level moderators with at least some empirical support concern participative management and organizational justice.

Regarding participative management, the Job Demand–Control model (Karasek, 1979) proposes that jobs vary in their levels of demands (i.e., stressors) and workers' level of control (Wall, Jackson, Mullarkey, & Parker, 1996). Probst (2005b) found that employees who perceived high control, defined as greater perceived input into organizational decision-making processes, experienced fewer negative outcomes from perceived job insecurity. Such findings suggest that participative decision making offers employees a chance to regain a sense of control that might be lost because of job insecurity.

The organizational justice literature concerns employees' perceived treatment at work, and thus reflects individuals' reactions to organizational policies and practices. Colquitt, Conlon, Wesson, Porter, and Ng (2001) described four components of organizational justice. *Distributive justice* refers to the fairness of outcomes that employees receive in comparison to their coworkers, personal standards, or their perceived contributions. *Procedural justice* describes the extent to which organizational procedures are applied consistently, are unbiased, and provide employees with opportunities for input. People tend to perceive higher levels of *interpersonal fairness* when they are treated respectfully during the implementation of procedures, and higher levels of *informational justice* when they receive timely explanations for decisions that affect them.

Justice can help both victims and survivors experience fewer adverse consequences from layoffs (e.g., Brockner, et al., 1994). For example, the effects of organizational change on employees may depend on the extent to which they receive sufficient and accurate information about the changes (Adkins, Werbel, & Farh, 2001). Regarding fairness and financial stress, research has shown that pay fairness predicts performance and well-being outcomes (e.g., Shaw & Gutpa, 2001) but further investigation of both direct and moderating effects is needed. Important questions remain about contemporary compensation issues such as furloughs (i.e., mandatory unpaid days off), cuts to health benefits, and disparities between executive and nonexecutive compensation.

The Macroeconomic Level

We define the macroeconomic level broadly to include economic systems, cultural issues, and industry-level influences. These factors influence economic growth and contraction through basic market forces such as supply and demand and include factors such as monetary policies, industry practices, and international trade/regulatory agreements. Macroeconomic health outcomes include objective economic well-being indicators such as gross domestic product and employment rates as well as subjective indicators such as consumer confidence (cf. www.confidence-board.org).

Macroeconomic forces affect individuals both directly and indirectly. The direct effects refer to individuals' reactions to macroeconomic conditions, such as when income-related stress stems from perceptions of regional or national economic conditions. Indirect effects operate through changes in organizational strategy, such as when organizations introduce furloughs as a strategic response to declining revenues. Finally, our model highlights the possibility of cross-level interactions. For example, reorganization may only lead to improved organizational health when there are concomitant macroeconomic improvements. Similarly, objective economic stressors might have stronger negative effects when employees anticipate that their organization's financial condition is likely to worsen in the future.

Macroeconomic antecedents

Both national/regional and industry-level unemployment rates provide useful indications of macroeconomic conditions related to employment (Reynolds, 1997). As unemployment rates rise, workers become more concerned about losing their jobs. Such changes should affect the perceived value of one's current job as they are associated with fewer employment alternatives and more competition for available openings. Organizations also typically change their staffing practices in a poor economic environment, employing more part-time/contingent workers or offering lower wages to new employees. Although we know of no research specifically on income-related stressors, macroeconomic conditions, such as real-estate or fuel costs, may also contribute to occupational health, particularly for lower income workers.

Macroeconomic moderators

Little research has examined the effects of cultural, socio-economic, and/or political systems on economic stress. However, cultural variables offer a promising direction for future research. Culture influences how people process information, specifying what people notice and how events are evaluated, and prescribing guiding principles and values (Triandis, 1995). Cultural values also influence job-related expectations (Hui, 1990) possibly influencing economic stress by shaping perceptions of and expectations about economic security.

Individualism/collectivism is perhaps the most frequently studied cultural dimension (Hofstede, 1980; Kagitcibasi & Berry, 1989; Triandis, 1995). Hofstede (1980) found that people from collectivist cultures place greater emphasis on job security and good working conditions (Oyserman et al., 2002), whereas people from individualistic cultures value autonomy and task variety. Because they value security, people from collectivistic cultures should be strongly threatened by employment and income-related stressors (cf. Probst & Lawler, 2006). Probst and Lawler (2006) suggest that the negative effects of job insecurity, long identified in the Western literature, may be exhibited to an even greater extent in the Chinese culture where expectations for job security were higher to begin with, but are no longer being met.

A less studied but equally pertinent cultural variable is uncertainty avoidance. According to Hofstede (2001), uncertainty avoidance (UA) reflects the society's level of tolerance for unstructured, unknown, or surprising situations. One might expect people in high UA cultures to react more negatively to economic insecurity. However, high UA societies also may craft public policies that emphasize uncertainty reduction. Thus, high UA societies may create stronger social safety nets to buffer workers from negative consequences of economic stressors. For example, the International Labour Organization (2004) research distinguishes countries in terms of their emphasis on labor market security. *Pacesetting countries* (e.g., EU countries, Canada, Israel, Japan) demonstrate a strong constitutional and policy commitment to social welfare, and protect their citizens' economic security. The United States is described as a *pragmatist country* because of its relatively limited attention to workers' economic security and failure to ratify ILO conventions. *Conventional countries* (e.g., Russia, Eastern bloc nations) have relevant governmental policies but little actual economic security because of other governmental challenges. Finally, *much-to-be-done countries* (e.g., many African and Middle Eastern nations) neither have policies to promote economic security, nor do they score well on economic indicators such as GDP and unemployment.

Although little research links socio-economic and political factors to economic stress, one recent study compared reactions to job insecurity in Switzerland and the United States (König, Probst, Staffen, & Graso, 2009). Switzerland and the United States have very different social safety nets for workers. For example, unemployed Swiss workers receive at least 70% of their normal income for up to two years and with a maximum yearly benefit of SFr.100,800 (US$89,300). Such strong benefits would be inconceivable in the United States, where unemployment benefits provide an income at or below the poverty threshold. In addition, in Switzerland, losing one's job does not affect health insurance, as health insurance is compulsory. Although König et al. (2009) found that the Swiss were less tolerant of uncertainty, U.S. participants reported more negative consequences from job insecurity. These findings are consistent with the idea that cultural differences shape public policy responses to economic insecurity, indicating the need for further attention to the socio-cultural context of economic stress.

Economic Stress Interventions

As with most areas of occupational health, there is a pressing need for empirically supported economic stress interventions. Table 1.1. depicts an organizational framework of interventions according to the type of prevention, the agent responsible for implementing the intervention, and the beneficiary of the intervention.

Table 1.1   A Multilevel Model of Economic Stress Interventions

Intervention level (goal)	Agent	Beneficiary	Example
Primary Promote employment and financial health	Organization	Individual	Financial education programs
		Organization	Employee furloughs
	Government	Individual	Government-sponsored skills development programs
		Organization	Economic development/ incentive programs
Secondary Promote coping in high-risk groups	Organization	Individual	Realistic merger & downsizing previews
		Organization	Downsizing/Restructuring
	Government	Individual	Targeted financial education for high risk groups
		Organization	Economic incentives (e.g., taxes) to support troubled local industries
Tertiary Restore health of the damaged	Organization	Individual	Psychological/Outplacement/ Financial counseling programs
		Organization	Reorganization (e.g., bankruptcy)
	Government	Individual	Unemployment benefits; Dislocated Worker Programs
		Organization	Bailout programs (e.g., the U.S. Troubled Asset Relief Program)

The prevention types include *primary prevention*, which concerns promoting employment and reducing income-related stress in the general population; *secondary prevention*, which includes efforts to encourage economic health in at-risk groups; and finally, *tertiary prevention*, which involves treatment to restore health among those who have experienced harm. We add intervention agents to the model to highlight the idea that while many interventions are implemented by management or its representatives (e.g., consultants, contractors), governments also shape economic health through regulation, public policy, and leadership. Finally, we distinguish between organizations and employees as the primary beneficiaries. Although some organizational changes may directly benefit employees (e.g., improved compensation), others cause considerable harm to a company's current workforce (e.g., when a company relocates overseas to save employment costs). Still other changes hurt employees in the short term while having long-term benefits (e.g., mandatory furloughs that reduce pay in the short term but possibly save jobs in the long run). We focus on three general clusters of economic stress interventions that require greater attention in OHP research: (1) financial education and counseling, (2) alternate staffing strategies, and (3) public policy interventions.

Financial education and counseling

Financial education and counseling programs may reflect primary, secondary, or tertiary prevention, depending on their focus. Francoeur (2001) notes the need for carefully planned proactive financial interventions that are tailored toward individuals' needs. Regarding primary prevention (e.g., teaching money management strategies), studies show that financial education can reduce financial stress (e.g., So-hyun & Grable, 2004) and have other benefits such as decreased absenteeism (Jacobson, Aldana, Goetzel, & Vardell, 1996), and increased employee satisfaction (Hira & Loibl, 2005). Less research has focused on secondary prevention, but some studies show the benefits of financial education interventions for high-risk groups (e.g., Lyons, Chang, & Scherpf, 2006 for low-income workers). Finally, people who are already in financial trouble or experiencing job insecurity may require tertiary prevention programs such as financial counseling or even general psychological counseling, given the links between economic stress and mental health (Chou & Chi, 1999; Mills, Grasmick, Morgan, & Wenk, 1992).

Alternate staffing strategies

Although restructuring and downsizing are the most familiar responses to performance downturns, organizations may use several other staffing strategies. Examples include hiring freezes, employee transfers, job sharing, temporary reductions in work hours, unpaid furloughs, part-time positions, early retirement, and sabbaticals. Each of these strategies may be regarded less negatively by employees when organizations seek employee participation as they consider options and seek fairness when programs are implemented. The Society for Human Resource Management (2009) conducted polls in October 2008 and March 2009 to determine how organizations were responding to the financial crisis. Along with budget cuts and attrition, layoffs were the most common initial reaction to the crisis. In October 2008, 48% of the firms had implemented layoffs, 48% had implemented hiring freezes, and only 3% had frozen wage increases. The March 2009 poll showed no change in the percentage of firms implementing layoffs (47%), but did reveal a 24% increase in retraining employees for new positions and a 46% increase in the use of freezing wages. While 44% of firms cut employee bonuses by March, only 18% had restructured executive compensation or severance packages. Creative solutions such as early retirement packages, furloughs, job sharing, or full-time telecommuting were instituted by 10% or less.

Irrespective of the strategy selected, organizations need to communicate effectively with their workforce about the nature of the changes (Bellarosa & Chen, 1997; Jones, 2003) to help reduce ambiguity and promote trust (Searle, & Ball, 2004). Human resources departments can help reduce employee strain during organizational change by encouraging effective organizational communication and ensuring that employees are treated with respect and dignity (Kickul, Lester, & Finkl, 2002; Teo & Waters, 2002). For example, Schweiger and DeNisi (1991) found that a "realistic merger preview" reduced the negative outcomes associated with a merger.

Public policy interventions

Public policy interventions may affect either individuals or organizations and may reflect primary, secondary, or tertiary prevention. Although OHP scholars encourage a focus on primary prevention, natural cyclical changes in local, national, and global economies preclude sole reliance on primary prevention. Additionally, unforeseen events such as natural disasters or large-scale terrorist attacks can wreak havoc on a nation's economy and require multifaceted responses. Therefore, public policy programs need to focus on all three forms of prevention.

At the primary level, many governments are developing and implementing "economic stimulus plans" to create employment and stem the tide of mass layoffs. Although some would argue that these are reactionary plans that respond to the current crisis, such plans could also be truly preventive in nature. Additionally, government entities often dedicate resources to attract individuals into high-demand and high-growth jobs that would, hopefully, be less susceptible to the vagaries of a poor economy. For example, the U.S. Department of Labor's (2009) *High Growth Job Training Initiative* targets worker training and career development resources to help workers gain skills needed for careers in growing industries such as health care, information technology, and advanced manufacturing. So-called "green jobs" programs (i.e., related to developing clean renewable energy) could be considered preventive as the green sector has experienced high rates of job growth over the past decade and seems to have been less affected by the current economic decline (The Pew Charitable Trusts, 2009). At the secondary level, governments can provide direct assistance to help individuals cope with economic stress. For example, the previous U.S. presidential administration sent several rounds of stimulus checks to families, hoping that consumers would use these funds to purchase goods, stimulating economic growth.

Such programs could be argued to represent either primary or secondary prevention, depending on a family's financial status. They also highlight the idea of interactions among the systems across levels of analysis, as the checks sent to individuals were anticipated to affect the health of the entire economy. Unfortunately, research suggests that tax rebates and tax cuts have relatively low return on investment (Zandi, 2008), highlighting the need for empirically supported approaches.

At the tertiary level, governments can develop programs to assist individuals who have lost their income source. For example, in the U.S., over 96% of waged and salaried civilian jobs are covered by unemployment insurance or unemployment compensation. Typically, 26 weeks of unemployment benefits are offered; however, in response to recent poor economic conditions, the federal government has extended these benefits by an additional 33 weeks and many states provide further coverage once workers have exhausted their federal benefits. As noted earlier, however, these benefits pale in comparison to those offered by most European countries. Moreover, most U.S. state and federal extended benefit programs are one-time programs that may not apply to future downturns. These differences between the U.S. and Europe are particularly notable because some research suggests that increasing unemployment benefits may be among the best ways to jump-start economic growth (Shapiro & Slemrod, 2003).

Governments can also provide retraining for laid-off workers to facilitate their entry into occupations with greater long-term growth potential. For example, the 1998 Workforce Investment Act provides block grants to U.S. states that target employment and training for dislocated workers, disadvantaged adults, and disadvantaged youth. Most of the dislocated worker funds go to local areas, which are responsible for providing re-employment services. A second example is the High Growth Job Training Initiative mentioned above that provides opportunities for dislocated workers by transitioning workers from declining industries into areas with future growth potential.

Research Directions

A multilevel approach raises interesting issues about the nature of economic stress as well as practical questions about the effects of economic stress on occupational health. We suggest three directions for future research that can contribute improved theory and help develop better interventions. These suggestions include (1) developing a better understanding of the mediating mechanisms that connect economic stressors to outcomes, (2) addressing methodological concerns in economic stress research, and (3) considering economic climate as an organizational construct.

Mediating mechanisms

Although not the explicit focus of this chapter, it is important to consider the mediating mechanisms that account for the negative outcomes individuals experience from economic stress. Organizations often lack feasible means to reduce job stress exposures (Schaubroeck & Merritt, 1997) and corporate downsizing is frequently a financial necessity. In addition, certain industries may be more vulnerable due to government deregulation, increasing globalization, and rapidly changing technology. Therefore, a better understanding of these mediating mechanisms might allow for the development of more effective interventions. Throughout this chapter we have discussed several theories and constructs that require more attention from economic stress researchers, including the Job Demand–Control model, core self-evaluations, and organizational justice. In this section, we discuss one additional model: Hobfoll's (2001) Conservation of Resources (COR) theory.

Hobfoll (2001) proposed that "people must invest resources in order to protect against resource loss, recover from losses, and gain resources" (p. 349). When their jobs are threatened, employees focus on (i.e., invest resources in) activities that best enable them to retain their job (i.e., protect against resource loss). For example, COR theory would predict that employees with high job insecurity will focus more on production and less on safety, because they perceive that investing effort in production is more likely to protect against further resource loss (i.e., job loss). Research largely supports this prediction, as several studies show that job insecurity is associated with negative safety attitudes, behaviors, and outcomes (Probst & Brubaker, 2001, 2007; Quinlan, 2005) and a greater focus on production at the expense of product quality (Probst, 2002). Interestingly, COR theory also provides an explanation for predicted employee withdrawal (lower commitment, higher absenteeism, etc.) in response to economic stress; under conditions of potential resource loss, withdrawal helps employees conserve psychological resources (cf. Grandey & Cropanzano, 1999; Leiter, 1991).

Methodological concerns

We see two primary methodological concerns for future economic stress research. First, a multilevel perspective on economic stress highlights the need for multilevel designs. Such designs have been used to model between and within individual differences simultaneously (e.g., Judge & Illes, 2004), and to study group-level aggregations of individual-level perceptions (e.g., Zohar & Luria, 2005). Economic stress research requires studies of different processes at each level, each of which is the domain of a different academic discipline. By highlighting the multilevel nature of economic stress, we have accomplished the easy task. Conducting multilevel studies is the harder challenge, as it involves a multidisciplinary approach as well as the ability to acquire distinctly different data at each level of analysis. However, one promising direction for such research would be studies that link large-scale survey data sets to other available data sources such as organizational records or government economic data.

A second issue concerns the need for better understanding of the relationships among economic stress measures. We have discussed several distinctions among economic stress measures, including employment versus income, future-oriented versus present-oriented, objective versus subjective, and wants versus needs. Other distinctions have been implied, such as direct (e.g., household income) versus indirect (e.g., composites of demographic variables). The need for greater conceptual clarity is a particularly vexing problem with regard to income-related stressors, as studies vary dramatically in the kinds of measures they use. Useful research directions include examining the relationship between measures of multiple economic stress constructs, accumulating data on single measures over several studies, and studying interactions between measures. This last issue presents a particularly interesting theoretical challenge, as it is unclear whether different kinds of economic measures function similarly for people in different economic circumstances. For example, do economic stressors lead to the same well-being outcomes for people in high- and low-income households?

Economic climate

OHP researchers have become increasingly interested in the effects of the shared perceptions of group members on outcomes in areas such as work stress (Tucker, Sinclair, & Thomas, 2005) and safety climate (Zohar, 2003). Future research could extend this idea to study the economic climate in an organization. Organizations often restructure by selling or otherwise disbanding large business units representing intact groups, such as by closing a factory or regional office or by selling a subsidiary. When organizations experience serious performance downturns, members of a business unit who share a common fate seem likely to form similar employment and income-related stress perceptions. We would refer to these shared perceptions as economic climate, defined as employees' shared concerns about their personal economic situation, to include both employment-related and income-related stressors.

Considering economic climate as a theoretical possibility raises interesting questions about how organizations manage meaning in relation to performance downturns. Economic research has long recognized the important role consumer confidence plays in economic health (www.confidence-board.org); confident consumers spend more and in doing so contribute to economic growth. But, what are the implications of such perceptual processes for how organizations respond to economic challenges? When organizations experience performance downturns should they be forthcoming and transparent about the negative state of the organization or should they continue to convey a sense of optimism about the future? Negative messages could be viewed as more credible, as employees are likely to recognize when their organization is in trouble. On the other hand, negative messages may create self-fulfilling prophesies, as employees who lose confidence in the organization are likely to consider other employment prospects and perhaps be less willing to exert extra effort on behalf of the organization. Literature on emotional contagion suggests that concerns about job insecurity or income-related stress are likely to spread through an organization through groups and informal networks (e.g., Hatfield, Cacioppo, & Rapson, 1994). Other research suggests such contagion effects at the industry level (Goins & Gruca, 2008) and family level (e.g., Mauno & Kinnunen, 2002). Organizational justice research on layoff survivors may provide some clues about these effects (cf., Skarlicki, Barclay, & Pugh, 2008), but there are clearly further opportunities to consider how people's optimism or pessimism fuels their future outcomes, as well as a need to consider how popular media messages may contribute to people's well-being at work.

Conclusion

Income is probably the strongest reason why people work and economic issues usually appear toward the top of lists of people's most important concerns. Thus, economic issues ought to be at the forefront of attention in OHP research. Our chapter highlights the idea that economic aspects of occupational health raise a complex set of concerns from multiple systems at different levels of analysis. However, our review barely scratched the surface of potentially relevant organizational theory and economics literature. The exciting part of this limitation is that it highlights the tremendous need for and potential benefits of multidisciplinary research in this interesting and important area of workplace health.

Note

1. Workers are considered "marginally attached" to the workforce if they want work, are available for work, and had searched for work in the past year but were not considered unemployed because they did not indicate searching for a job in the last four weeks because they believe no jobs are available for them or because of other reasons such as attending school, family responsibilities, or transportation issues (BLS, 2009a).

References

Adebayo, D. O. (2006). The moderating effect of self-efficacy on job insecurity and organisational commitment among Nigerian public servants. *Journal of Psychology in Africa, 16,* 35–43.

Adkins, C. L., Werbel, J. D., & Farh, J. (2001). A field study of job security during a financial crisis. *Group & Organization Management, 26,* 463–483.

Ahuja, G., & Katila, R. (2001). Technological acquisitions and the innovation performance of acquiring firms: A longitudinal study. *Strategic Management Journal, 22,* 197–220.

Anderson, C. L., & Nevitte, N. (2006). Teach your children well: Values of thrift and saving. *Journal of Economic Psychology, 27,* 247–261.

Ashford, S. J., Lee, C., Bobko, P. (1989). Content, causes, and consequences of job insecurity: A theory-based measure and substantive test. *Academy of Management Journal, 32,* 803–829.

Bellarosa, C., & Chen, P. Y. (1997). The effectiveness and practicality of occupational stress management interventions: A survey of subject matter expert opinions. *Journal of Occupational Health Psychology, 2,* 247–262.

Brett, J., Cron, W., & Slocum, J., Jr., (1995). Economic dependency on work: A moderator of the relationship between organizational commitment and performance. *The Academy of Management Journal, 38,* 261–271.

Brockner, J., Konovsky, M., Cooper-Schneider,R., Folger, R., Martin, C., & Bies, R. J. (1994). Interactive effects of procedural justice and outcome negativity on victims and survivors of job loss. *Academy of Management Journal, 13*, 397–409.

Brotheridge, C. M. (2003). The role of fairness in mediating the effects of voice and justification on stress and other outcomes in a climate of organizational change. *International Journal of Stress Management, 10*, 253–268.

Bureau of Labor Statistics. (2009a). Employment situation summary: May 2009 (U.S. Department of Labor Economic News Release 09-0588). Retrieved from www.bls.gov/news.release/empsit.nr0.htm

Bureau of Labor Statistics. (2009c). Mass layoffs summary: Extended mass layoffs in the first quarter of 2009 (U.S. Department of Labor Economic News Release 09-0506). Retrieved from www.bls.gov/news.release/mslo.nr0.htm

Cascio, W. F. (2002). *Responsible restructuring: Creative and profitable alternatives to layoffs.* San Francisco: Berrett-Koehler.

Cheng, G. H.-L., & Chan, D. K.-S. (2008). Who suffers more from job insecurity? A meta-analytic review. *Applied Psychology: An International Review, 57*, 272–303.

Chou, K., & Chi, I. (1999). Determinants of life satisfaction in Hong Kong Chinese elderly: A longitudinal study. *Aging and Mental Health, 3*, 328–335.

Colquitt, J. A., Conlon, D. E., Wesson, M. J., Porter, C. O. L. H., Ng, K. Y. (2001). Justice at the millennium: A meta-analytic review of 25 years of organizational justice research. *Journal of Applied Psychology, 86*, 425–445.

Conger, R., Elder, G., Jr., Lorenz, F., Conger, K., Simons, R., Whitbeck, L., ... Melby, J. N. (1990). Linking economic hardship to marital quality and instability. *Journal of Marriage and the Family, 52*, 643–656.

Creed, P. A., & Bartrum, D. A. (2008). Personal control as a mediator and moderator between life strains and psychological well-being in the unemployed. *Journal of Applied Social Psychology, 38*, 460–481.

Crosier, T., Butterworth, P., & Rodgers, B. (2007). Mental health problems among single and partnered mothers: The role of financial hardship and social support. *Social Psychiatry and Psychiatriatric Epidemiology, 42*, 6–13.

Dackert, I., Jackson, P. R., Brenner, S., & Johansson, C. R. (2003). Eliciting and analyzing employees' expectations of a merger. *Human Relations, 56*, 705–725.

Daft, R. L. (1995). *Organizational theory and design* (5th ed.). New York: West.

Department of Labor (2009). High growth job training initiative. Retrieved June 22, 2009 from www.doleta.gov/Brg/JobTrainInitiative.

Department of Trade and Industry. (2006). *Success at work: Protecting vulnerable workers, supporting good employers.* London: U.K. Department of Trade and Industry.

Doran, L., Stone, V., Brief, A., & George, J. (1991). Behavioral intentions as predictors of job attitudes: The role of economic choice. *Journal of Applied Psychology, 76*, 40–45.

Elliot, M. (2001). Gender differences in causes of depression. *Women & Health, 33*, 163–177.

Feldman, D. C. (1996). The nature, antecedents, and consequences of underemployment. *Journal of Management, 22*, 385–407.

Ferraro, K. F. & Su, Y.-P. (1999). Financial strain, social relations, and psychological distress among older people: A cross-cultural analysis. *Journals of Gerontology: Series B: Psychological Sciences and Social Sciences, 54*, S3–S15.

Finegold, D., Mohrman, S., & Spreitzer, G. M. (2002). Age effects on the predictors of technical workers' commitment and willingness to turnover. *Journal of Organizational Behavior, 23*, 655–674.

Fox, J., Bartholomae, S., & Lee, J. (2005). Building the case for financial education. *Journal of Consumer Affairs, 39*, 195–214.

Francoeur, R. B. (2001). Reformulating financial problems and interventions to improve psychosocial and functional outcomes in cancer patients and their families. *Journal of Psychosocial Oncology, 19*, 1–20.

Goins, S., & Gruca, T. S. (2008). Understanding competitive and contagion effects of layoff announcements. *Corporate Reputation Review, 11*, 12–34.

Gong, Y., & Chang, S. (2008). Institutional antecedents and performance consequences of employment security and career advancement practices: Evidence from the People's Republic of China, *Human Resource Management, 47*, 33–48.

Grandey, A., & Cropanzano, R. (1999). The conservation of resources model applied to work–family conflict and strain. *Journal of Vocational Behavior, 54*, 350–370.

Hanisch, K. (1999). Job loss and unemployment research from 1994 to 1998: A review and recommendations for research and intervention. *Journal of Vocational Behavior, 55*, 188–220.

Hatfield, E., Cacioppo, J., & Rapson, R. L. (1994). *Emotional contagion*. New York: Cambridge University Press.

Hira, T. K., & Loibl, C. (2005). Understanding the impact of employer-provided financial education on workplace satisfaction. *Journal of Consumer Affairs, 39*, 173–194.

Hobfoll, S. E. (2001). The influence of culture, community, and the nested-self in the stress process: Advancing conservation of resources theory. *Applied Psychology: An International Review, 50*, 337–421.

Hofstede, G. (1980). *Culture's consequences*. Beverly Hills, CA: Sage.

Hofstede, G. (2001). *Culture's consequences: Comparing values, behaviors, institutions, and organizations across nations*. Thousand Oaks, CA: Sage.

Howlett, E., Kees, J., & Kemp, E. (2008). The role of self-regulation, future orientation, and financial knowledge in long-term financial decisions. *The Journal of Consumer Affairs, 42*, 223–242.

Hui, C. H. (1990). Work attitudes, leadership styles, and managerial behaviors in different cultures. In R. W. Brislin (Ed.) *Applied cross-cultural psychology* (pp. 186–208). Thousand Oaks, CA: Sage.

International Labour Organization. (2004). *Economic security for a better world*. Geneva, Switzerland: ILO.

International Labour Organization. (2009). Global employment trends: May 2009 update (ILO Publication – Geneva). Retrieved from www.ilo.org/wcmsp5/groups/public/—dgreports/—dcomm/documents/publication/wcms_106504.pdf

Jacobson, B. H., Aldana, S. G., Goetzel, R. Z., & Vardell, K. D. (1996). The relationship between perceived stress and self-reported illness-related absenteeism. *American Journal of Health Promotion, 11*, 54–61.

Jimmieson, N. L., Terry, D. J., & Callan, V. J. (2004). A longitudinal study of employee adaptation to organizational change: The role of change-related information and change-related self-efficacy. *Journal of Occupational Health Psychology, 9*, 11–27.

Jones, A. M. (2003). Managing the gap: Evolutionary science, work/life integration, and corporate responsibility. *Organizational Dynamics, 32*, 17–31.

Judge, T. A. & Bono, J. E. (2001). Relationship of core self-evaluations traits—self-esteem, generalized self-efficacy, locus of control, and emotional stability–with job satisfaction and job performance: A meta-analysis. *Journal of Applied Psychology, 86*, 80–92.

Judge, T. A., Hurst, C., & Simon, L. S. (2009). Does it pay to be smart, attractive, or confident (or all three)? Relationships among general mental ability, physical attractiveness, core self-evaluations, and income. *Journal of Applied Psychology*, 94, 724–755.

Judge, T. A., & Ilies, R. (2004). Affect and job satisfaction: a study of their relationship at work and at home. *Journal of Applied Psychology*, 89, 661–73.

Kagitcibasi, C., & Berry, J. W. (1989). Cross-cultural psychology: Current research and trends. *Annual Review of Psychology, 40*, 493–532.

Karasek, R. A. (1979). Job demands, job decision latitude, and mental strain: Implications for job redesign. *Administrative Science Quarterly, 24*, 285–309.

Kickul, J., Lester, S. W., & Finkl, J. (2002). Promise breaking during radical organizational change: Do justice interventions make a difference? *Journal of Organizational Behavior, 23*, 469–488.

König, C. K., Probst, T. M., Staffen, S., & Graso, M. (2009, May). *Do people in Switzerland react differently to job insecurity compared to people in the US?* Paper presented at the FourteenthEuropean Congress of Work and Organizational Psychology, Santiago de Compostela, Spain.

Lee, C., Bobko, P., & Chen, Z. X. (2006). Investigation of the multidimensional model of job insecurity in China and the USA. *Applied Psychology: An International Review, 55*, 512–540.

Leiter, M. (1991). Coping patterns as predictors of burnout: The function of control and escapist coping patterns. *Journal of Organizational Behavior, 12*, 123–144.

Lim, V. K. G. (1997). Moderating effects of work-based support on the relationship between job insecurity and its consequences. *Work & Stress, 11*, 251–266.

Love, E. G., & Kraatz, M. (2009). Character, conformity, or the bottom line? How and why downsizing affected corporate reputation. *Academy of Management Journal, 52*, 314–335.

Lyons, A. C., Chang, Y., Scherpf, E. M. (2006). Translating financial education into behavior change for low-income populations. *Financial Counseling and Planning, 17*, 27–45.

Mauno, S., & Kinnunen, U. (2002). Perceived job insecurity among dual-earner couples: Do its antecedents vary according to gender, economic sector and the measure used? *Journal of Occupational and Organizational Psychology, 75*, 295–314.

McKee-Ryan, F., Song, Z., Wanberg, C., & Kinicki, A. (2005). Psychological and physical well-being during unemployment: A meta-analytic study. *Journal of Applied Psychology, 90*, 53–76.

McKinley, W., Sanchez, C., & Schick, A. (1995). Organizational downsizing: Constraining, cloning, learning. *Academy of Management Executive, 9*, 32–42.

Mills, R., Grasmick, H., Morgan, C., & Wenk, D. (1992). The effects of gender, family satisfaction, and economic strain on psychological well-being. *Family Relations, 41*, 440–445.

Norvilitis, J. M., Merwin, M. M., Osberg, T. M., Roehling, P. V, Young, P., & Kamas, M. M. (2006). Personality factors, money attitudes, financial knowledge, and credit-card debt in college students. *Journal of Applied Social Psychology, 36*, 1395–1413.

Oyserman, D., Coon, H. M., & Kemmelmeier, M. (2002). Rethinking individualism and collectivism: Evaluation of theoretical assumptions and meta-analyses. *Psychological Bulletin, 128*, 3–72.

Pearlin, L., Lieberman, M., Menaghan, E., & Mullan, J. (1981). The stress process. *Journal of Health and Social Behavior, 22*, 337–356.

Probst, T. M. (2002). Layoffs and tradeoffs: Production, quality, and safety demands under the threat of job loss. *Journal of Occupational Health Psychology, 7*, 211–220.

Probst, T. M. (2005a). Economic stressors. In J. Barling, K. Kelloway, & M. Frone (Eds.) *Handbook of work stress*, (pp. 267–297). Thousand Oaks, CA: Sage.

Probst, T. M. (2005b). Countering the negative effects of job insecurity through participative decision making: Lessons from the demand–control model. *Journal of Occupational Health Psychology, 10*, 320–329.

Probst, T. M. & Brubaker, T. L. (2001). The effects of job insecurity on employee safety outcomes: Cross-sectional and longitudinal explorations. *Journal of Occupational Health Psychology, 6*, 139–159.

Probst, T. M., & Brubaker, T. L. (2007). Organizational safety climate and supervisory layoff decisions: Preferences versus predictions. *Journal of Applied Social Psychology, 37*, 1630–1648.

Probst, T. M., & Lawler, J. (2006). Cultural values as moderators of employee reactions to job insecurity: The role of individualism and collectivism. *Applied Psychology: An International Review, 55*, 234–254.

Quinlan, M. (2005). The hidden epidemic of injuries and illness associated with the global expansion of precarious employment. In C. L. Peterson & C. Mayhew (Eds.), *Occupational Health and Safety: International Influences and the New Epidemics*. Amityville, NY: Baywood Publishing.

Reisel, W. D., Probst, T. M., Chia, S-L., Maloles, C. M., Brown, J. W., & Hazen, J. (2007, April). The effects of job insecurity on job satisfaction, organizational citizenship behavior, deviant behavior, and negative emotions of employees. Paper presented to the annual conference of the Society for Industrial/Organizational Psychology, New York.

Reynolds, J. R. (1997). The effects of industrial employment conditions on job-related distress. *Journal of Health and Social Behavior, 38*, 105–116.

Rugulies, R., Aust, B., Burr, H., & Bültmann, U. (2008). Job insecurity, chances on the labour market and decline in self-rated health in a representative sample of the Danish workforce. *Journal of Epidemiology & Community Health, 62*, 245–250.

Said, T., Le Louarn, J., Tremblay, M. (2007). The performance effect of major workforce reductions: Longitudinal evidence from North America. *International Journal of Human Resource Management, 18*, 2075–2094.

Schaubroeck, J., & Merritt, D. E. (1997). Divergent effects of control on coping with work stressors: The key role of self-efficacy. *Academy of Management Journal, 40*, 738–754.

Schweiger, D. M., & Denisi, A. S. (1991). Communication with employee following a merger: A longitudinal field experiment. *Academy of Management Journal, 34*, 110–135.

Searle, R. H., & Ball, K. S. (2004). The development of trust and distrust in a merger. *Journal of Managerial Psychology, 19*, 708–721.

Sears, L. (2008). *Work-related outcomes of financial stress: Relating perceived income adequacy and financial strain to job performance and well-being*. Unpublished master's thesis. Department of Psychology, Portland State University, Portland, OR.

Shapiro, M, & Slemrod, J. (2003). Consumer response to tax rebates. *American Economic Review, 93*, 281–396.

Shaw, J., & Gupta, N. (2001). Pay fairness and employee outcomes: Exacerbation and attenuation effects of financial need. *Journal of Occupational and Organizational Psychology, 74*, 299–320.

Simons, R., Lorenz, F., Conger, R., & Wu, C. (1992). Support from spouse as mediator and moderator of the disruptive influence of economic strain on parenting. *Child Development, 63*, 1282–1301.

Sinclair, R. R., & Martin, J. E. (2006). *Examining some assumptions about lower income entry-level workers*. Paper presented at the Annual conference of the Society for Industrial and Organizational Psychology, Dallas, TX.

Skarlicki, D. P., Barclay, L. J., & Pugh, D. S. (2008). When explanations for layoffs are not enough: Employer's integrity as a moderator of the relationship between informational *justice* and retaliation. *Journal of Occupational and Organizational Psychology, 81*, 123–146.

Skinner, M. A., Zautra, A. J., & Reich, J. W. (2004). Financial stress predictors and the emotional and physical health of chronic pain patients. *Cognitive Therapy and Research, 28*, 695–713.

Society for Human Resource Management. (2009). *SHRM poll: Financial challenges to the U.S. and global economy and their impact on organizations*. March 11, 2009. Alexandria, VA: SHRM.

So-hyun, J. & Grable, J. E. (2004). An exploratory framework of the determinants of financial satisfaction. *Journal of Family and Economic Issues, 25*, 25–50.

Stuckler, D., Basu, S., Suhrcke, M., Coutts, A., & McKee, M. (2009). The public health effect of economic crises and alternative policy responses in Europe: An empirical analysis. *Lancet, 374*, 315–323.

Sverke, M., Hellgren, J., & Näswell, K. (2002). No security: A meta-analysis and review of job insecurity and its consequences. *Journal of Occupational Health Psychology, 7*, 242–264.

Teo, C., & Waters, L. (2002). The role of human resources practices in reducing occupational stress and strain. *International Journal of Stress Management, 9*, 207–226.

The Pew Charitable Trusts (2009). *The clean energy economy: Repowering jobs, business, and investments across America*. Retrieved June 22, 2009 from www.pewcenteronthestates. org/uploadedFiles/Clean_Economy_Report_Web.pdf

Tivendell, J., & Bouronnais, C. (2008). Job insecurity in a sample of Canadian civil servants as a function of personality and perceived job characteristics. *Psychological Reports, 87*, 55–60.

Triandis, H. C. (1995). *Individualism and collectivism*. Boulder, CO: Westview.

Tucker, J. S., Sinclair, R. R., & Thomas, J. L. (2005). The multilevel effects of occupational stressors on soldiers' well-being, organizational attachment, and readiness. *Journal of Occupational Health Psychology, 10*, 276–299.

van Hooft, E. A. J., & Crossley, C. D. (2008). The joint role of locus of control and perceived financial need in job search. *International Journal of Selection and Assessment, 16*, 258–271.

Voydanoff, P. (1990). Economic distress and family relations: A review of the eighties. *Journal of Marriage and the Family, 52*, 1099–1115.

Wadsworth, M. E., & Santiago, C. D. (2008). Risk and resiliency processes in ethnically diverse families in poverty. *Journal of Family Psychology, 22*, 399–410.

Wall, T. D., Jackson, P. R., Mullarkey, S., & Parker, S. K. (1996). The demands-control model of job strain: A more specific test. *Journal of Occupational and Organizational Psychology, 69*, 153–166.

Zandi, M. M. (2008). *Assessing the Macro Economic Impact of Fiscal Stimulus 2008*. Retrieved June 22, 2009 from www.economy.com/mark-zandi/documents/assissing-the-impact-of-the-fiscal-stimulus.pdf

Zohar, D. (2003). Safety climate: Conceptual and measurement issues. In J. C. Quick and L. Tetrick (Eds), *Handbook of Occupational Health Psychology* (pp. 123-142). Washington, DC: APA Books.

Zohar, D., & Luria, G. (2005). A multilevel model of safety climate: cross-level relationships between organization and group-level climates. *Journal of Applied Psychology, 90*, 616–628.

2

Developing New Ways of Evaluating Organizational-Level Interventions

Karina Nielsen
National Research Centre for the Working Environment, Denmark

Raymond Randall
University of Leicester, U.K.

Karl Bang Christensen
University of Copenhagen, Denmark

Although there is an increasing interest in combining process and effect evaluation using mixed methods there has to date been very little discussion and empirical research that demonstrates how this may be done. This chapter discusses the key challenges in linking process evaluation and effect evaluation and describes an empirical study that attempts to meet some of these challenges. The study was carried out during the implementation of teamwork in the elderly care sector. It used mixed methods (both qualitative and quantitative) to determine whether different types of team training, when coupled with a teamwork intervention, enhanced employee well-being and satisfaction. The effects of team implementation were examined alongside the effects of facilitating and hindering factors surrounding the intervention. Results indicated that training employees and team managers (the intervention process) was linked to intervention effects. However, it was also found that other aspects of the intervention processes and context (e.g., organizational turbulence and the perceptions of managers and staff) had been less positive and had blunted the effects of the intervention. The study illustrates how a detailed examination of intervention processes can be carried out, and how the results of this process evaluation can be used to draw valid inferences from effect evaluation.

Introduction

The traditional quasi-experimental approach has dominated the research on the effects of organizational-level interventions within occupational health psychology

(Semmer, 2006; Randall, Cox, & Griffiths, 2007). This research has focused on effect evaluation and has produced some positive results that show that some interventions can be very effective. However, it also shows that many organizational change initiatives fail to meet expectations (Herold, Fedor, & Caldwell, 2007). Some argue that too few intervention studies are the well-designed quasi-experiments needed for valid evaluation (e.g., Richardson & Rothstein, 2008). Others point out that this body of research focuses on effect evaluation (i.e., what works) at the expense of a thorough analysis of intervention processes (i.e., why it works) and that there is a need to break away from the natural science paradigm in evaluation research (Cox, Karanika, Griffiths, & Houdmont, 2007). The focus on effect evaluation means that factors in the intervention context and the change processes that influence intervention effects are not well-understood (Semmer, 2006).

This chapter has three aims. The first is to discuss the need for a better understanding of both intervention context and intervention processes when assessing the effectiveness of interventions. The second is to provide an example of how mixed methods research and an expanded nexus of data collection may be used to strengthen the evaluation of multi-faceted interventions in complex functioning work environments. The third is to provide an example that shows how these methodological approaches can be used in combination with effect evaluation to enhance the evaluation of a complex organizational intervention (team implementation combined with employee training).

The Challenges of Evaluating Organizational-Level Interventions

The organizational environment can place significant constraints on evaluation research designs (Cox et al., 2007). These constraints place limits on the validity of studies that rely upon strong study design and controlled manipulation of intervention exposure for their explanatory power (Cox et al., 2007; Randall, Griffiths, & Cox, 2005). However, even when strong study designs can be achieved, organizational-level interventions rarely resemble the simple manipulations of conditions seen in controlled experimental research. Most such change initiatives are complex. In participative action research, for example, change processes often involve many people in the implementation of change, and interventions tend to be multi-faceted and delivered in intervention "packages" (Parkes & Sparkes, 1998).

This complexity makes it difficult to obtain valid results by using a single level of analysis that looks for links between changes in outcome variables (such as job satisfaction or well-being) and patterns of planned, carefully controlled, intervention exposure. In functioning organizations, because interventions cannot be considered in isolation from the context in which they occur and the processes that make them happen, explanations for effects are likely to be holistic with change being driven by complex mechanisms (Semmer, 2006). This may mean that evaluating interventions with functioning organizations requires the use of research methods that examine not only the impact of the intervention itself, but also intervention processes and the intervention context (Randall et al., 2007). Reviewers of intervention studies have suggested that process evaluation and effect evaluation need to be combined to get a complete picture of the effects of organizational-level interventions (Egan, Bambra, Petticrew, & Whitehead, 2009; Murta, Sanderson, & Oldenburg, 2007). In summary, intervention researchers need to better document and analyze why change takes place (Semmer, 2003, 2006) and cannot simply rely on experimental control to isolate intervention effects (Randall, Nielsen, & Tvedt, 2009).

This represents a significant shift in thinking. Rather than viewing the organizational context as a source of confounding variables (or threats to validity), researchers are starting to consider the influence of the intervention context as an integral part of the change process (Nielsen, Fredslund, Christensen, & Albertsen, 2006; Randall et al., 2007; Randall et al., 2009). Looking at interventions in this way may help to produce more powerful and valid intervention research from organizational settings, but it does add complexity to the research process. For example, it is possible that various levels of the intervention context may be important (i.e., the context at both the upper and lower levels in the organization, and the context external and internal to the organization [Pettigrew, 1990; Randall et al., 2007]). This means that analyzing intervention data is likely to include an analysis of the cross-level linkages between each of the levels of the context, and between the context and the key evaluation variables (Herold et al., 2007).

In a recent review of organizational-level interventions Bambra, Egan, Thomas, Petticrew, and Whitehead (2007) highlight the impact of many different contextual factors on intervention outcomes: a variety of factors have been implicated when interventions fail to find positive effects. Concurrent organizational events such as mergers, downsizing or large-scale reorganizations are often mentioned as possible explanations for poor intervention outcomes. Bambra et al. (2007) also highlight another important failing of intervention research: too little attention has been paid to the examination of change processes. There is growing evidence that the way an intervention is implemented—and not just the content of the intervention—is an important determinant of its effectiveness. Factors such as employee participation, involvement in the intervention design, line manager support (Randall et al., 2009), the availability of information about interventions, and perceptions of intervention quality (Nielsen et al., 2007) have been shown to influence intervention outcomes.

Semmer (2003, 2006) has emphasized the importance of monitoring carefully implementation fidelity and intervention mechanisms. Randall et al. (2002, 2005) showed that, because of implementation problems, the effects of intervention were closely related to participants' reported exposure to it: the effectiveness of the intervention was seriously underestimated if it was assumed that all employees had experienced it. Argyris (1992) proposed that change only really occurs when the espoused theory (i.e., the intervention plan) is seen to be happening in the workplace through, for example, changes in behavior (i.e., theories-in-use). Training interventions are a good example of the importance of gathering data about intervention mechanisms so that intervention outcomes can be understood. Measuring the degree to which training participants learn something they can use is more important than simply measuring employee involvement in the training (Campbell & Kuncel, 2005).

Furthermore, training evaluation then needs to consider training transfer if its impact on organizational outcomes is to be understood (Kraiger, 2003).

In this opening section we have identified two neglected areas of intervention research: measurement of the intervention context and measurement of intervention processes. Researchers are also faced with the challenge that, once gathered, such data needs to be linked to intervention outcomes. In the next section of this chapter we discuss how such challenges may be partly met by the use of two methodological innovations: the use of a mixed methods methodology (combining quantitative and qualitative research methods) and the application of a "bracketing" philosophy to widen the field of enquiry.

Meeting the Challenges of Evaluation: Bracketing and Mixed Methods

The organizational context of intervention studies has usually been studied using qualitative methods (e.g., Saksvik, Nytrø, Dah-Jørgensen, & Mikkelsen, 2002). Given that every organizational context is unique, qualitative methods offer a flexibility of enquiry which makes them particularly suited to gathering data about the intervention context (Cook & Shadish, 1994; Miles & Huberman, 1994). It is also true that quasi-experimental quantitative research methods focused on intervention outcomes have a lot to offer (Richardson & Rothstein, 2008). Therefore, one way of carrying out strong evaluation research (especially when the organization setting places constraints on, or precludes, controlled exposure studies[1]) is to use mixed methods research designs (Johnson, Onwuegbuzie, & Turner, 2007):

> Mixed methods research is a type of research in which a researcher or a team of researchers combines elements of qualitative and quantitative research approaches (e.g. use of qualitative and quantitative viewpoints, data collection, analysis, inference techniques) for the broad purposes of breath and depth of understanding and corroboration. (p. 123)

Mixed methods research is a new paradigm with a history that goes back to Campbell and Fiske's (1959) concept of triangulation, an approach that draws upon two or more methods as a way of testing the validity of research results. They argued that convergence of research findings stemming from two or more methods enhances the validity of results and minimizes the risk of methodological bias. Mixed method researchers emphasize several other advantages of combining qualitative and quantitative methods. Greene, Caracelli, and Graham (1989) identified five specific uses of mixed methods approaches:

1. triangulation: to corroborate and validate the results using different methods
2. to enhance and illustrate the results of one method using the results of another method (i.e., the use of complementary methods)

3. to use the results from one method to help develop or inform other methods (i.e., where one method is used to inform the choice of sampling and implementation of other methods)
4. to use multiple methods to discover paradoxes and new perspectives through recasting questions from one method with the questions or results from other methods (i.e., to initiate)
5. to extend the breadth and range of enquiry by using different methods for different inquiry components.

To date, there have been very few mixed method intervention studies in occupational health psychology (Nastasi, Hitchcock, Sarkar, Varjas, & Jayasana, 2007). Greene et al.'s (1989) analysis shows that evaluation research can be enhanced in many ways by the use of mixed methods. For example, triangulation of qualitative and quantitative methods can be used to examine the acceptability, integrity, and effectiveness of interventions within the same study. Mixed methods research also facilitates concurrent effect and process evaluation so that research can determine the effectiveness of the intervention but also deal with questions about why the intervention works or fails in a particular organizational context. Because of this, mixed methods may provide information on how intervention programs can be modified and which elements are transferable to other settings. There are other important potential gains: the mixed methods approach allows us to draw conclusions on the applicability of interventions to daily working life, on cultural specificity, e.g., the relevance and appropriateness of the intervention to a given context and the experiences of participants, and on the immediate and long-term outcomes of interventions (Nastasi et al., 2007). In summary, the mixed methods approach offers strength of study design, but also the breadth and flexibility of data collection methods needed to link intervention processes, organizational context, and intervention outcomes to each other.

Very little quasi-experimental research has to date used a mixed methods approach; in a review of the organizational research literature, Bryman (2006) found that only five studies out of a total of 232 mixed method studies had used a quasi-experimental design. In this chapter we present an example of how qualitative and quantitative methods were used to enrich the evaluation of team implementation in the elderly care sector.

Mixed methods allow researchers to widen the field of enquiry and this may be particularly important when attempting to make sense of various contextual influences on an intervention. Hackman (2003) suggested the concept of "bracketing" (i.e., defining the boundaries of data capture *outside* of the intervention itself in order to better understand change *within* the intervention group). Hackman argued that to understand the dynamics of the focal level of the change, researchers must also consider the context at least one level above as well as one level below the focal level of the change. In this chapter we use Hackman's bracketing concept to present a comprehensive evaluation of the implementation of a complex and multi-faceted teamwork intervention in a complex organizational setting. In this example, the focal level of analysis was at the team level with several levels of analysis being used within the "brackets" of the evaluation. These levels were:

1. the organizational context (e.g., events impacting upon the organization as a whole)
2. the context of each team (e.g., how team members and managers perceived themselves as a team and the role of the manager in team organization)
3. the individual context (e.g., team members' and managers' accounts of their experiences during the intervention).

Combining this wider field of enquiry with a mixed methods approach also allowed the impact of intervention context on intervention processes and intervention outcomes to be examined. This simple framework could be easily modified for other interventions or to fit with other organizational structures (e.g., if teams did not exist). Randall et al. (2007) provide an example of how the various components of intervention context can be identified in the evaluation process.

In summary, bracketing allows the collection of data that lies outside of the range of traditional quasi-experimental designs: pre-post measurements of outcome variables offer little information about the upper and lower levels of the intervention context. Mixed methods research can then be used to link the rich data collected to the analysis of intervention outcome.

Case Study: Teamwork Evaluation Using Mixed Methods and Bracketing

There are several papers that point to the weaknesses of traditional evaluation research; few, however, provide detailed guidance on how researchers should proceed in a way that addresses these weaknesses, and fewer still supply researchers with a "worked example" of how new evaluation methods can be applied in practice. The remainder of this chapter describes the evaluation of a complex, multifaceted intervention (the implementation of teamwork combined with employee or manager training—or both) showing how the evaluation methods we propose can be applied in practice. Complex interventions like this (e.g., those involving participative action research) are common in the intervention literature.

It is important to highlight that the approach need not be confined to teamwork interventions, but teamwork is chosen as an example because it is a common intervention in organizations that is implemented in different ways, and one that is likely to be heavily influenced by contextual factors. In this chapter it is used to illustrate how data about intervention processes and intervention context can be collected and analyzed to understand better how intervention processes and context can be linked to intervention outcomes.

Most teamwork research shows that organizing work this way is likely to have a positive effect (Rasmussen & Jeppesen, 2006). However, implementing teams does not always bring about these positive effects, and previous research has generally failed to consider how the method of implementing teamwork and the organizational context influence intervention outcomes (Bambra et al., 2007). This means that there is a gap in information for organizations: It appears that implementing teams can be a good thing to do, but there is little guidance on how to manage the implementation process to maximize its impact. In this chapter we present research that examines one potentially important aspect of the implementation process, i.e., whether teamwork is facilitated by training those involved. It has been suggested that training employees and managers such that they are capable of implementing change and working in the new organizational structure is one of the factors which may have a positive impact on the effects of organizational-level interventions (Becker-Reims, 1994). Team organization puts new demands on group members with regard to the ability to do the task and work with others, and the ability of the team members to communicate, coordinate, and adopt positive attitudes towards colleagues and working in a team. Team members might not possess these skills before the implementation of teams and may therefore require training if implementation is to be effective (Kraiger, 2003). There is some evidence to suggest that training may provide positive support to team implementation.

The existing research that has been carried out confounded the implementation of teams with training provided to the employees. For example, in the studies by Wall, Kemp, Jackson, and Clegg (1986) and Cordery, Mueller, and Smith (1991) employees received training; however, the impact of the training remains uncertain because its relationship to the outcome variables was not isolated from the effects of the team implementation itself. Morgeson, Johnson, Campion, Medsker, and Mumford (2006) did formally test the moderating effect of training on changes in effort, skills usage, and problem solving. No significant effects were found, but the questions asked focused on existing general employee training programs rather than training specifically aimed at team implementation and the skills required to work in teams. Therefore there is a need to examine whether specific employee and manager training is linked to the effective implementation of teams. This chapter examines the facilitating role of several different forms of training: team manager training and team member training, tailored training and off-the shelf training, mandatory training and voluntary training.

A teamworking intervention was also suitable for the application of these evaluation methods because teams are subject to the influence of many different "contexts" within organizations. Some of these are external to the teams (since a single team is nested within the contexts provided by groups of teams, the organization, the economy, and the wider political context [Matheiu, Heffner, Goodwin, Salas, & Cannon-Bowers, 2007]). Marks, Mathieu, and Zaccaro (2001) found that the extent to which the larger organizational environment was supportive of teamwork was linked to employee motivation to participate in interpersonal processes within a team. Nielsen et al. (2006) found that managerial turnover, budget cuts and conflicts at the workplace had a significant negative impact on intervention effects. There is also a context within the team that is heavily influenced by the individual members and their managers (Hackman, 2003; Kozlowski & Bell, 2003). Nielsen, Randall, & Albertsen (2007) found that employees' appraisal of various aspects of a variety of interventions and the way these were delivered (e.g., the quality of the intervention) were significantly linked to intervention outcomes.

The evaluation presented in this chapter is a natural field experiment. This has been identified as a desirable research strategy for obtaining knowledge about a variety of organizational-level interventions (Saksvik et al., 2002). The advantages are many: (a) It strengthens the causal inferences where random assignment and controlled manipulation is not possible, (b) it minimizes the ethical dilemmas of inequity and deception, (c) it can use the context to explain conflicting findings, (d) it offers the opportunity to examine the sustainability of interventions over a longer period of time, and (e) finally, it offers an opportunity for researchers to collaborate with practitioners thus bridging the gap between theory and practice (Grant & Wall, 2008). The study used a six-group longitudinal research design including a control group: this was possible because of the naturally occurring variance between teams in terms of the delivery of the training intervention: all groups were involved in the team implementation intervention.

The team intervention

The study presented in this chapter was carried out in Danish elderly care centers. The local government organization running the centers had made the decision to implement teamwork in all of them. The aim was to develop teams that all had at least some degree of self-management. An elderly care center manager, who had previous experience with implementing teamwork, worked as a full-time team consultant to develop and roll out a top-down strategy for implementing teams. In total 17 elderly care center managers participated in meetings where they were told about teamwork to ensure their involvement and participation in the intervention. The implementation of teams was supported by the team consultant who held after-work meetings where managers and employees were told about the advantages and the challenges of implementing and working in teams. Staff newsletters also carried information about the intervention on a regular basis.

Employee and manager training

The organization recognized that the introduction of teamwork would place different demands on employees and their managers. In order to support the managers, two different kinds of managerial training courses were completed during the intervention process. A *tailored training programme* for all managers (n = 12 managers) was put in place in one of the elderly care centers. This consisted of a six-day training course where managers would learn about team characteristics and team processes and how to plan and implement team organization. As part of the training course, managers were split into three network groups that would meet in between training modules and were given homework related to the content of the module. This was designed to help the group of managers themselves function as a team and develop a shared strategy for the implementation of teamwork. The decision to participate in training was made by the elderly care center manager and it was mandatory for all managers to participate.

An *off-the shelf-training course* (i.e., not a bespoke course) was applied for managers. This involved eight training days ending with a combined written and oral exam (n = 7 managers). The off-the-shelf manager training course was designed to train the managers in post-modern management styles including self-management, communicative competencies, coaching (narrative models) and team implementation. All managers in the local government department were invited to join this training (seven out of eighteen participated).

Training was also offered to all employees. Team managers and team members decided at a team level whether they wanted to participate. Only whole teams of employees, and not parts of teams could participate as the training was delivered to whole teams (while temporary staff or other teams covered the shift). The training focused on educating employees about the characteristics of good teams and the factors that make teams function effectively. As part of the training, team members would participate in exercises that helped them to reflect on how well they worked together. Whole-team training such as this has been found to enhance team coordination, communication and cooperation (Kozlowski & Bell, 2003) with these issues also being dealt with during the training. The courses were offered by different agencies but all courses shared the same characteristics and objectives. Most courses lasted approximately four days.

The exposure of the six different groups to the different training interventions is summarized in Figure 2.1.

Grouping	Category
Group 1: NT	No training courses (5 teams)
Group 2: ET	Only employees received training (2 teams)
Group 3: OMT	Managers: off-the-shelf training course (1 team)
Group 4: TMT	Managers received tailored training course (6 teams)
Group 5: EOMT	Managers: off-the-shelf and employee training (6 teams)
Group 6: ETMT	Managers: tailored and employee training (3 teams)

Figure 2.1   Grouping of Teams Based on Participation in Training

As can be seen from the description of the intervention and its context, the team implementation study presented several methodological challenges. It is a longitudinal between-groups natural experiment in which groups varied in the degree of training they received. Three different kinds of training were evaluated: a tailored training course for team managers, an off-the-shelf training course for team managers, and off-the-shelf employee training courses. There was also the challenge of linking training exposure to intervention outcomes and disentangling its impact from the various intervention contexts. For the analyses we used exposure to the training to establish the study design. Process evaluation was needed to identify the incremental impact of the training from the impact of the implementation of teams.

Therefore, the study design allowed us to test for the facilitating role of team and team manager training, and the facilitating (or hindering role) of intervention context through two hypotheses:

Hypothesis 1: Training team employees and managers will bring about improvements in team inputs, processes and outputs over and above those found in teams where training is not used to facilitate the implementation of teams.

We also tested whether the tailored training course for managers had more positive effects than an off-the-shelf training course. This is due to the fact that a tailored training course is based on a needs analysis and because participation in the development of the training course can motivate participants to fully participate in the training (Argyris, 1977, 1992). In addition, we examined whether a combination effect occurs such that teams where *both* the manager and the team members receive training do better during the intervention than teams where only either managers or team members experience training. This is because both parties will be better equipped to understand how the teams work and how they may work with team implementation (Latham & Saari, 1979). To enable us to determine the effects of the intervention we used a bracketing approach to examine the impact of intervention processes and context on interventions outcomes.

Hypothesis 2: We predict that such factors will influence both the impact of the training and the processes and outcomes of the team implementation.

Sample

In Denmark, the elderly care sector is organized into units where some staff provide care to elderly who are still in their own home and others provide care in elderly care homes. Two units, each including both types of staff were included (in this sample 51% of the healthcare staff worked in the homecare and the remainder in the elderly care homes). All staff from the centers were affected by the implementation of teamwork. The sample included different groups of staff ranging from cleaning personnel, canteen personnel, healthcare assistants, nurses, physiotherapists, and maintenance staff. Staff were organized in groups, e.g., home care staff covering a geographical area or staff covering a nursing home would constitute a team. Each

Table 2.1   Participant Demographics

Participants	Baseline			Follow-up		
	N	*%*	*M(SD)*	*N*	*%*	*M(SD)*
Response rates	447/551	81%		280/280	55%	
Team size	15			2		
Age			44(11.1)			45(10.9)
Tenure (in years)			11.6(10.2)			7.6(7.8)
Gender (% women)		93%			91%	
Healthcare assistants		62%			65%	
Nurses		12%			10%	
Other healthcare-related education		8%			6%	
No healthcare-related education		18%			19%	

team had a formal, external leader with managerial responsibilities—this was the manager that participated in training. The majority of employees were nurses or healthcare assistants who spent the majority of their working time delivering care to clients.

Twenty-three managers and their teams were included in our analysis. Senior-level managers (e.g., the elderly care center manager and the manager of the home-care group managers) were not included in our analysis as they do not have their own separate teams. Only data from those managers who remained in the unit throughout the study were included.

Design and procedure

Outcome evaluation was conducted using quantitative data: a questionnaire survey distributed to managers and employees both before and after training with an 18-month interval between measures. On both occasions, participants were asked questions about their perceptions of team organization (input), team functioning (process) and team performance and well-being (output). Three months prior to follow-up, a qualitative process evaluation was conducted: this gathered data about the process and context surrounding the intervention. All managers (n = 28) were interviewed individually and employee representatives (n = 94) from all teams participated in 24 focus groups. From each team at least two employees participated in the group interview.

Methods and measures

Effect evaluation. Team interdependence (the extent that team members are mutually responsible for a shared task, depend on each other to complete this task, and have complementary skills) was one team input that was expected to change as a result of the team implementation. A second input factor, autonomy, was also examined as a marker of the successful formation of teams (Campion, Papper, & Medsker, 1996; Cohen & Bailey, 1997). Team *output* concerns the team's effectiveness in terms of team performance and team members' involvement at work (Cohen, Ledford, & Spreitzer, 1996; Guzzo & Dickson, 1996; Parker & Williams, 2000). An overview of the measures used in the effect evaluation can be found in Table 2.2.

Multilevel analyses were used to analyze data from individuals nested within teams, and from measurement occasions nested within individuals (Bryk & Raudenbush, 1992; Hox, 2002). At baseline there were significant between-team differences on all measured variables (except age): therefore these were controlled for in the analyses.

Qualitative evaluation of context and processes. The results of previous papers on intervention process evaluation were used to construct semi-structured interview guides (Nielsen et al., 2006; Nytrø, Saksvik, Mikkelsen, Bohle, & Quinlan, 2000; Saksvik et al., 2002). Semi-structured interviews were conducted with managers, and focus groups were conducted with employee representatives from all teams. Organizational material regarding the type and content of training was also included. In the collection and analysis of data, four themes were explored:

Table 2.2   Key Measures Used in the Study

Measure	Wording	Source
Team interdependence Cronbach's a T1 = .80, T2 = .78	An example of an item is: *"Members of my team have skills and abilities that complement each other".*	Sprigg, Jackson, & Parker, 2000
Autonomy Cronbach's a T1 = .79, T2 =.78	An example of an item is: *We decide as a team who will do what in the team.*	West et al., 2004
Team effectiveness Cronbach's a T1 = .69, T2 =.72	An example of an item is: The team is consistently told that it achieves or exceeds its goals.	West et al., 2004
Involvement Cronbach's a T1 = .71, T2 =.85	An example of an item is: *"Do you feel that your place of work is of great personal importance to you?"*	West et al., 2004

1.   *Intervention Context.* Change occurs in turbulent settings characterized by many other distractions and (conflicting) changes that influence change outcomes (Herold et al., 2007). Previous studies have shown how the *context*—downsizing, restructuring, lay offs, manager turnover—has had an impact on both the interventions themselves and intervention outcomes (Saksvik et al., 2002; Nielsen et al., 2006). Furthermore, situational factors have been found to exert an influence on the transfer of training (Baldwin & Ford, 1998; Campbell & Kuncel, 2005). We therefore asked employees and managers to identify factors in the context that may have hindered and facilitated team implementation.

2.   *Description of the intervention and its implementation.* We asked employees and managers to describe the team activities that had taken place during the implementation phase to test whether anything had been done to implement teams.

3.   *Managers' mental models and teams' mental models.* Data was collected on the subjective interpretations of team managers and team members in order to examine how they perceived, understood, and remembered the intervention process (Pettigrew, 1990). We used the theory of mental models (Druskat & Pescosolido, 2002; Mathieu, Heffner, Goodwin, Salas, & Cannon-Bowers, 2000) to explore how managers and teams perceived working in teams and the management of the team. This was examined because shared mental models in team training have been shown to lead to a shared understanding of team processes and functioning (Cannon-Bowers, Salas, & Converse, 1991). To do this we asked team members and managers about how they saw the role of the manager and the team members in team implementation and whether they saw themselves as a (well-functioning) team.

4.   *Organizational learning.* We asked about whether actual work practices had changed to detect whether employees reported working in teams either (a) without significant actual change in how they worked together, or (b) whether they had actually altered their daily practices to teamwork. If participants' accounts revealed that they had changed working practices such that they now had joint responsibility for their task and experienced higher levels of autonomy it would a sign that they now worked in teams. After matching data from employees to the data from their manager, template analysis (Patton, 2002) was applied to detect response patterns showing how the context had influenced the intervention and its outcomes.

Results

Effect evaluation. Table 2.3. shows the complex array of changes that emerged from the effect evaluation. Small decreases were found in team interdependency in group 1 (no training), in group 4 (where managers had been on a tailored training course) and group 6 (where managers had been on the tailored training course and employees had also received training); however, these were not significant. Groups 2 (where only employees had been on training), and 3 (where the team manager had been on off-the-shelf training) experienced significant increases in interdependency while

Table 2.3   Changes over Time Input Factors Controlled for Baseline Team Levels

Variable	Group	Baseline Mean (SD)	Follow-up Mean (SD)	Change	CI
Interdependency	1	67.8(14.0)	63.2(13.8)	−4.33	(−10.05; 1.39)
	2	64.4(14.9)	71.5(14.7)	6.83[†]	(−0.43; 14.10)
	3	39.2(12.4)	57.2(11.4)	16.56[*]	(2.51; 30.61)
	4	66.6(15.0)	63.5(14.6)	−3.56	(−8.60;1.49)
	5	61.6(14.3)	61.9(15.9)	0.27	(−5.09; 5.63)
	6	67.8(14.1)	63.6(18.4)	−4.45	(−10.95;2.04)
Autonomy	1	65.8(12.1)	66.0(11.0)	0.46	(−5.22; 6.13)
	2	53.6(13.2)	67.5(14.6)	12.84[**]	(4.09; 21.58)
	3	58.0(15.2)	62.1(18.2)	5.08	(−6.06; 16.21)
	4	63.1(15.7)	65.5(10.3)	1.21	(−4.16; 6.59)
	5	57.3(20.1)	63.3(15.9)	5.29[†]	(−0.24; 10.82)
	6	56.5(18.7)	59.9(17.7)	2.41	(−4.61; 9.44)
Team effectiveness	1	55.2(19.8)	48.5(16.8)	−6.72[*]	(−13.35; −0.10)
	2	49.0(16.4)	60.6(18.0)	11.89[**]	(3.19; 20.59)
	3	38.9(18.8)	53.8(20.9)	14.58[†]	(−2.09; 31.25)
	4	55.3(16.1)	58.8(18.2)	1.18	(−4.82; 7.18)
	5	55.1(19.1)	50.9(18.4)	−4.30	(−10.59; 1.99)
	6	60.0(18.6)	56.6(21.1)	−3.67	(−11.38; 4.04)
Involvement	1	61.3(15.2)	53.6(15.4)	−7.50[**]	(−13.11; −1.89)
	2	56.8(19.9)	62.7(15.1)	3.93	(−4.02; 11.88)
	3	47.5(16.4)	50.3(14.9)	2.86	(−8.08; 13.79)
	4	60.3(14.2)	62.2(13.3)	1.27	(−4.02; 6.55)
	5	51.7(17.9)	53.1(16.6)	1.57	(−3.73; 6.87)
	6	53.1(14.9)	61.3(15.4)	7.83[*]	(0.91; 14.74)

[†] = p<.10 [*] = p < .05, [**] = p < .01. CI = Confidence Interval

group 5 (where team managers had been on the off-the-shelf training course and employees also had received training) remained stable (Table 2.3.). In group 2 there was a tendency towards significant change on these variables (p = .07), whereas the increase was significant in group 3. With regards to autonomy, group 2 reported a significant increase and there was a tendency towards higher autonomy in group 5.

We found a tendency towards a significant increase in group 2 and a tendency in group 3 (p = .08) with regards to team effectiveness. Group 1 experienced a decrease in team effectiveness. The increased involvement in group 6 was significant as was the decrease in group 1.

Previous research on the implementation of teams suggests that positive change should have occurred in these situations in all groups, with the largest changes being in the groups receiving training. The group of teams where neither employees nor team managers had been on a training course either remained stable or reported some decreases when supposedly exposed to the implementation of teams. This suggests that without some training, team implementation is likely to be less effective than it could be (hypothesis 1). The largest improvements were found in groups 3 and 5 where team managers had participated in an off-the-shelf training course (and employees had been on a training course). This is in contrast with hypothesis 1 where we predicted that tailored training would have a greater impact due to it being more appropriately developed to fit the group's need. Interestingly, positive effects were found where only employees received training (group 2) and there were no additional positive effects to be found when team and manager training were combined.

A conclusion from the quantitative effect evaluation could be that implementing teams was ineffective or potentially damaging unless it was supported by training (based on the findings from group 1). We might also conclude that if team managers or employees (but not both) participated in an off-the-shelf training program the intervention would be more effective. The results also suggest that tailoring a training programme for managers offers no significant gains. We then used the qualitative process evaluation to test the validity of these interim conclusions.

Process evaluation

Training process evaluation. All managers, both those participating in the tailored and the off-the-shelf training course, reported that they had felt the training course to be very useful. This was partly because the tools provided could be used in their daily work as a team manager responsible for implementing teamwork. They also reported that the training course had given them the opportunity to discuss their experiences of implementing teams with colleagues in the same situation. Furthermore, managers that had participated in the tailored training course were all from the same elderly care center and saw the training as an opportunity to develop a shared strategy for team implementation. This appeared to rule out the possibility that some forms of the training (i.e., tailored training, or combining employee and manager training) had in some way hindered the effectiveness of the team implementation.

Organizational context evaluation. During the project some organizational-wide changes took place that influenced the implementation process. The local government had overspent and paid a financial penalty to the government. This led to downsizing and reorganization in the local government's elderly care. Managers

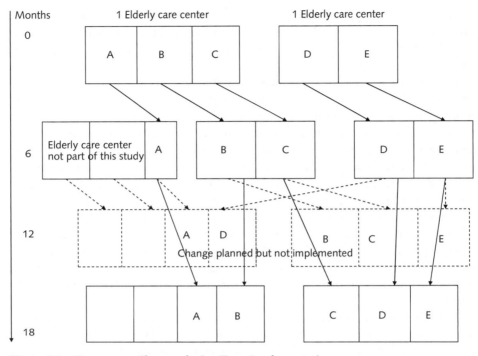

Figure 2.2   Concurrent Changes during Team Implementation

were no longer allowed to use temporary staff from agencies: this represented a serious problem as the elderly care sector has a high absence rate and has problems maintaining and recruiting staff. Most teams in this study had vacant positions they could not fill. As a result, hardly any shifts had full coverage. Both employees and managers reported this made it difficult to devote time and energy to work on team implementation. Also, changes specific to each elderly care center were detected: six months after baseline it was decided to merge part of one of the elderly care centers with another so the center participating in our study became smaller. This meant that one team consisting of both homecare and elderly care home staff was separated from one of the two participating elderly care centers. However, they still participated in this study (from group 2, see Figure 2.2.). It also meant that some of the kitchen team and the activity team (consisting of ergonomic therapists and physiotherapists) became smaller. Twelve months after the baseline survey (and six months before follow-up) it was decided that the other elderly care center had to merge with another elderly care center and it was made clear that the number of line managers would have to be reduced. Functional managers (managers of the activity team, the kitchen team, the homecare manager and the elderly care center manager) had to re-apply for their jobs in competition with managers from the other elderly care center. Six months went by without any clarification of the future and then with a month's notice it was decided that the other elderly care center would be split up between this elderly care center and another not participating in our study. This happened as we sent out the follow-up questionnaire. Naturally these changes created turbulence among both employees and managers in all six study groups. Many found it difficult to focus on their daily work let alone the team implementation. Figure 2.2. provides an overview of this merger process.

This overall analysis of the intervention process strengthened the effect evaluation. Further analysis was then carried out within the six groups to test further the validity of the effect evaluation.

Group 1: no training (5 teams)

The context of this group provided a number of explanations for the drop in team effectiveness and involvement. It had been difficult to retain and recruit staff and positions had been vacant for long periods of time. Managers reported a lack of support from the elderly care center manager in implementing teams. Employees reported being skeptical about the introduction of teams, believing there to be a hidden management agenda i.e., a way of getting team members to pressure each other to come to work and thus reduce absenteeism. Analysis of mental models in two out of the five teams in group 1 indicated that employees believed they had worked in teams before the intervention. In two teams they reported wanting to work with teams but felt that the team manager did not support teamwork and that they had no time to work on team implementation. Only in the last team had changes taken place (where team members were made responsible for planning meetings and rosters) but the process had stagnated when the team manager went on sick leave. With regards to learning, the last team (where the manager was on sick leave and some changes had been implemented prior to her absence) reported that they had learnt to use each others' skills and had experienced a synergy effect due to team implementation.

Group 2: only employee training (2 teams)

All reported that the elderly care center manager did not support team implementation. Turnover had been high in these teams. One team manager had taken a sabbatical and team members themselves were responsible for daily management and team implementation. In effect, in this team, two employees had been "designated" as team leaders. As a result the team functioned as two separate "subteams". The idea of teams had been welcome in one subgroup and they shared responsibility for the roster and for the planning of tasks and the budgets. There was evidence that they had developed a psychological contract on collaboration and cooperation within the team. The designated leader of this subgroup leader felt that the group had embraced the idea of teams and all had worked hard to implement teamwork. Employees also expressed great enthusiasm for the team idea, and that the training course had helped give them an idea of what a team is and how they could go forward. It was reported that employees who had previously been quiet had grown with the task; they were more outspoken and eager to take responsibility. Where they were responsible for financial issues they also had greater insight into the team's role in the organization. In the other sub-group there was very little change.

The team manager who was not on sick leave and the other designated subgroup leader found it difficult to implement teams: both felt that employees wanted a strong manager. Employees managed by these people reported less enthusiasm and much disappointment with the leader. These differences within Group 2 help to explain why the overall effects for this group are modest, but also suggest that the significant improvements in interdependency, autonomy, and effectiveness came from the group that had embraced team implementation and had therefore been able to transfer the employee training to the working environment.

Group 3: only off-the-shelf manager training course (1 team)
Here budget cuts were not a problem as the team had its own group of temporary staff consisting of students that were paid the same as staff (not the higher rate of pay that agency staff received). No support had been needed from the elderly care center manager. As a result of the implementation of teams, employees had been split into two subgroups that were each responsible for a smaller group of clients and were now responsible for planning team meetings. There was evidence that they had become responsible for the roster, and several teambuilding initiatives had been initiated. They also had more direct responsibility for patient care and contact. Team members indicated that working in a team was an opportunity to have more autonomy and know the clients better. The team manager welcomed the team idea and was aware of her role in developing the team and its members (as a coach and a source of inspiration for staff). She did not feel that the context had been a problem during team implementation and she had perceived the lack of support from upper management as freeing her to implement teams. The team members perceived themselves as functioning well together, collaborating and supporting each other. They also perceived the team manager as being very supportive. Both the team manager and employees reported that they were now able to discuss and solve problems and they had developed an understanding of a shared purpose and joint responsibility. Taken together this is consistent with the significant gains in autonomy and effectiveness reported by the group. It was surprising that such gains were not also found in the other outcome variables.

Group 4: only tailored manager training course (6 teams)
This group had experienced a great deal of turbulence. 5 out of 6 managers in group 4 would have to apply for their own position because of the imminent merger. In several teams people had been made redundant (25% in one team). Only in one team had any changes occurred that were related to the implementation of teams—here they developed a psychological contract and conducted a competency mapping exercise to ensure efficient task completion. The mental models of team managers revealed that they saw employees as working in a team pre-intervention. Although they all felt the training programme had been useful, they had not used the tools provided in their daily work. They felt pressured by the imminent merger and found it difficult to implement changes when they had to make staff redundant. One manager even said she felt it unethical to talk about teams in such difficult times. 4 out of 6 teams also reported that they already worked as a team and that the organizational

changes made it very difficult to work with a team structure. No examples were given of learning in this group. Therefore it would not be appropriate to conclude the tailored training was ineffective. In a more stable intervention context, such training may transfer better to the work environment.

Group 5: off-the-shelf manager training course and employee training (6 teams)
There appeared to be significant problems with implementation in this group. It was perceived that the elderly care center manager was not supportive of team implementation, and that one team had experienced significant redundancies (10% of all staff). Another team had been without a manager for a couple of months. In five out of the six teams the group of employees had been divided into two "subteams". All teams were now responsible for the roster and work planning. All held regular team meetings. The leaders' mental models revealed that they saw their teams as competent and they were aware of their role in supporting the team. The teams' mental models supported this. Most teams saw the team manager as supportive of them and the team implementation, and all felt they worked well together. Two teams reported that older employees had found the transition difficult. With regards to learning, four teams reported that team members now took more responsibility and two teams reported that employees who had previously been very quiet were now participating and contributing to the joint task of the team. Therefore, it would not be reasonable to conclude that combining employee and manager training was ineffective. The impact of intervention within this group appeared to be blunted by the lack of support from senior managers.

Group 6: Tailored team manager training course and employee training (3 teams)
Two out of three team managers were newly appointed (but are included in this group as the previous manager had been on training and thus had the opportunity to implement changes before s/he left). All managers agreed that the management team supported each other in making changes and the elderly care center manager was supportive as well. In two groups team meetings had been introduced and in the third (although employees had been split into two groups that each covered their own geographical area) employees still held meetings together. In one team employees were responsible for roster planning but in another they had this responsibility pre-intervention. In the third team they developed an explicit psychological contract—an agreement on how they worked together including rules for "good" behaviour. Managers saw teams as working well together, but two team managers did not feel they had progressed well although teams were very motivated and in the third team the manager felt her employees had always worked as a team. This was supported by the team members who felt that they worked well together but not much had happened. In one team this was attributed to the fact they had always worked in teams, while another team indicated that the manager now delegated more to them. With regards to learning, it was reported that one team now took more responsibility and another team reported that they used each other more. The relative stability in effect evaluation measures in this group appears to be explained

by the finding that employees considered themselves to be working in a team before the intervention: this is supported by the relatively high baseline levels of the various effect evaluation measures (Table 2.3.).

Summary of findings
As can be seen above, the four themes shaping our process evaluation had a great impact on how managers and their subordinates had worked with team implementation. Organizational turbulence meant that, in some groups, managers and subordinates had felt it inappropriate to work with team implementation. Also the mental models meant that managers and their subordinates already felt they worked in teams and saw little need to change their working practices. Where changes in quantitative outcomes variables were found, changes had taken place: managers and subordinates had bought into the idea of teamwork and had not felt constrained by the organizational turbulence.

Discussion

We have reported here the findings of a longitudinal intervention study of the effects of supporting team implementation by use of training. Hypothesis 1 was supported: beneficial effects were found when team implementation was supported through some forms of training. For the group that received no training at all, no changes, or even decreases were found. Those that received training remained stable, or in some cases increased (i.e., positive changes in team inputs, processes and outcomes). This is contrary to other studies that have found beneficial effects of team implementation (Cordery et al., 1991; Terra, 1995; Wall & Clegg, 1981; Wall et al., 1986). When looking at our process evaluation we see much turbulence that may very well have caused the decreases found in group 1. Terra (1995) and Elo, Ervasti, Kuosma, and Mattila (2008) have previously talked about protective interventions. It may be the case here that, where managers and employees have been on a training course, it is possible that they are given the motivation and skills to work with team implementation that serve them well in times of turbulence.

Interestingly, the tailored team manager training course brought about fewer changes than the off-the shelf team manager training course. It has previously been argued that it is important to consider how individual characteristics influence training outcomes, i.e., the degree to which employees are ready for training can enhance motivation to learn and learning itself (Kraiger, 2003). In this study the tailored training course was mandatory. It is possible that these team managers were less motivated to implement changes that those that went on off-the-shelf training (a course that was voluntary). In addition, a large proportion of the team managers that went on the tailored training course felt that, pre-intervention, their employees worked in teams. Finally, the context had a significant impact on this group: managers went for a long time not knowing whether they had to apply for their own position and not knowing how many and whom they had to make redundant. Therefore, differential effects of the two types of management training may be due to situational factors (Baldwin & Ford, 1998) rather than actual effect of the training itself. However, it could also be that participation in training creates unrealistic expectations, thus damaging motivation and lower achievement of training goals (Baldwin & Magjuka, 1997).

It was also found that the largest improvements took place in the team where only employees had been on training or where only the team manager had been on the off-the-shelf training course. Smaller improvements were found where team training had been combined with either kind of team manager training. Process evaluation again helped to explain this finding. In one place the team had taken responsibility themselves for implementing teams in the absence of a formal team manager. In addition, the team manager in group 3 had felt very strongly about the implementation of teamwork and had worked hard to make changes. Also, the team in group 3 had very low baseline scores and it is possible that there was more room for improvement (Nielsen et al., 2006).

As can be seen, the mixed methods approach and bracketing proved invaluable in the evaluation process. For example, even if managers reported they found the course useful they sometimes reported difficulties working with the implementation of teamwork because of the uncertainty caused by downsizing and the imminent merger. In addition, analysis of the mental models of team members and managers showed that few changes had taken place in teams where managers and employees had been suspicious of the local government's motive for implementing teams or where they thought they already worked in teams.

Aside from these specific examples, the use of mixed methods and bracketing enriched understanding of the intervention in several ways. First, it served as a validity check for the results of the quantitative effect evaluation e.g., that the no-training group had made little progress towards team implementation. Second, it illustrated how teams were actually implemented in terms of changes in responsibilities and working more closely together as a close-knit unit. Third, it served to expand the breadth and range of the results of the quantitative effect evaluation by increasing our understanding of how the context had influenced team implementation.

Had we only used a traditional before and after measurement approach using survey data we would have been unable to distinguish between theory and program failure (Kristensen, 2005; Lipsey & Cordray, 2000). When looking at the process evaluation there was a strong indication that it may be program failure rather than theory failure that accounts for the results of the effect evaluation. Both managers and employees evaluated the courses to be useful. However, when it came to transfer of learning this was perceived to be problematical due to the turbulence.

We were not able to determine whether tailored training was better than off-the shelf training because the tailored training was compulsory and the off-the shelf training course was voluntary. This means that those attending off-the-shelf training were highly committed whereas in some cases the managers on the tailored training course may have felt pressured to attend. However, we would argue that rather than dismissing the study as unscientific we should be focusing on the strengths of the study and the conclusions that can be made based on the mixed methods approach.

The study meets Semmer's call (2003, 2006) to extract the most knowledge possible from "lesser" designs. By using the naturally occurring intervention and control groups we were able to make tentative conclusions that training does have an effect, it may even buffer the negative consequences of concurrent and competing change initiatives. The study had several strengths: the sample size was relatively large, there was a high level of documentation of both effect and process, the process evaluation was integrated with the outcome evaluation (Semmer, 2006), and pretest levels of study variables were controlled to rule out many of the threats to internal validity (Cook & Campbell, 1979).

Implications for Process Evaluation

This study has three important implications. First, it appears that using training to facilitate the implementation ensured good effects, even, or perhaps especially, in times of turbulence (mergers and downsizing). Second, it also shows the importance of careful documentation of the implementation processes to understand changes. Without such careful documentation we would not have been able to interpret the changes found. Intervention evaluation frameworks need to consider the realities of the intervention context and process: individual perceptions and attitudes and concurrent changes influence the outcomes of a given intervention. And finally, it shows how valuable knowledge may be extracted from less-than-optimal designs.

Note

1. Or even when controlled manipulation and good study design is possible, mixed methods can add significant value to evaluation research (see Cook & Shadish, 1994).

References

Argyris, C. (1977). Double loop learning in organizations: Continuity and change. *Harvard Business Review, 55*, September–October.

Argyris, C. (1992). *On organizational learning*. Malden, MA: Blackwell.

Baldwin, T. T., & Ford, J. K. (1998). Transfer of training: A review and directions for future researcher. *Personnel Psychology, 41*, 63–105.

Baldwin, T. T., & Magjuka, R. J. (1997). Organizational context and training effectiveness. In J. K. Ford, W. J. Kozlowski, K. Kraiger, E. Salas, & M. S. Teachout (Eds.), *Improving training effectiveness in work organizations* (pp. 99-128). Mahwah, NJ: Erlbaum.

Bambra, C., Egan, M., Thomas, S., Petticrew, M., & Whitehead, M. (2007). The psychosocial and health effects of workplace restructuring. 2. A systematic review of task restructuring interventions. *Journal of Epidemiology and Community Health, 61*, 1028–1037.

Becker-Reims, E. D. (1994). *Self-managed work teams in health care organizations*. San Francisco: Jossey-Bass.

Bryk, A., & Raudenbush, S. (1992). *HLM: Applications and data analysis methods*. Newbury Park, CA: Sage.

Bryman, A. (2006). Integrating quantitative and qualitative research: How is it done? *Journal of Mixed Methods Research, 6*, 97–113.

Campbell, D. T., & Fiske, D. W. (1959). Convergent and discriminant validation by the multitrait-multimethod matrix. *Psychological Bulletin, 56*, 81–104.

Campbell, J. P., & Kuncel, N. R. (2005). Individual and team training. In N. Anderson, D. S. Ones, H. S. Sinanagil, & C. Viswesvaran (Eds.), *Handbook of industrial, work & organizational psychology* (pp. 278–312). London: Sage.

Campion, M., Papper, E., & Medsker, G. (1996). Relations between work team characteristics and effectiveness: A replication and extension. *Personnel Psychology, 49*, 429–453.

Cannon-Bowers, J. A., Salas, E., & Converse, S.A. (1991). Cognitive psychology and team training: Shared mental models of complex systems. *Human Factors Society Bulletin, 33*, 1–4.

Cohen, S., & Bailey, D. (1997). What makes teams work: Group effectiveness research from the shop floor to the executive suite. *Journal of Management, 23*, 239–290.

Cohen, S., Ledford, G., & Spreitzer, G. (1996). A predictive model of self-managing work team effectiveness. *Human Relations, 49*, 643–676.

Cook, T. D. & Campbell, D. T. (1979). *Quasi-experimentation: Design and analysis issues for field settings*. Chicago: Rand McNally.

Cook, T. D. & Shadish, W. R. (1994). Social experiments: Some developments over the last fifteen years. *Annual Review of Psychology, 45*, 545–580.

Cordery, J., Mueller, W., & Smith, L. (1991). Attitudinal and behavioral effects of autonomous group working: a longitudinal field study. *Academy of Management Journal, 34*, 464–476.

Cox, T., Karanika, M., Griffiths. A., & Houdmont, J. (2007). Evaluating organisational-level work stress interventions: Beyond traditional methods. *Work & Stress, 21*, 348–362.

Druskat, V. U., & Pescocolido, A. T. (2002). The content of effective teamwork mental models in self-managing teams: Ownership, learning and heedful interrelating. *Human Relations, 55*, 283–314.

Egan, M., Bambra, C., Petticrew, M., and Whitehead, M. (2009). Reviewing evidence on complex social interventions: appraising implementation in systemic reviews of the health effects of organisational-level workplace interventions. *Journal of Epidemiology & Community Health. 63*, 4–11.

Elo, A., Ervasti, J., Kuosma, E., & Mattila, P. (2008). Evaluation of an organizational stress management program in a municipal public works organization. *Journal of Occupational Health Psychology, 13*, 10–23.

Grant, A. M., & Wall, T. D. (2008). The neglected science and art of quasi-experimentation: Why-to, when-to, and how-to advice for organizational researchers. *Organizational Research Methods*, doi:10.1177/1094428108320737

Greene, J. C., Caracelli, V. J., & Graham, W. F. (1989). Toward a conceptual framework for mixed-method evaluation designs. *Educational Evaluation and Policy Analysis, 11*, 255–274.

Guzzo, R., & Dickson, M. (1996). Teams in organizations: Recent research on performance and effectiveness. *Annual Review of Psychology, 47*, 307–338.

Hackman, J. R. (2003). Learning more by crossing levels: Evidence from airplanes, hospitals, and orchestras. *Journal of Organizational Behavior, 24*, 905–922.

Herold, D. M., Fedor, D.B., & Caldwell, S. D. (2007). Beyond change management: a multi-level investigation of contextual and personal influences on employees' commitment to change. *Journal of Applied Psychology, 92*, 942–951.

Hox, J. J. (2002). *Multilevel analysis: Techniques and applications*. Mahwah, NJ: Erlbaum.

Lipsey, M. W., & Cordray, D. S. (2000). Evaluation methods for social intervention. *Annual Review of Psychology, 51,* 345–375.

Johnson, R. B., Onwuegbuzie, A. J., & Turner, L. A. (2007). Toward a definition of mixed methods research. *Journal of Mixed Methods Research, 1,* 112–133.

Kozlowski, S. W. J., & Bell, B. S. (2003). Work groups and teams in organizations. In W. C. Borman, D. R. Ilgen, & J. R. Klimoski (Eds.), *Handbook of psychology: Industrial and organizational psychology* (pp. 333–375). London: John Wiley & Sons.

Kraiger, K. (2003). Perspectives on training and development. In W. C. Borman, D. R. Ilgen, & J. R. Klimoski (Eds.), *Handbook of psychology: Industrial and organizational psychology* (pp. 171–192). Hoboken, NJ: John Wiley & Sons.

Kristensen, T. (2005). Intervention studies in occupational epidemiology. *Occupational and Environmental Medicine, 62,* 205–210.

Latham, G..P., & Saari, L.M. (1979). The application of social learning theory to training supervisors through behavioral modelling. *Journal of Applied Psychology, 64,* 239–246.

Lipsey, M., & Cordray, D. (2000). Evaluation methods for social intervention. *Annual Review of Psychology, 51,* 345–375.

Marks, M., Mathieu, J., & Zaccaro, S. (2001). A temporally based framework and taxonomy of team processes. *Academy of Management Review, 26,* 356–375.

Mathieu, J. E., Heffner, T. S., Goodwin, G. F., Salas, E., & Cannon-Bowers, J. A. (2000). The influence of shared mental models on team process and performance. *Journal of Applied Psychology, 85,* 273–283.

Miles, M. B., & Huberman, M. A. (1994). *Qualitative data analysis: An expanded sourcebook*. Thousand Oaks, CA: Sage.

Morgeson, F. P., Johnson, M. D., Campion, M. A., Medsker, G. J., & Mumford, T. V. (2006). Understanding reactions to job redesign: A quasi-experimental investigation of the moderating effects of organizational context on perceptions of performance behavior. *Personnel Psychology, 59,* 333–363.

Murta, S. G., Sanderson, K., & Oldenburg, B. (2007). Process evaluation in occupational stress management programs: A systematic review. *American Journal of Health Promotion, 21,* 248–254.

Nastasi, B. K., Hitchcock, J., Sarkar, S., Burkholder, G., Varjas, K., & Jayasena, A. (2007). Mixed methods in intervention research: Theory to adaptation. *Journal of Mixed Methods Research, 1,* 164–182.

Nielsen, K., Fredslund, H., Christensen, K. B., & Albertsen, K. (2006). Success or failure? Interpreting and understanding the impact of interventions in four similar worksites. *Work & Stress, 20,* 272–287.

Nielsen, K., Randall, R., & Albertsen, K. (2007). Participants' appraisals of process issues and the effects of stress management interventions. *Journal of Organizational Behavior, 28,* 793–810.

Nytrø, K., Saksvik, P. Ø., Mikkelsen, A., Bohle, P., & Quinlan, M. (2000). An appraisal of key factors in the implementation of occupational stress interventions. *Work & Stress, 14,* 213–225.

Parker, S., & Williams, H. (2001). *Effective teamworking: reducing the psychosocial risks*. Norwich, UK: HSE Books.

Parkes, K. R., & Sparkes, T. J. (1998). *Organizational interventions to reduce work stress: Are they effective? A review of the literature*. Sudbury, UK: HSE Books.

Patton, M. Q. (2002). Qualitative research & evaluation methods. Thousand Oaks, CA: Sage.

Pettigrew, A. M. (1990). Longitudinal field research on change: Theory and practice. *Organization Science, 1*, 267–292.

Randall, R., Cox, T., and Griffiths, A. (2007). Participants' accounts of a stress management intervention. *Human Relations, 60,* 1181–1209.

Randall, R., Griffiths, A., & Cox, T. (2005). Evaluating organizational stress-management interventions using adapted study designs. *European Journal of Work and Organisational Psychology, 14,* 23–41.

Randall, R., Nielsen, N., & Tvedt, S. (2009). The development of five scales to measure participants' appraisals of organizational-level stress management interventions. *Work and Stress, 23,* 1–23.

Rasmussen, T. H., & Jeppesen, H. J. (2006). Teamwork and associated psychological factors: A review. *Work & Stress, 20,* 105–128.

Richardson, K. M., & Rothstein, H. R. (2008). Effects of occupational stress management intervention programs: A meta-analysis. *Journal of Occupational Health Psychology, 13,* 69–93.

Saksvik, P. Ø., Nytrø, K., Dahl-Jørgensen, C., & Mikkelsen, A. (2002). A process evaluation of individual and organizational occupational stress and health interventions. *Work & Stress, 16,* 37–57.

Semmer, N. K. (2003). Job stress interventions and organization of work. In L. Tetrick & J. C. Quick (Eds.), *Handbook of occupational health psychology* (pp. 325–353). Washington, DC: APA.

Semmer, N. K. (2006). Job stress interventions and the organization of work. *Scandinavian Journal of Work and Environmental Health, 32,* 515–527.

Sprigg, C., Jackson, P., & Parker, S. (2000). Production teamworking: The importance of interdependence and autonomy for employee strain and satisfaction. *Human Relations, 53,* 1519–1543.

Terra, N. (1995). The prevention of job stress by redesigning jobs and implementing self-regulating teams. In L. Murphy, J. Hurrell, S. Sauter, & G. Keita (Eds.), *Job stress interventions* (pp. 265–281). Washington DC: APA.

Wall, T. D. & Clegg, C. (1981). A longitudinal field study of group work redesign. *Journal of Occupational Behavior, 2,* 3149.

Wall, T. D., Kemp, N. J., Jackson, P. R., & Clegg, C. W. (1986). Outcomes of autonomous workgroups: a long-term field experiment. *Academy of Management Journal, 29,* 280–304.

West, M., Markiewicz, L., & Dawson, J.F. (2004). *TPI: The Team Performance Inventory: User guide.* Birmingham. Aston Organisation Development.

3

Leadership and Employee Health
A Challenge in the Contemporary Workplace

Töres Theorell, Peggy Bernin, Anna Nyberg,
Gabriel Oxenstierna, Julia Romanowska,
and Hugo Westerlund
Stress Research Institute, Stockholm University, Stockholm[1]

This chapter describes scientific discussions about leadership in Sweden during the past two decades and sets them against the historical background. One of the main themes in this discussion has been participatory leadership. While this kind of managerial leadership seems to have many advantages, it may also have the disadvantage that laissez faire patterns—though still rare—are becoming relatively more common. The scientific literature suggests that such a leadership style may be bad for employee health and should therefore be addressed in management education. Three empirical examples serve as illustrations of research on the relationship between managerial leadership and employee health. The first example, which comes from a cross-sectional epidemiological study of Swedish workers, shows that employee descriptions of their leader are related to their own absence on grounds of sickness and sickness presenteeism patterns. The second example is based upon a prospective study of the risk of developing hard endpoint coronary heart disease in male employees in relation to their descriptions of the leadership that they experience in their work. The findings show that men who describe their managers as psychosocially competent have a decreased risk of developing a myocardial infarction during follow-up, after adjustment for accepted cardiovascular risk factors. The third example is based upon a year-long randomized controlled intervention study, with follow-up at 18 months, of managers (who were randomly assigned to two manager education programs) and their subordinates. Preliminary results show that an intervention based upon artistic sessions followed by ethical/moral discussions influenced self-rated mental health favourably and that the blood concentration of a regenerative hormone (which protects against the adverse health effects of long-lasting stress) is also favourably influenced in this group after follow-up.

General Conditions for Management in Sweden

In this contribution we use Sweden and its recent dynamic developments in working life as a background for a discussion of some central aspects of managerial leadership. In all the Nordic countries there is a strong emphasis on democracy and this also means that Scandinavian leadership has its particular traditions. This emphasis on democracy has a long historical tradition, and it is an important background in our discussions regarding the leadership and management of work. Such a discussion will be of interest to researchers and practitioners in many other countries, both those who are in the same developmental phase as Sweden and those who will face a similar development in the future. As our country is going through a transition, the democratic discourse regarding leadership and management may be changing character. This also means that we need a thorough discussion regarding desired management techniques that are adapted to a new working world.

In Sweden serfdom was abolished early, to a great extent because it was not economically feasible in a sparsely populated country. From the 16th century farmers had considerable influence over national policy through the parliament. Sweden was relatively slow in adopting industrialization, but when it happened our country was rapidly industrialized. Mining, forestry, and industry brought Sweden to the forefront of international development, particularly in heavy industry. The labour movement became strong and the social democratic party held uninterrupted political power in parliament and local government for four decades. Similar developments happened in the other Nordic countries. However, Sweden did not participate in the two world wars, and this saved our country from the halt in material progress that its neighbours experienced during the 1940s, 1950s, and 1960s. It may also have contributed to the development of laws to govern the participation of employees in decisions regarding their work and also to protect their employment security. Accordingly, it could be argued that the democracy movement was particularly strong in Sweden for historical reasons.

An active national economic policy in Sweden since the Second World War has been focused mainly on keeping unemployment rates low. However, this changed at the beginning of the 1990s when politicians (a broad majority from right to left) decided that the overriding aim of national economic policy should be to keep inflation low. This drastic change was prompted by a national financial crisis that occurred when Sweden made preparations for entering the European Union. One of the concrete consequences of this sudden shift in national financial policy was a very rapid threefold rise in unemployment over a two-year period, 1990–1991. Many parallel developments coinciding with those in other similar countries have been observed. However, many of the changes that took place over a short period of ten years in our country had been progressing at a slower pace for decades in other highly industrialized countries such as the United States, Great Britain, and the Netherlands. The rapid pace of the changes that took place in Sweden may have contributed to a common feeling of crisis.

There were other changes too. During a period from the mid 1980s to the mid 2000s the number of employees in farming and forestry, industry, and health care decreased. A corresponding increase in numbers of employees in knowledge production, information distribution, teaching, services, and administration took place during the same period. The level of education was rising steadily at the same time.

Information technology, automation of heavy industry, and new management traditions gained ground. Perhaps the most important change, particularly during the latter half of the 1990s and the early 2000s, was that a pronounced downsizing during the first half of the 1990s was followed by repeated reorganizations, with an increasing feeling of insecurity and lack of control. This development was particularly pronounced among women in the public sector. As in most European countries, several indicators used in national surveys showed that work intensity increased steadily in all branches of the Swedish labour market. The strongest increase was observed among employees in counties and municipalities ("the public sector") and particularly among women. In addition, an increasing feeling that control of work had been lost was reported among women in this sector from 1997 onwards, and this feeling became more and more common until a plateau was reached in the mid 2000s. These feelings of increasing loss of control among women in the public sector were paralleled by an increased incidence of work-related mental ill health, long-term sick leave, and retirement on a disability pension in this group. This development reached its peak in the early 2000s.

The increased incidence of long-term absence due to sickness and early retirement starting during the latter half of the 1990s was associated with a large increase in societal public insurance costs. Sweden, Norway, and the Netherlands had the highest rates of sick leave in the world. A number of changes instituted in the insurance system as well as a new law (July 2008) have aimed at a tightened application of rules for paying sickness benefits. These changes have been followed by a considerable decrease in long-term sick leave. Discussions about the responsibilities of companies in this development have been intense. For reviews of this development in Sweden, see Palme et al. (2003) and Theorell (2004).

Leadership in the Scandinavian Context

In studies of preferred management styles, a participatory leadership style, with its emphasis on democracy, has traditionally been favoured in Sweden. During the 1980s the emphasis on employee participation was particularly strong, and this triggered a movement towards "removing middle management". The underlying concept was increased employee participation by means of "flattened hierarchies". Scientific follow-up of employees in companies that had followed this strategy showed (Le Grand, Szulkin, & Tåhlin, 1996) that the effect of removing middle managers was not increased perceived improvement of decision authority for employees, but frequently the opposite. This may have contributed to a backlash against the "participation" movement. Managers following this development observed that companies adopting the "removal of middle management" philosophy did not experience an improved psychosocial work environment, nor a decrease in sick leave rates. It is possible that many of them may have reached the conclusion—erroneously—that it had now been proved that increased employee participation would not lead to improved conditions. However, from the researcher's point of view it was not the theory of the benefits of employee participation to health that was wrong. There is a vast scientific literature confirming the theory that a high level of decision latitude for employees benefits their health (available reviews include Karasek and Theorell, 1990; Theorell, 2008). It was the application of the theory that was wrong. Taking away middle managers may not give employees more decision authority. It is easy to imagine how a large or middle-sized worksite that has no middle management may suffer serious problems. The remaining top-level managers may have too many decisions to make, and the subordinates may experience a great deal of frustration when they are waiting for decisions from their overburdened managers.

The reduction in the number of middle managers also represents a development in the organization of work that took place internationally—from hierarchic organizations to project-based temporary structures and the individualization of work tasks. The individual becomes more and more responsible for his or her own situation (Allvin, 2004), and this frequently induces a "boundaryless" work situation in which leisure and work hours become mixed and the number of working hours tends to increase in an increasingly intensive work situation (Allvin 2008). In addition, temporary employment is rapidly becoming more common and long-term contracts less so. Although the effect of this varies for different groups of employees, this development has bad consequences for the health of many of them (for a review, see Quinlan, Mayhew, & Bohle, 2001).

The strong emphasis on employee participation in Scandinavia became particularly clear in the GLOBE study which examined preferred management styles among managers in European countries (Brenk et al., 2000; Hanges & Dickson, 2004; House, Hanges, Javidan, Dorfman, & Gupta, 2004) but has also emerged as a clear theme in other research (Holmberg & Åkerblom, 2005). Although in the GLOBE study it was clear that there was a "Nordic cluster" of "participatory" styles, there were some differences among the Nordic countries. The preferred form of leadership was even more participatory in Sweden than in Finland, for instance, and this difference was also observed in a direct comparison between employee descriptions of leadership in Finland and Sweden within one large international forestry and paper pulp corporation (Hyde, Jappinen, Theorell, & Oxenstierna, 2006). This survey included a question on typical ways of solving conflicts in the workplace: Is the problem typically solved by means of participatory discussion (democratic), or by having the superior decide (autocratic), or is the problem never solved (laissez faire)? This large international company has units in many countries, and, according to employees across the corporation, the typical problem-solving patterns differed strikingly between countries. Sweden led in the "democratic" style and the Finnish experiences were clearly less "democratic" and also clearly more "autocratic". The "laissez faire" pattern was, on the whole, less common than the other patterns in all countries, but in Sweden "laissez faire" was relatively common compared to other countries and clearly more common than in Finland. In cross-sectional analyses of the relationship between these patterns and self-reported mental health, employees who reported that the democratic style was common in their workplace had a greater likelihood of reporting good mental health and low absence rates for sickness than other employees in the company in the same country. The "laissez faire" pattern was clearly the worst alternative with regard to self-rated health in all countries—employees who reported this pattern were more likely to report poor self-rated health than others. Our conclusion from these analyses has been that a democratic and participatory leadership/management style has many benefits, but that it may also have disadvantages if the "laissez faire" approach is allowed to operate in an uncontrolled fashion.

In a country where participatory management has been instituted for a long time both in practice and in law, many oblique adaptation processes may arise. Not all managers may like participatory processes since these take time and energy and may cause emotional reactions that are difficult to handle. Therefore situations may arise in many work places where the participatory processes "look fine on printed documents" but are not really applied in practice. The following may serve as an example of this:

> All the teachers in a school are participating in a weekend conference, organized by the principal, on an upcoming organizational change. The event takes place in a beautiful conference facility situated in the countryside. Good food and spa activities are offered between the work sessions. Two consultants have been engaged and they form groups in which the teachers are allowed to formulate their views on the need for organizational changes. Everything is carefully noted down in the protocols, and the groups gather and make a joint analysis, which is also taken into the protocol.
>
> When the teachers come back to work after the weekend it becomes obvious to them that the principal has already made decisions regarding organizational changes and that these decisions were taken before the weekend conference.

The example illustrates a situation which is characterized by a glossy "participatory" surface which does not correspond to any real influence for the employees. A growing concern in our country is the counterpart of this among employees—a coping pattern which our research group labels "covert coping". This pattern has been assessed in situations where participants have been exposed to unfair treatment at work. Covert coping corresponds to a passive behavior in this situation—the aggressor (the one carrying out the unfair treatment) will not be confronted with the fact that the employee has been humiliated, and associated emotions fail to find expression. This behavior is more frequent among women in our studies and it is associated with poor health. In men it is associated with high blood pressure (at least in middle age) and prospectively with long-term sick leave (Theorell, Westerlund, Alfredsson, & Oxenstierna, 2005). We do not know whether such behaviors are more frequent in Swedish working life than in other countries, although the study of the international forestry corporation showed that laissez faire was more common in Sweden. "Laissez faire" could be related to covert coping, however, in the sense that a general feeling of negative expectation could result both in "laissez faire" and covert coping—"what I do will not matter in the end". This relates to the cognitive activation theory of stress, abbreviated CATS (Ursin & Eriksen 2004) that emphasizes the important role that expectation plays in stress reactions. According to this theory adverse stress reactions are less likely to occur when there are positive expectations and vice versa.

Hypothesized Desirable Management Styles

With this general background, what might be required of managers and leaders in the present Swedish working situation? On the basis of recent developments the following hypotheses could be formulated:

1.   One of the most prominent features of the present situation is lack of stability and predictability. The work situation would have to compensate for this. Accordingly, *structure and stability* would be required to create systems for *fairness and justice*. This has considerable support in recent literature which has identified *social justice* as a feature favouring employee health (Judge, Piccolo, & Ilies, 2004; Kivimäki, Elovainio, Vahtera, & Ferrie, 2003; Kivimäki et al., 2005; Väänänen et al., 2004).

2.   One related feature would be *willingness to take responsibility* in crisis situations. In a work culture that favours participation, superiors may not realize when it is necessary for them to take personal responsibility in ethically critical situations. This means that avoidance of "laissez faire" attitudes and efforts to stimulate openness should be correlated with good employee health. This hypothesis has been supported by recent studies (Hetland, Sandal, & Johnsen, 2007; Skogstad, Einarsen, Torsheim, Aasland, & Hetland, 2007; Nyberg, Bernin, & Theorell, 2005; Hyde et al., 2006).

3.   *Willingness to cooperate* and to solve conflicts which arise easily during a period of financial crisis with frequent reorganization and downsizing experiences. A popular name for this in management research is *teambuilding*. This aspect of leadership is typical of the Scandinavian leadership style (Brenk et al., 2000; Hanges & Dickson, 2004; Holmberg & Åkerblom, 2005). Social support at work is a prominent feature of teambuilding. It is also a characteristic of work environments that are associated with good employee health.

4.   Since competition is a prominent feature of modern industry and service production, *inspirational behavior* could be assumed to be an important component in leadership. This has been identified as a prominent feature in successful leadership, so-called *transformational leadership*, which has also been shown to be related to good employee health (Berson & Avolio, 2004; DeGroot, Kiker, & Cross, 2000; Fuller, Patterson, Hester, & Stringer, 1996; Howell & Avolio, 1993; Lowe, Kroeck, & Sivasubramaniam, 1996).

Empirical Tests in Our Own Research

How do the crucial elements in leadership described in the hypotheses outlined above relate to employee health? Empirical studies performed by our research group will illustrate how such leadership/management variables relate to various aspects of employee health.

The first example illustrates how leadership characteristics (as perceived by employees) relate to sickness absence statistics in public statistics for the 12 months preceding the survey in the same individuals. This study (Nyberg, Westerlund, Magnusson Hanson, & Theorell, 2008) was based upon a large epidemiological survey in our country. The participants answered a questionnaire on work environment and management dimensions as well as on health, including sickness presenteeism (after Aronsson and Gustafsson, 2005) and sick leave.

The survey covered 5,141 Swedish employees, 56% of the participants in a nationally representative sample of the Swedish working population. The leadership dimensions measured were five subscales of a standardized leadership questionnaire based on a European leadership survey (Hanges & Dickson, 2004): integrity, team integration, inspirational leadership, autocratic leadership, and self-centred leadership. Multiple logistic regression analyses were conducted, adjusting for factors in private life, employment category, labour market sector, working conditions, self-reported general health, and satisfaction with life in general.

Inspirational leadership was associated with a lower rate of short spells of sickness absence (< 1 week) for both men and women. Autocratic leadership was related to a greater number of total sick days taken by men. *Sometimes* showing integrity was associated with higher sickness absence > 1 week among men, and *rarely* showing integrity was associated with more sickness presenteeism among women. Managers *sometimes* seeking team integration was associated with women taking less short (< 1 week) and long (> 1 week) spells of sickness absence. Adjustment for self-reported general health did not alter these associations for men, but did so to some extent for women.

Some of these results were more difficult to interpret than we had expected. First of all, they are based upon employee views reported in self-administered questionnaires and our outcome measures are retrospective 12-month sick leave data supplemented with self-reported sickness presenteeism reports. This means that the directions of the associations are not known. For instance, it is not known whether a high total number of sick leave days over a 12-month period stimulates an *autocratic leadership style* or vice versa. Intuitively the second alternative (autocratic leadership causing a high total number of days of sick leave) seems more likely than the first one, because an autocratic leadership style is likely to be based upon uninformed decisions and lack of flexibility which may be of utmost importance for employees with partial work capacity returning to work after an episode of illness. Work flexibility in this sense has been emphasized by several authors as an important factor in explaining long-term sick leave (Johansson, 2007). Autocratic behavior is the opposite of what was labelled *willingness to cooperate* under point three above.

The variable *integrity* relates to structure and stability as well as fairness and justice. The finding that among women, managers seldom showing integrity may give rise to a greater frequency of sickness presenteeism makes sense intuitively. If it is impossible to trust the manager, there may be a feeling that one has to be present even during illnesses—because an absent worker may lose ground in an insecure situation with a boss who is not trustworthy. The finding among men that the worst alternative was the middle one (manager sometimes showing integrity) in relation to a high rate of sickness absence lasting for at least a week could perhaps be explained if lack of structure and stability is considered to be the crucial dimension. It may be easier to adapt to a situation with a manager who never shows integrity (or always does) than to one with a manager who sometimes does so!

That *inspirational* leadership was associated with low rates of short spells of sick leave was exactly what could be predicted both for historical reasons and according to the scientific literature (see also the discussion regarding effectiveness in relation to transformational and transactional leadership, Lowe et al., 1996). It was interesting, however, that the findings only applied for short spells, not for longer spells of absence through sickness. One interpretation of this is that an inspirational climate is more important for the social climate and may not have far-reaching consequences for more serious forms of ill health. This is entirely speculative, however, and the interpretation requires more research.

The second example shows how one objective and dramatic health outcome, the incidence of hard endpoint ischemic heart disease, relates to leadership dimensions as they are perceived by the employees. The aim of the study (Nyberg et al., 2009) was to investigate the association between managerial leadership and hard endpoint ischemic heart disease (IHD) among employees. The examination was based upon a prospective cohort study (WOLF: Work, Lipids and Fibrinogen, risk factors in relation to ischemic heart disease) and included 3,239 Swedish male employees. The baseline examination was carried out between 1992 and 1995. Managerial leadership variables (provision of clear work objectives, sufficient power in relation to responsibilities, feedback and support—all of which relate to the hypotheses listed above) were rated by subordinates. The items were summarized into a total "good manager" score. Records of hospital admissions with a diagnosis of acute myocardial infarction or unstable angina and deaths from ischemic heart disease or cardiac arrest up to the end of 2003 (average 9.7 years) were obtained from national registers and were used to ascertain episodes of IHD which occurred in 74 men. Age-adjusted likelihood of incident IHD per one standard deviation increase in standardized leadership score was calculated by means of Cox regression which takes into account the fact that individual follow-up periods varied in length. A higher leadership score was associated with lower IHD risk. The inverse association was stronger the longer the participant had worked at the same workplace [hazard ratio if employed for at least 1 year: 0.76 (95% CI 0.61–0.96), 2 years: 0.77 (0.61–0.97), 3 years: 0.69 (0.54–0.88), 4 years: 0.61 (0.47–0.80)], and robust to adjustments for socioeconomic factors and conventional risk factors. This dose-response association was also evident in analyses with only acute MI and cardiac death (even "harder" outcomes) as the outcome.

An interesting aspect of the findings in this study was that there were a total of 10 items included in the leadership score. In separate analyses each one was related to the outcome in the predicted direction, albeit only seven of them significantly so. The two items that seemed to be the most important ones were the leader's ability to "push through" and to "explain goals". These seem to relate in general to a manager's psychosocial competence. The two next in terms of importance were first whether the manager gave "the employee sufficient power to manage his/her tasks" and "the information needed". Both of these are closely related to the employee's decision latitude in the demand-control model (Karasek, 1979, Karasek & Theorell, 1990). The three items following in importance, "manager takes time over my professional development", "shows that he/she cares about me", and "praise from my boss" are all related to the reward dimension in the effort–reward imbalance model (Siegrist, 1996) as well as the social support dimension of the demand–control–support model (for a review, see Theorell, 2008). Accordingly, the two psychosocial work environment theories that have dominated studies of the relationship between psychosocial factors and work and health are both represented but the most important factor is psychosocial "general competence".

The most important aspect of the second example, however, is that the employee's rating of the manager relates to as important a health outcome as ischemic heart disease, even prospectively, and that there may be an element of dose-response in this relationship. It should be borne in mind that the information is based upon employee ratings and could have a subjective bias—influenced by factors related to the employee rather than to the manager.

The third example shows that the way in which leadership education is conducted may be of great importance and that a manager's emphasis on moral obligations, ethical awareness, and willingness to take personal responsibility may be of profound importance in a Scandinavian setting. Such aspects may have been underestimated in a long-lasting process intended to facilitate employee participation. Laissez faire patterns may have to be addressed more directly than hitherto in management programs. The importance of ethical considerations in management training has been emphasized by Brown and Treviño (2006), and Skogstad et al. (2007).

Managers who were given the opportunity to participate in a one-year managerial training program were randomized to two different programs, one "artistic" and one "traditional." Leader competence was defined as the ability to make judgments and to take action. It was hypothesized that the "artistic" program would have a stronger beneficial effect on leader competence. The program participants and four subordinates for each one of them, as well as a manager colleague and a manager supervisor (the latter two only for a few variables), had their assessments before commencement, a year later (when the programs had ended) and a further half a year later (18 months after the start). Participants and subordinates were asked to deliver a morning blood sample as well as to fill out questionnaires focused on mental health (emotional exhaustion, depressive symptoms, and sleep disturbance). Blood samples were analyzed with regard to the serum concentration of cortisol (a raised level of which mirrors energy mobilization) and DHEA-s (a raised level of which mirrors regeneration/anabolism). In both groups there were 12 training sessions during the study year.

The "traditional program" built upon practical experiences in Scandinavian leadership training. This emphasizes group functioning and communication and the educational method builds upon lectures and group discussions as well as the sharing of group experiences. An evaluation in a previous Swedish study (Theorell, Emdad, Arnetz, & Weingarten, 2001) showed that employees whose managers attended a program similar to that of the traditional program in the present study had significantly decreased serum cortisol levels in the morning (under circumstances interpreted to indicate a lower level of energy mobilization in the morning). No such development was seen in the comparison group of employees followed during the same period in the same company. Similarly the employees with managers who attended that program reported a higher level of decision authority after the study year than before, whereas the opposite tendency was seen in the comparison group. For both these analyses the two-way interactions (time·group) were statistically significant. Thus there was support from the previous study for the hypothesis that this program may have beneficial effects on employee health.

The "artistic program" built on performances of poetry and music in combination, followed by discussions about themes raised in the performances. These were focused on existential problems related to moral responsibilities as well as ethical decision making and judgments. This program has not been evaluated in relation to employee health. However, it was hypothesized that it would have stronger effects on employee health than the traditional program because it addresses crucial aspects of manager behavior related to laissez faire, which has turned out in other research to be a crucial negative management style.

The results are preliminary and no details can be given. However, with regard to the health of managers and their subordinates (the groups were combined) there were no consistent differences between the groups after one year although—consistent with previous research—the serum cortisol levels tended to decrease in the traditional group but increase in the artistic group, possibly indicating stress/energy mobilization in the latter. After 18 months, however, there were several changes in self-reported mental health (sleep disturbance, depressive symptoms, and emotional exhaustion) with statistically significant two-way interactions in the direction of benefit for the artistic group compared to the traditional group. The same statistically significant tendency was observed for the regenerative/anabolic hormone DHEA-s. Analyses of employee ratings of managers before, after one year, and after 1.5 years in both groups indicated that laissez faire became less common and "responsibility taking" more common in the artistic group's managers. These preliminary results seem to confirm our hypothesis. They also illustrate that it may be beneficial to address "laissez faire" patterns directly. Another important aspect of these findings is that psychosocial processes often take a long time. It is not possible to achieve profound effects within days or weeks; intervention processes often take months and years. In addition it may often be necessary to pass through distressing stages that both the managers and their employees would prefer to avoid.

Conclusion

The Swedish situation shows that our historical tradition may have been an important background to our strong emphasis on participatory managerial leadership. This has many advantages and is a beneficial factor in employee health. However, albeit uncommon, a laissez faire leadership style may arise in some workplaces partly as a consequence of a strong participatory emphasis. The risk of this style is that "nobody takes responsibility in difficult situations". Such a climate seems to have adverse effects on employee health. Preliminary results point towards the possible beneficial effects of managerial education aimed at this problem. However, in order to translate such results into managerial training it is necessary to apply educational principles other than those commonly used in that field. It is suggested that artistic components may be useful.

Note

1. Töres Theorell and Anna Nyberg are also affiliated to the Department of Public Health Sciences, Karolinska Institute, Stockholm.

References

Allvin, M. (2004). The individualisation of labour. In C. Garsten & K. Jacobsson (Eds.). *Learning to be employable: New agendas on work, responsibility and learning in a globalizing world*. Houndsmills: Palgrave Macmillan.

Allvin, M. (2008). New rules of work: Exploring the boundaryless job. In K. Näswall, J. Hellgren, & M. Sverke (Eds.), *The individual in the changing working life.* (pp. 19–45) Cambridge: Cambridge University Press.

Aronsson, G., & Gustafsson, K. (2005). Sickness presenteeism: Prevalence, attendance-pressure factors, and an outline of a model for research. *Journal of Occupational and Environmental Medicine, 47*, 958–66.

Berson, Y., & Avolio, B. (2004). Transformational leadership and the dissemination of organizational goals: A case study of a telecommunication firm. *Leadership Quarterly, 15*, 625–646.

Brenk, K., Castel, P., Papalexandris, A., Hartog, D., Papalexandris, N., Donnelly-Cox, G., … Booth, S. (2000). Cultural variation of leadership prototypes across 22 European countries. *Journal of Occupational and Organizational Psychology, 73*, 1–29.

Brown, M., & Treviño, L. (2006). Ethical leadership: A review and future directions. *Leadership Quarterly, 17*, 595–616.

DeGroot, T., Kiker, D., & Cross, T. (2000). A meta-analysis to review organizational outcomes related to charismatic leadership. *Canadian Journal of Administrative Sciences, 13*, 356–371.

Fuller, J., Patterson, C., Hester, K., & Stringer, D. (1996). A quantitative review of research on charismatic leadership. *Psychological Reports, 78*, 271–287.

Hanges, P., & Dickson, M. (2004). The development and validation of the GLOBE culture and leadership scales. In R. House, P. Hanges, M. Javidan, P. Dorfman, & V. Gupta (Eds.). *Culture, leadership, and organizations: The GLOBE study of 62 societies* (pp.122–151). Thousand Oaks, CA: Sage.

Hetland, H., Sandal, G., & Johnsen, T. (2007). Burnout in the information technology sector: Does leadership matter? *European Journal of Work and Organizational Psychology, 16*, 58–75.

Holmberg, I., & Åkerblom, S. (2001). The production of outstanding leadership—An analysis of leadership images in the Swedish media. *Scandinavian Journal of Management, 17,* 67–85.

House, R., Hanges, P., Javidan, M., Dorfman, P., & Gupta, V. (Eds.). *Culture, leadership, and organizations: The GLOBE study of 62 societies.* Thousand Oaks, CA: Sage.

Howell, J., & Avolio, B. (1993). Transformational leadership, transactional leadership, locus of control, and support for innovation: key predictors of consolidated business unit performance. *Journal of Applied Psychology, 78,* 891–902.

Hyde, M., Jappinen, P., Theorell, T., & Oxenstierna, G. (2006). Workplace conflict resolution and the health of employees in the Swedish and Finnish units of an industrial company. *Social Science and Medicine, 63,* 2218–2227.

Johansson, G. (2007). *The illness flexibility model and sickness absence.* Sweden: Karolinska Institutet.

Judge, T., Piccolo, R., & Ilies, R. (2004). The forgotten ones? The validity of consideration and initiating structure in leadership research. *Journal of Applied Psychology, 89,* 36–51.

Karasek, R. (1979). Job demands, job decision latitude and mental strain: Implications for job redesign. *Administrative Sciences Quarterly, 24,* 285–307.

Karasek, R., & Theorell, T. (1990). *Healthy work: Stress, productivity, and the reconstruction of working life.* New York: Basic Books.

Kivimäki, M., Elovainio, M., Vahtera, J., & Ferrie, J. (2003). Organisational justice and health of employees: prospective cohort study. *Occupational and Environmental Medicine, 60,* 27–33.

Kivimäki, M., Ferrie, J., Bruner, E., Head, J., Shipley, M., Vahtera, J., & Marmot, M. (2005). Justice at work and reduced risk of coronary heart disease among employees: The Whitehall II Study. *Archives of Internal Medicine, 165,* 2245–2251.

Le Grand, C., Szulkin, R., & Tåhlin, M. (Eds.) (1996). Sveriges Arbetsplatser—Organisation, Personalutveckling, Styrning [Swedish workplaces—Organization, staff development and leadership]. Stockholm: SNS.

Lowe, K., Kroeck, K., & Sivasubramaniam, N. (1996). Effectiveness correlates of transformational and transactional leadership: A meta-analytic review of the MLQ literature. *Leadership Quarterly, 7,* 385–425.

Nyberg, A., Alfredsson, L., Theorell, T., Westerlund, H., Vahtera, J., & Kivimäki, M. (2009). Managerial leadership and ischemic heart disease among employees: The Swedish WOLF study. *Occupational and Environmental Medicine, 66,* 51–55.

Nyberg, A., Bernin, P., & Theorell, T. (2005). *The impact of leadership on the health of subordinates.* Stockholm: National Institute for Working Life.

Nyberg, A., Westerlund, H., Magnusson Hanson, L., & Theorell, T. (2008). Managerial leadership is associated with self-reported sickness absence and sickness presenteeism among Swedish men and women. *Scandinavian Journal of Public Health, 36,* 803–811.

Palme, J., Bergmark, Å., Bäckman, O., Estrada, F., Fritzell, J., Lundberg, O., … Szebehely, M. (2003). A welfare balance sheet for the 1990s. Final report of the Swedish Welfare Commission. *Scandinavian Journal of Public Health: Supplement, 60,* 7–143.

Quinlan, M., Mayhew, C., & Bohle, P. (2001). The global expansion of precarious employment, work disorganization, and consequences for occupational health: A review of recent research. *International Journal of Health Services, 31,* 335–414.

Siegrist, J. (1996). Adverse health effects of high-effort/low-reward conditions. *Journal of Occupational Health Psychology, 1,* 27–41.

Skogstad, A., Einarsen, S., Torsheim, T., Aasland, M., & Hetland, H. (2007). The destructive-ness of laissez-faire leadership behavior. *Journal of Occupational Health Psychology, 12*, 80–92.

Theorell, T. (2004). Democracy at work and its relationship to health. In M. Perrewé, & D. Ganster (Eds.). *Research in occupational stress and well-being. Vol. 3*, (pp. 323-357). Oxford: Elsevier.

Theorell, T. (2008). After 30 years with the demand-control-support model—How is it used today? *Scandinavian Journal of Work, Environment and Health, Supplement, 6*, 3–5.

Theorell, T., Emdad, R., Arnetz, B., & Weingarten, A-M. (2001). Employee effects of an edu-cational program for managers at an insurance company. *Psychosomatic Medicine, 63*, 724–733.

Theorell, T., Westerlund, H., Alfredsson, L., & Oxenstierna, G. (2005). Coping with critical life events and lack of control—The exertion of control. *Psychoneuroendocrinology. 30*, 1027–32.

Ursin, H., & Eriksen, H. (2004). The cognitive activation theory of stress. *Psycho-neuroendocrinology, 29*, 567–92.

Väänänen, A., Kalimo, R., Toppinen-Tanner, S., Mutanen, P., Peiró, J.M., Kivimäki, M., & Vahtera, J. (2004). Role clarity, fairness, and organizational climate as predictors of sick-ness absence: a prospective study in the private sector. *Scandinavian Journal of Public Health, 32*, 426–34.

4

Employee Burnout and Health
Current Knowledge and Future Research Paths

Arie Shirom
Tel-Aviv University, Israel

The major objective of this chapter is to integrate and summarize what is already known about burnout and certain aspects of physical health. Another objective is to provide a roadmap depicting promising future research directions on employee burnout and health. The major sections of the review focus on burnout and health behaviors, burnout and self-rated health, and burnout and chronic disease. The chronic diseases that I focus on are cardiovascular disease and its major risk factors, diabetes, and musculoskeletal disorders, primarily because there is a significant body of evidence on each of them. In the final section, I suggest several promising future research paths on employee burnout and health. Given the complexity of the burnout construct and the controversy over its operational definition (e.g., Kristensen, Borritz, Villadsen, & Christensen, 2005), I first provide a conceptual analysis of the phenomenon of burnout.

The literature on burnout is now vast; a bibliography covering the period 1990–2002 (Boudreau & Nakashima, 2002) identified 2,138 distinct items, while a more recent (March 2009) search of Google Scholar—under the key term *burnout*—yielded more than 260,000 entries. Given the amount of time most adults spend on work-related activities, and the wealth of literature pointing to the pivotal importance of one's job characteristics to one's self-identity (Bandura, 2002), the focus on burnout is understandable. A number of comprehensive reviews of various aspects of burnout at work have been published in recent years (e.g., Halbesleben, 2006; Halbesleben & Buckley, 2004; Melamed, Shirom, Toker, Berliner, & Shapira, 2006; Schaufeli & Buunk, 2003). The current review, however, does not overlap with any of these; instead, it attempts to discuss themes and topics that have not yet been systematically reviewed in prior studies.

Burnout is viewed as an affective reaction to ongoing stress whose core content is the gradual depletion over time of individuals' intrinsic energy resources, including, as the major types of energy resource depletion, emotional exhaustion, physical fatigue, and cognitive weariness (cf. Shirom, 2003). This review focuses on employee burnout in work organizations, excluding research that deals exclusively with nonwork-related settings.

Why Use Burnout Rather Than Stress Exposure?

It could be argued that if burnout reflects and summarizes individuals' experiences of work-related stress—as posited above—researchers could focus on work-related stress as a major predictor of subsequent health impairments. Why do we need the construct of burnout to better understand the impact of the work context on employee health?

To demonstrate the relevance of focusing on burnout rather than on stress at work, I would like to present the case of stress, burnout, and cardiovascular disease (CVD). There is a substantial body of empirical evidence linking each of a large number of work-related stresses to CVD morbidity and mortality (Belkic, Landsbergis, Schnall, & Baker, 2004; Rozanski, Blumenthal, Davidson, Saab, & Kubzansky, 2005). However, there have been very few attempts to study the effects of combined exposure to these stresses on CVD risk factors (Belkic, Schnall, Savic, & Landsbergis, 2000). Such attempts often encounter basic problems which are very difficult to solve in any study. These basic problems include identifying the most relevant subset of stresses to be covered by any given study, how to represent both contextualized (idiographic) and noncontextualized (nomothetic) types of stress, which types of stress to cover (namely, chronic stress, critical work events, hassles), whether to combine the impact of the specific stresses covered by a study in a linear or nonlinear manner, and how to account for dose-response relationships (Zapf, Dormann, & Frese, 1996). A major limitation of past attempts to use stress inventories (e.g., Belkic, Schnall, Savic, & Landsbergis, 2000) is the lack of theoretical and empirical consideration of the actual reality of work environments, characterized by nonlinear relationships and complex interactions among types of stress (Cummings & Cooper, 1998). Burnout develops after an extended period of exposure to job stress, and therefore could be viewed as a major manifestation of stress consequences (Melamed et al., 2006). I regard burnout as a proxy variable that may be used to assess the extent to which individuals have experienced work-related stresses that deplete their energy resources.

On the Conceptual Meaning of Burnout

When measured on several occasions in longitudinal studies, burnout was found to have moderate to high stability coefficients. In longitudinal studies on burnout, the across-time correlations (also referred to as stability coefficients) were found to range from .50 to .60, regardless of the measure of burnout used (for references to these longitudinal studies, please see Melamed et al. 2006). This suggests that, regardless of the sample makeup, the cultural context, and the length of time of the follow-up survey, the phenomenon of burnout exhibits stability, attesting to its chronic nature. Other types of affective states have been found to exhibit the same degree of stability over time (Conley, 1984; Luthans, Avolio, Avey, & Norman, 2007), so burnout is not exceptional in its chronic nature. Below, I review three major conceptualizations of burnout.

The Maslach Burnout Inventory (MBI)

The MBI (or any of its more recent versions, such as the MBI-General Survey) has been the most popular instrument for measuring burnout in empirical research (for a review of studies using this measure see Collins, 1999; Lee & Ashforth, 1996; Schaufeli & Enzmann, 1998). The MBI contains items purportedly assessing each of the three clusters of symptoms included in the syndrome view of burnout, which are emotional exhaustion, cynicism or depersonalization, and reduced effectiveness or lowered professional efficacy. It asks respondents to indicate the frequency over the work year with which they have experienced each feeling on a 7-point scale ranging from 0 (never) to 6 (every day). Kristensen et al. (2005) provide a description of the way the BMI was constructed: by collecting a large pool of items, subjecting them to an exploratory data analytic technique (exploratory factor analysis), and labeling the resultant factors as per the three components of the MBI, claiming that these factors represent the range of experiences associated with the phenomenon of burnout (see also Maslach, 1998, p. 68; Schaufeli & Enzmann, 1998, p. 51). As Kristensen et al. (2005) and others (e.g., Shirom, 2003) point out, the MBI was not constructed based on an underlying theory explaining why the three factors should belong to the phenomenon of burnout rather than, say, to its immediate consequences (such as depersonalization or reduced personal accomplishments, two components of the MBI).

The factorial validity of the MBI has been extensively studied (for a recent meta-analysis of validation studies, see: Worley, Vassar, Wheeler, & Barnes, 2008). Most of the researchers examining this aspect of MBI validity have reported that a three-factor solution better fits their data than does a two-dimensional or a one-dimensional structure. Researchers using the MBI have most often constructed three different scales corresponding to the three dimensions of emotional exhaustion, cynicism, and reduced personal effectiveness, and have used them as three separate scales, following the specific recommendation included in the MBI manual *not* to use the MBI's total score (Maslach, Jackson, & Leiter, 1996). Several authors interpreted this instruction from the MBI manual and empirical evidence as indicating that, conceptually, the aggregation of the three MBI dimensions is meaningless, and therefore an overall score of the MBI should not be used (Kristensen et al., 2005). The emotional exhaustion dimension has been consistently viewed as the core component of the MBI, predicting the other two components in longitudinal studies (Taris, Le Blanc, Schaufeli, & Schreurs, 2005). Most studies have shown it to be the most internally consistent and stable component, relative to the other two (Schaufeli & Enzmann, 1998). In meta-analytic reviews, the emotional exhaustion dimension has been shown to be the one that is most responsive to the nature and intensity of work-related stress (Lee & Ashforth, 1996; Schaufeli & Enzmann, 1998).

Pines's burnout model and measure

Pines and colleagues defined burnout as a state of physical, emotional, and mental exhaustion caused by long-term involvement in emotionally demanding situations (for references, see Pines, 1993). Pines and colleagues (e.g., Pines, Aronson, & Kafry, 1981) view burnout as applicable to all life domains, including, for example, marital relationships (Pines, 1987). Much like the MBI, their conceptualization of burnout emerged from clinical experiences and case studies. In the process of actually con-structing a measure that purported to assess burnout—dubbed the *burnout measure* (BM)–Pines and her colleagues moved away from the definition offered previously. In the BM, Pines and her colleagues viewed burnout as a syndrome of co-occurring symptoms that include helplessness, hopelessness, entrapment, decreased enthusi-asm, irritability, and a sense of lowered self-esteem (Pines, 1993). None of these symptoms, however, is anchored in the context of work or employment relation-ships. The BM is considered a one-dimensional measure yielding a single-composite burnout score. Evidently, the overlap between the conceptual definition and the operational definition is minimal (cf. Schaufeli & Enzmann, 1998, p. 48). In addi-tion, the discriminant validity of burnout, as assessed by the BM, relative to depres-sion, anxiety, and self-esteem is impaired (Shirom & Ezrachi, 2003). This has led researchers to describe the BM as an index of psychological strain that encompasses physical fatigue, emotional exhaustion, depression, anxiety, and reduced self-esteem (e.g., Schaufeli & Dierendonck, 1993, p. 645).

The Shirom–Melamed Burnout Model and Measure

The conceptualization of burnout that underlies the Shirom–Melamed Burnout Measure (SMBM: freely downloadable from www.shirom.org) was inspired by the work of Maslach and colleagues and Pines and colleagues, as described earlier. Burnout is viewed as an affective state characterized by one's feelings that one's physical, emotional, and cognitive energies are depleted. Theoretically, the SMBM was based on Hobfoll's (Hobfoll, 1989, 2002) Conservation of Resources (COR) theory. The basic tenets of COR theory state that people are motivated to obtain, retain, and protect that which they value. The things that people value are called *resources*, of which there are several types, including material, social, and energy resources. The conceptualization of burnout formulated by Shirom (1989) on the basis of COR theory (Hobfoll & Shirom, 2000) relates to energy resources only, and covers physical, emotional, and cognitive energies (for the theoretical rationale of focusing on energy resources, see Shirom, 2003). COR has often been used in past research to explain burnout (e.g., Halbesleben & Rathert, 2008; Neveu, 2007; Wright & Cropanzano, 1998). Burnout is most likely to occur in situations where there is an actual resource loss, perceived threat of resource loss, or when one fails to obtain resources to offset lost resources—situations defined as being stress-related in COR (Hobfoll & Shirom, 2000).

Burnout, based on COR and as operationally defined by the SMBM, was conceptualized as a multidimensional construct whose three facets were physical fatigue (feelings of tiredness and low energy) emotional exhaustion (lack of the energy to display empathy to others), and cognitive weariness (feelings of reduced mental agility). There were several theoretical reasons for focusing on these three facets. First, physical, emotional, and cognitive energy are individually possessed, and are expected to be closely interrelated (Hobfoll & Shirom, 2000). COR theory postulates that personal resources affect one another and exist as a resource pool—lacking one is often associated with lacking another. Furthermore, COR theory argues that these resources represent a set of resources internal to the self that facilitates the development and use of other resources (Hobfoll, 2002). Third, the conceptualization of the SMBM clearly differentiates burnout from stress appraisals anteceding burnout, from coping behaviors that individuals may engage in to ameliorate the negative aspects of burnout—like distancing themselves from client recipients—as well as from probable consequences of burnout—like performance decrements similar to reduced personal accomplishments in the MBI. Using confirmatory structure analysis, empirical research conducted using the SMBM confirmed the tri-component view of the construct (cf. Melamed et al., 2006; Shirom, Nirel, & Vinokur, 2006; Shirom, Vinokur, & Nirel, in press). The MBI was found (Shirom & Melamed, 2006) to be comparable in terms of construct validity to the conceptualization of burnout used in this study. A series of studies that confirmed expected relationships between the SMBM and physiological variables have lent support to its construct validity (for a review of these studies, please see Melamed et al., 2006).

Burnout and Health Behaviors

The theoretical perspective on burnout proposed above, based on the Conservation of Resources theory (Hobfoll & Shirom, 2000) leads to the expectation that people experiencing a loss of resources will try to limit further losses and thus engage in poor health behaviors. People often distract themselves from situations that cause them distress, like burnout, by engaging in health-impairing activities such as smoking, consuming alcohol, or eating high-sugar food—health behaviors that may alleviate their distress in the short run, but at the expense of a deteriorating state of health in the long run (Schwarzer & Fuchs, 1995). There is a body of evidence documenting negative associations between denial and avoidance types of coping, such as those represented by the above health behaviors, and health status (Penley, Tomaka, & Wiebe, 2002). For example, there is a widespread belief that high job-stress can lead to high levels of alcohol consumption, a paradigm known as the "tension reduction model" (Cooper, Russell, & Frone, 1990). However, recent evidence has substantiated the theoretical argument that the relationship between work stress and alcohol consumption is mediated by impoverished worker resources, among other vulnerabilities of workers (Frone, 2003).

The relationships between burnout and health behaviors have hardly been subjected to empirical scrutiny (Schaufeli & Enzmann, 1998, pp. 87–89). For example, we could not identify any prior study that related burnout to nutrition habits, weight control, and physical exercise. Schaufeli and Enzmann (1998, p. 88) found four studies that investigated the linkages among health behaviors (coffee consumption, alcohol consumption, caloric intake, substance abuse, and smoking) and emotional exhaustion or burnout, all of which reported null or very small correlations. However, their review did not cover burnout as defined by the vital exhaustion construct as a measure of burnout (Appels, 2004). Appels (for references, see Appels, 2004) introduced the construct of *vital exhaustion*, abbreviated as VE, which refers to a state characterized by excess fatigue, lack of energy, increased irritability, sleep disturbances, and feelings of demoralization. VE is considered to be a measure conceptually akin to burnout, but differing from it because it includes items gauging sleep disturbances, anxiety and depression; therefore, it was not included among the major approaches toward the conceptualization of burnout described in an earlier section. Several studies reported that burnout, as assessed by the VE measure, was closely correlated with smoking (Bages, Falger, Perez, & Appels, 2000). A large-scale epidemiological study of males and females in Denmark (Prescott, Holst, Gronbaak, Schohr, Jensen, & Barefoot, 2003) found VE to be closely correlated with two measures of obesity (waist-hip ratio and body mass index), smoking, leading a physically inactive life, and alcohol consumption. None of the above studies controlled for depression, which conceptually (Suls & Bunde, 2005) and empirically (Schaufeli & Enzmann, 1998) partially overlaps burnout regardless of the measure used to assess either. Based on the above body of evidence and theoretical reasoning, I would like to suggest that future research examine if, and under what conditions, burnout would be positively associated with adverse health behaviors, including smoking, lack of exercise, and excessive caloric intake leading to obesity.

The importance of new knowledge about burnout–health behaviors relationships is highlighted by a recent study that indicated that they may synergistically interact in influencing CVD risk. A follow-up study of a large cohort of initially healthy individuals uncovered a synergistic effect of smoking and VE on ischemic stroke risk. In a multivariate analysis, current smoking and high burnout were found to be independent risk factors for ischemic stroke, with the corresponding hazard ratios of 1.76 and 1.94, respectively. However, in combination they yielded a hazard ratio of 2.71 (Schwartz, Carlucci, Chambless, & Rosmand, 2004).

Burnout and Self-Rated Health

I have chosen to focus on self-rated health (SRH) for several reasons. First, several meta-analytic studies have concluded that SRH predicts mortality and survival after adjusting for traditional risk factors, sociodemographic characteristics, and objective measures of health status (Benyamini & Idler, 1999; DeSalvo, Bloser, Reynolds, He, & Muntner, 2006; Idler & Benyamini, 1997). Second, SRH has also been demonstrated to predict a variety of outcomes related to healthcare utilization and costs (DeSalvo et al., 2009). Third, the predictive power of SRH with respect to subsequent survival possibly reflects its ability to cover a wide spectrum of health conditions and attests to its validity as a global health status measure (McGee, Liao, Cao, & Cooper, 1999). Corresponding to the literature (e.g., DeSalvo et al., 2004), SRH was conceptualized to reflect a person's global assessment of his or her general state of health. Qualitative (Benyamini, Leventhal, & Leventhal, 2000) and quantitative (Singh-Manoux et al., 2006) studies found that SRH represents a holistic summary of how individuals perceive their overall health status.

Good health, as indexed by SRH, should be negatively linked to burnout because it represents a pivotal coping resource, reducing the impact of individuals' exposure to stressors on their burnout, and allowing individuals to recover from situations of depleted energy resources (Hobfoll, 2002). Additionally, burnout signifies that one's energy resources in an important life domain have depleted, and this should lead to a decrement in one's SRH.

The VE measure has been linked to self-reported ill-health or disease states. Using a measure of self-reported general health in a two-wave study of healthy males in Sweden, Halford, Anderzen, & Arnetz, (2003) found this measure to correlate negatively with VE. Self-rated health has also been found to be closely correlated with burnout in other studies (Gorter, Eijkman, & Hoogstraten, 2000; Soderfeldt, Soderfeldt, Ohlson, Theorell, & Jones, 2000). In a longitudinal study of staff burnout in a psychiatric hospital, self-reported frequency of serious illness shared 10% of the variance with burnout, as measured by emotional exhaustion, after controlling for social support and other confounders (Corrigan et al., 1994); a similar result was obtained for the relationship of these variables in another study (Bhagat, Allie, & Ford, 1995). Vinokur, Pierce, & Lewandowski-Romps (2009) made a unique contribution to the study of the effects of burnout on health by viewing SRH as a health-related outcome being impacted by burnout. They assessed burnout based on the Conservation of Resources (COR) theory as referring to individuals' affective reactions to the gradual depletion of their energy resources (cf. Shirom, 2003). These represent important and basic coping resources; therefore, a feeling that one's physical, cognitive and emotional or interpersonal resources have been depleted is likely to impact one's SRH. The obverse may also be correct: one's perceived state of health is an important resource, therefore, any changes in it are likely to have an impact on one's level of burnout. Based on a longitudinal design and using structural equation modeling, Vinokur et al. (2009) were able to demonstrate that across time, perceived health predicted a decrease in burnout and burnout predicted a decrease in perceive health, providing support for the coexistence of both types of effects. However, they were also able to find considerable support for their expectation that the effect of perceived health on burnout is stronger than the effects of burnout on perceived health. Furthermore, when they applied a one-item measure of SRH widely used in past studies, rather than the four-item measure of perceived health that they used themselves, only the effect of SRH on burnout turned out to be significant. This finding provides support for the COR-based theoretical view of burnout.

The effects of burnout on SRH could be moderated by self-efficacy, social support, and proactive coping. Personal and social resources are regarded as mitigating the impact of burnout on distress and well-being (Hobfoll & Shirom, 2000) and this proposition has been supported by empirical evidence (Schaufeli & Enzmann, 1998). Among the many coping resources, there are two that play a key role in social cognitive theories which explain human development, adaptation and change (Bandura, 2002). These two coping resources have received the most empirical support in terms of their effects on health and health behaviors: social support (Uchino, 2006) and self-efficacy (Bandura, 2002). Coping strategies represent behavioral and cognitive efforts to manage external and internal demands that are perceived as taxing or exceeding a person's resources (Lazarus, 1999). Self-efficacy and proactive coping represent fundamental components of individual adaptability (Bandura, 2002).

Proactive coping represents yet another important mediational link in the burnout–health behaviors relationship. A recent review of the burnout literature reported that burnt-out individuals tend to cope with stressful situations or events by utilizing a rather defensive and passive coping style (Schaufeli & Enzmann, 1998, p. 78). Following the theoretical lead of Knoll, Rieckmann, & Schwarzer (2005), I too argue that coping mediates burnout–health behaviors relationships.

Burnout and Cardiovascular Disease (CVD)

The body of evidence linking burnout with the subsequent incidence of CVD is primarily based on studies that used the VE measure to predict the incidence of CVD. This body of evidence suggests that, even after adjusting for potential confounding variables, the relative risk associated with burnout and the VE approach was equal to and sometimes, depending on the outcome studied, even exceeded the risk conferred by classical risk factors, such as age, body mass index (BMI), smoking, blood pressure and lipid levels.

Using VE as a predictor variable, Appels et al. (2003) conducted the first systematic research study in this area using objective indicators of physical morbidity. VE was predictive of future MI in apparently healthy men and women, independent of the classic risk factors (Appels, Falger, & Schouten, 1993; Appels & Mulder, 1988). To illustrate, in a 4.2-year follow-up of apparently healthy men, VE was predictive of future MI, even after controlling for blood pressure, smoking, cholesterol levels, age and use of antihypertensive drugs (Appels & Mulder, 1988). In a prospective study of adults (41–66 years of age), VE was found to be associated with the triple risk of fatal and nonfatal MI (new cases as well as recurrent MI), after controlling for a host of potential confounding variables, including previous MI (Schuitemaker, Dinant, Van der Pol, & Appels, 2004). In another prospective study of a community sample, VE was found to be a risk factor for ischemic heart disease (with an RR ranging between 1.36 and 2.10, depending on the questionnaire items selected), and with all-cause mortality (Prescott et al., 2003). VE was also found to be associated with excess CHD mortality, with adjusted Rate Ratio = 2.07 (Cole, Kawachi, Sesso, Paffenbarger, & Lee, 1999). In other studies, VE was also found to be associated with a 1.3-1.9-fold increased risk of incident stroke (Schuitemaker, Dinant, Van Der Pol, Verhelst, & Appels, 2004; Schwartz et al., 2004), and to be a precursor of sudden cardiac death, with an RR = 2.28 or 2.81, depending upon the reference group (Appels, Golombeck, Gorgels, De Vreede, & Van Breukelen, 2002).

Other studies have also indicated that burnout may be a risk factor for coronary heart disease (CHD). In a recent case-control study, women with CHD reported a higher level of burnout compared with matched controls. The CHD women also showed a lower level of coping abilities (Hallman, Thomsson, Burell, Lisspers, & Setterlind, 2003), replicating an earlier case-control study in which burnout was found to be associated with increased risk of CHD for both men (RR = 3.1) and women (RR= 3.4) (Hallman, Burell, Setterlind, Oden, & Lisspers, 2001). Using data from the prospective study of healthy men mentioned above, Appels & Schouten (1991) found that a single question measuring burnout, "Have you ever been burned out?", was found to be predictive of MI risk (RR = 2.13). It should be noted that the reliability of this burnout measure is unknown.

In sum, there is sufficient evidence from several prospective cohort studies linking burnout and VE with risk of CVD and cardiovascular related events. The relative risk associated with burnout and VE is of similar magnitude to that of the classical risk factors for CVD.

Organizational-Level Burnout

To date, the literature on burnout has dealt almost exclusively with the individual level of analysis. With few exceptions (Leiter & Maslach, 1988; O'Driscoll & Schubert, 1988), the potentialities of investigating group or organizational burnout have not yet been systematically explored. It is plausible that burnout as analyzed on the individual level has its organizational counterpart. There may be parallel processes operating at the individual and organizational levels. The open-systems approach postulates that there is a dynamic interplay and interconnectedness among elements of any system, its subsystems, and within the more inclusive system. Focusing on organizational burnout may entail a much higher system complexity than the extant focus on individual burnout.

A process of depletion of organizational resources may be self-imposed by those at the helm of the organization, like setting unrealistic production targets that overload and overuse the employees' available energy resources, eventually also exacerbating their level of burnout. This process may be externally imposed by stakeholders' excessive demands for product or service quality that continuously deplete the organization's energy resources. For example, it was shown that resource scarcity, on the collective level, influences intergroup cooperation and conflict (Kramer, 1991). Organizational behavior has imported the resource-based model of the firm from the field of economics as a major theoretical framework. Within this resource-based view of organizations, issues like resource mobility and heterogeneity have been applied to explain firms' competitive advantage (Barney, 1991).

Indirect evidence from several studies indicates that concentration of burned-out employees in certain work groups is an existent phenomenon. In a relevant study (Roundtree, 1984), task groups in organizations were investigated for the prevalence of individual level burnout: it was found that almost 90% of those high on burnout were members of work groups in which at least 50% of all their members suffered from advanced burnout. In a series of studies, Bakker and colleagues (Bakker, Demerouti, & Schaufeli, 2003, 2005; Bakker, Demerouti, Taris, Schaufeli, & Schreurs, 2003; Bakker, Le Blanc, & Schaufeli, 2005) found evidence for burnout contagion processes among teachers, nurses, and other occupational categories. Still, the evidence is largely indirect and does not clarify whether the concentration of burned-out employees in certain work groups is a result of common exposure to stress, contagion processes that operate within these work groups, or other possible alternative explanations.

Approaches to Reducing Burnout

In this section, I review studies that evaluate interventions designed to reduce burnout. It has been argued that workplace-based interventions, aimed at reducing stress and modifying some of the maladaptive responses to stress, often have little or no effect (Briner & Reynolds, 1999). Is this conclusion also relevant to interventions designed to ameliorate burnout? Most of the burnout interventions reported in the literature are individual-oriented and provide treatment, not prevention, much like other stress interventions (Nelson, Quick, & Simmons, 2001). There are hardly any existing reports on interventions that were based on a systematic audit of the structural sources of workplace burnout with the objectives of alleviating or eliminating the stresses leading to burnout. One possible explanation could be that employees with burnout are more often targets of individual-focused than occupational-focus intervention, as found in Finland (Ahola et al., 2007). A review of this issue (Schaufeli & Enzmann, 1998) noted that there are more than two dozen different approaches suggested as being useful for ameliorating burnout levels among employees. The burnout literature does not include reports of testing the vast majority of these approaches in research using a randomized control design. Using randomized control design is considered as the gold standard for testing the effectiveness of any therapeutic agent, including psychosocial interventions.

One type of intervention frequently used by organizations attempting to ameliorate burnout among their employees is that of peer support groups. The theoretical perspective offered in this chapter may explain the focus of many interventions on enriching and strengthening the social support available to or used by burned-out employees. According to the predictions of COR theory, the depletion of one's energy resources and impoverished social support are closely related (Hobfoll, 1989). Those lacking a strong resource pool, including those with impoverished social support, are more likely to become burned-out or to go through cycles of resource loss when they cope with work-related stress. In addition, people with depleted energy resources who complain of physical fatigue, emotional exhaustion, and cognitive weariness may appear less attractive to their significant others at work and therefore become less likely to have access to social support. There is considerable support for these arguments. A review of the area of social support and stress (Curtona & Russell, 1990) included four studies that investigated the effects of social support on burnout among public school teachers, hospital nurses, therapists, and critical care nurses, respectively. In all four studies, negative associations between social support and burnout were found. For reasons explained earlier, these negative relationships may be reciprocal.

The peer social support intervention is particularly popular in educational institutions (Vandenberghe & Huberman, 1999). Such peer-based support groups provide their members with informational and emotional support, and in some cases, instrumental support as well. Because social support is a major potential route to resources that are beyond those that individuals possess directly, it is a critical resource in many employment-related stressful situations (Hobfoll & Shirom, 2000), and may help these individuals to replenish their depleted energy resources. However, how social support is actually used depends on several factors, including one's sense of mastery and environmental control. Several examples of past interventions that used peer-based support groups in the prevention of burnout were recently described by Peterson, Bergstrom, Samuelsson, Asberg, & Nygren (2008). Interventions based on different forms of group therapy (Salmela-Aro, Naatanen, & Nurmi, 2004) also found favorable effects of intra-group social support facilitated by the intervention on measures of burnout. Some interventions (Le Blanc, Hox, Schaufeli, Taris, & Peeters, 2007) combined staff support groups with a participatory action research approach and found the levels of emotional exhaustion in the experimental groups to be favorably influenced by the intervention.

In a longitudinal research of burnout among teachers, Brouwers and Tomic (2000) found that emotional exhaustion had a negative effect on self-efficacy beliefs, and that this effect occurred simultaneously, rather than over time. Hence, they reasoned that interventions that incorporate enactive mastery experiences—the most important source of self-efficacy beliefs—were likely to have an ameliorative effect on teachers' emotional exhaustion. An example would be having teachers learn and experiment with skills aimed at helping them cope with disruptive student behavior. In the same vein, environmental sense of control is another important stress management resource (Fisher, 1984). Those with a high sense of control tend to use their resources judiciously, relying on themselves when this is deemed most appropriate, and using available social support when this is the more effective coping route (Hobfoll & Shirom, 2000).

It follows from the above that interventions that combine social support and bolstering of control, such as the participatory approach of increasing employee involvement in decision-making processes, may be more efficacious in reducing burnout in organizations. For example, a multifaceted intervention combining peer social support and bolstering of professional self-efficacy was found to reduce burnout (measured by the SMBM), relative to a control group of nonparticipants (Rabin et al.,

2000). Another example is the study by Freedy and Hobfoll (1994), who enhanced nurses' coping skills by teaching them how to use their social support and individual mastery resources and found a significant reduction in emotional exhaustion in the experimental group, relative to the nontreated control group.

Senior management has a role to play in instituting preventive measures, including steps to ameliorate chronic work-related stress, particularly overload, as well as training programs designed to promote effective stress management techniques and on-site recreational facilities. Organizational interventions to reduce burnout have great potential, but are complex to implement and costly in terms of required resources. The changing nature of employment relationships, including the transient and dynamic nature of employee–employer psychological contact, entails putting more emphasis on individual-oriented approaches to combat burnout. The role of individual coping resources, including self-efficacy, hardiness, and social support from friends and family, may become more important in future interventions.

Yet another major approach used in experimental studies whose objective was to reduce burnout among employees is that of cognitive-behavioral therapy. In a cognitively oriented intervention designed to reduce feelings of inequity and ameliorate burnout in professional social workers (Van Dierendonck, Schaufeli, & Buunk, 1998) —an intervention based on one experimental group and two control groups, with two follow-ups, 6 months and 1 year later—it was found that the intervention was indeed effective in reducing emotional exhaustion (assessed based on the MBI). This intervention, as well as some of its predecessors (cf. Schaufeli & Entzmann, 1998), provided additional support for the view, expressed above, that the three facets of the MBI are influenced by different sets of antecedents.

Future Research

An important area for future research lies in determining the validity of burnout, according to either of its different operational definitions, and distinguishing it from other types of emotional distress, particularly anxiety and depression. I have argued that burnout, anxiety, and depression are conceptually distinct emotional reactions to stress. Still, the overlap found in several studies (Schaufeli & Enzmann, 1998) between depression and the emotional exhaustion scale of the MBI—the most robust and reliable out of the three scales that make up the MBI—is a cause for concern. The propositions that early stages of individual burnout are more likely to be accompanied by heightened anxiety, while more progressive stages of burnout may be linked to depressive symptoms need to be tested in longitudinal research.

The plausibility of the proposition that burnout, as conceptualized in terms of its core meaning, will overlap, to some extent, with the disease state of chronic fatigue syndrome (CFS) or with its immediate precursor, chronic fatigue, has yet to be tested. In future investigations, individuals who score highest on burnout measures should be followed up for possible development of CFS.

A further important area of research concerns burnout as a possible precursor of cardiovascular disease. Early in the 1960s and 1970s, prospective studies found that being tired on awakening or being exhausted at the end of the day were possible antecedents of cardiovascular heart disease (Appels & Mulder, 1988, 1989). Appels and Mulder (1988, 1989) discovered that those initially high on their measure of vital exhaustion (a combination of burnout, anxiety, and depression) were significantly more at risk of developing myocardial infarction within four years, after controlling for known risk factors such as blood pressure, smoking, cholesterol, and age. In cross-sectional studies that tested the associations among cardiovascular risk factors and burnout, Melamed et al. (2006) found evidence linking the two entities. Longitudinal studies of fairly large and occupationally representative samples should be conducted to cross-validate these findings.

Conclusion

Advances in our knowledge are unlikely to result from research using fuzzy concepts and relying on instruments whose construct validity is in doubt. For this reason, in this review I have selectively focused on theoretical and conceptual issues in burnout research.

Burnout is likely to represent a pressing social problem in the years to come. Competitive pressures in manufacturing industry that originate in the global market, the continuing process of consumer empowerment in service industries, and the rise and decline of the high-tech industry are among the factors likely to affect employees' levels of burnout in different industries. In addition, employees in many advanced market economies experience heightened job insecurity, demands for excessive work hours, the need for continuous retraining in the wake of the accelerating pace of change in informational technologies, and the blurring of the line separating work and home life. In many European countries, employers are enjoined by governmental regulations on occupational health to implement preventive interventions that concern job stress and burnout. This review is an attempt to steer future research on burnout along the lines suggested earlier to make future preventive interventions more effective.

References

Ahola, K., Honkonen, T., Virtanen, M., Kivimaki, M., Isometsa, E., Aromaa, A., & Lönnqvist, J. (2007). Interventions in relation to occupational burnout: The population-based health 2000 study. *Journal of Occupational and Environmental Medicine, 49*(9), 943–952.

Appels, A. (2004). Exhaustion and coronary heart disease: The history of a scientific quest. *Patient Education and Counseling, 55*(2), 223–229.

Appels, A., Falger, P. R. J., & Schouten, E. G. W. (1993). Vital exhaustion as risk indicator for myocardial infarction in women. *Journal of Psychosomatic Research, 37*(8), 881–890.

Appels, A., Golombeck, B., Gorgels, A., De Vreede, J., & Van Breukelen, G. (2002). Psychological risk factors of sudden cardiac arrest. *Psychology & Health, 17*(6), 773.

Appels, A., & Mulder, P. (1988). Excess fatigue as a precursor of myocardial infarction. *European Heart Journal, 9*, 758–764.

Appels, A., & Mulder, P. (1989). Fatigue and heart disease: The association between "vital exhaustion" and past, present and future coronary heart disease. *Journal of Psychosomatic Research, 33*, 727–738.

Appels, A., & Schouten, E. G. W. (1991). Burnout as a risk factor for coronary heart disease. *Behavioral Medicine, 17*, 53–59.

Bages, N., Falger, P. R., Perez, M. G., & Appels, A. (2000). Vital exhaustion measures and their association with coronary heart disease risk factors in a sample of Spanish-speakers. *Psychology and Health, 15*, 787–799.

Bakker, A. B., Demerouti, E., & Schaufeli, W. B. (2003). The socially induced burnout model. In S. P. Shohov (Ed.), *Advances in psychology research* (Vol. 25, pp. 13–30). New York, New York: Nova Science Publishers.

Bakker, A. B., Demerouti, E., & Schaufeli, W. B. (2005). The crossover of burnout and work engagement among working couples. *Human Relations, 58*(5), 661–689.

Bakker, A. B., Demerouti, E., Taris, T. W., Schaufeli, W. B., & Schreurs, P. J. G. (2003). A multigroup analysis of the job demands-resources model in four home care organizations. *International Journal of Stress Management, 10*(1), 16–38.

Bakker, A. B., Le Blanc, P. M., & Schaufeli, W. B. (2005). Burnout contagion among intensive care nurses. *Journal of Advanced Nursing, 51*(3), 276–287.

Bandura, A. (2002). Social cognitive theory in cultural context. *Applied Psychology, 51*(2), 269–290.

Barney, J. (1991). Special theory forum on the resource-based model of the firm: Origins, implications, and prospects. *Journal of Management, 17*, 97–98.

Belkic, K. L., Landsbergis, P. A., Schnall, P. L., & Baker, D. B. (2004). Is job strain a major source of cardiovascular disease risk? *Scandinavian Journal of Work Environment & Health, 30*(2), 85–128.

Belkic, K. L., Schnall, P. L., Savic, C., & Landsbergis, P. A. (2000). Multiple exposures: Toward a model of total occupational burden. *Occupational Medicine, 15*(1), 94–105.

Benyamini, Y., & Idler, E. L. (1999). Community studies reporting association between self-rated health and mortality- additional studies. *Research on Aging, 21*(3), 392–401.

Benyamini, Y., Leventhal, E. A., & Leventhal, H. (2000). Gender differences in processing information for making self-assessments of health. *Psychosomatic Medicine, 62*(3), 354–364.

Bhagat, R. S., Allie, S. M., & Ford, D. L. (1995). Coping with stressful life events: An empirical analysis. In R. C. P. L. Perrewe (Ed.), *Occupational Stress.* Philadelphia, PA: Taylor and Francis.

Boudreau, R., & Nakashima, J. (2002). *A bibliography of burnout citations, 1990–2002.* Winnipeg, CA: ASAC.

Briner, R. B., & Reynolds, S. (1999). The costs, benefits, and limitations of organizational level stress interventions. *Journal of Organizational Behavior, 20*(5), 647–664.

Brouwers, A., & Tomic, W. (2000). A longitudinal study of teacher burnout and perceived self-efficacy in classroom management. *Teaching and Teacher Education, 16*(2), 239–253.

Cole, S. R., Kawachi, I., Sesso, H. D., Paffenbarger, R. S., & Lee, I.-M. (1999). Sense of exhaustion and coronary heart disease among college alumni. *The American Journal of Cardiology, 84*(12), 1401–1405.

Collins, V. A. (1999). *A meta-analysis of burnout and occupational stress.* Unpublished doctoral dissertation, University of North Texas, Texas, USA.

Conley, J. J. (1984). Longitudinal consistency of adult personality: Self-reported psychological characteristics across 45 years. *Journal of Personality and Social Psychology, 47*(6), 1325–1333.

Cooper, M. L., Russell, M., & Frone, M. R. (1990). Work stress and alcohol effects: A test of stress-induced drinking. *Journal of Health and Social Behavior, 31*(3), 260–276.

Corrigan, P. W., Holmes, E. P., Luchins, D., Buican, B., Basit, A., & Parkes, J. J. (1994). Staff burnout in a psychiatric hospital: A cross-lagged panel design. *Journal of Organizational Behavior, 15*, 65–74.

Cummings, T. G., & Cooper, C. L. (1998). A cybernetic theory of organizational stress. In C. L. Cooper (Ed.), *Theories of organizational stress* (pp. 101–122). Oxford: Oxford University Press.

Curtona, C. E., & Russell, D. W. (1990). Types of social support and specific stress: Toward a theory of optimal matching. In B. R. Sarason, I. G. Sarason & G. R. Pierce (Eds.), *Social support: An interactional view* (pp. 319–361). New York: Wiley.

DeSalvo, K. B., Bloser, N., Reynolds, K., He, J., & Muntner, P. (2006). Mortality prediction with a single general self-rated health question. A meta-analysis. *Journal of General Internal Medicine, 21*(3), 267–275.

DeSalvo, K. B., Jones, T. M., Peabody, J., McDonald, J., Fihn, S., Fan, V., … Muntner, P. (2009). Health care expenditure prediction with a single item, self-rated health measure. *Medical Care, 47*(4), 440–447.

Dierendonck, D., & Schaufeli, W.B. (1993). Burnout en organisatie betrokkenheid bij leerling-verpleegkundigen: De rol van billijkheid, sociale steun en probleemhantering [Burnout and organizational commitment among student nurses: About the role of inequity, social support and coping]. *Tijdschrift voor Sociale Gezondheidszorg, Gezondheid & Samenleving, 71*, 339–244.

Fisher, S. (1984). *Stress and the perception of control.* London: Lawrence Erlbaum.

Freedy, J. R., & Hobfoll, S. E. (1994). Stress inoculation for reduction of burnout: A conservation of resources approach. *Anxiety, Stress and Coping, 6*, 311–325.

Frone, M. R. (2003). Predictors of overall and on-the-job substance use among young workers. *Journal of Occupational Health Psychology, 8*(1), 39–54.

Gorter, R. C., Eijkman, M. A. J., & Hoogstraten, J. (2000). Burnout and health among Dutch dentists. *European Journal of Oral Sciences, 108*(4), 261–267.

Halbesleben, J. R. B. (2006). Sources of social support and burnout: A meta-analytic test of the conservation of resources model. *Journal of Applied Psychology, 91*(5), 1134–1145.

Halbesleben, J. R. B., & Buckley, M. R. (2004). Burnout in organizational life. *Journal of Management, 30*(6), 859–879.

Halbesleben, J. R. B., & Rathert, C. (2008). Linking physician burnout and patient outcomes: Exploring the dyadic relationship between physicians and patients. *Health Care Management Review, 33*(1), 29–39.

Halford, C., Anderzen, I., & Arnetz, B. (2003). Endocrine measures of stress and self-rated health: A longitudinal study. *Journal of Psychosomatic Research, 55*(4), 317–320.

Hallman, T., Burell, G., Setterlind, S., Oden, A., & Lisspers, J. (2001). Psychosocial risk factors for coronary heart disease, their importance compared with other risk factors and gender differences in sensitivity. *Journal of Cardiovascular Risk, 8*(1), 39–49.

Hallman, T., Thomsson, H., Burell, G., Lisspers, J., & Setterlind, S. (2003). Stress, burnout and coping: Differences between women with coronary heart disease and healthy matched women. *Journal of Health Psychology, 8*(4), 433–445.

Hobfoll, S. E. (1989). Conservation of resources: A new attempt at conceptualizing stress. *American Psychologist, 44*(3), 513–524.

Hobfoll, S. E. (2002). Social and psychological resources and adaptation. *Review of General Psychology, 6*(4), 307–324.

Hobfoll, S. E., & Shirom, A. (2000). Conservation of resources theory: Applications to stress and management in the workplace. In R. T. Golembiewski (Ed.), *Handbook of organization behavior* (2nd revised ed., pp. 57–81). New York: Dekker.

Idler, E. L., & Benyamini, Y. (1997). Self-rated health and morbidity: A review of twenty-seven community studies. *Journal of Health and Social Behavior, 38*(1), 21–37.

Knoll, N., Rieckmann, N., & Schwarzer, R. (2005). Coping as a mediator between personality and stress outcomes: A longitudinal study with cataract surgery patients. *European Journal of Personality, 19*(3), 229–247.

Kramer, R. M. (1991). Intergroup relations and organizational dilemmas: The role of categorization processes. In B. M. Staw & L. L. Cummings (Eds.), *Research in organizational behavior* (Vol. 13, pp. 191–228). London: JAI Press.

Kristensen, T. S., Borritz, M., Villadsen, E., & Christensen, K. B. (2005). The Copenhagen Burnout Inventory: A new tool for the assessment of burnout. *Work & Stress, 19*(3), 192–208.

Lazarus, R. S. (1999). *Stress and emotion.* New York: Springer.

Le Blanc, P. M., Hox, J. J., Schaufeli, W. B., Taris, T. W., & Peeters, M. C. W. (2007). Take care! The evaluation of a team-based burnout intervention program for oncology care providers. *Journal of Applied Psychology, 92*(1), 213–227.

Lee, R. T., & Ashforth, B. E. (1996). A meta-analytic examination of the correlates of the three dimensions of job burnout. *Journal of Applied Psychology, 81*(2), 123–133.

Leiter, M. P., & Maslach, C. (1988). The impact of interpersonal environment on burnout and organizational commitment. *Journal of Organizational Behavior, 9*(4), 297–308.

Luthans, F., Avolio, B. J., Avey, J. B., & Norman, S. M. (2007). Positive psychological capital: Measurement and relationship with performance and satisfaction. *Personnel Psychology, 60*(3), 541–572.

Maslach, C. (1998). A multidimensional theory of burnout. In C. L. Cooper (Ed.), *Theories of organizational stress* (pp. 68–85). Oxford: Oxford University Press.

Maslach, C., Jackson, S. E., & Leiter, M. P. (1996). *Maslach Burnout Inventory manual* (3rd ed.). Palo Alto, CA: Consulting Psychologists Press.

Maslach, C., Schaufeli, W. B., & Leiter, M. P. (2001). Job burnout. *Annual Review of Psychology, 52*, 397–422.

McGee, D. L., Liao, Y., Cao, G., & Cooper, R. S. (1999). Self-reported health status and mortality in a multiethnic US cohort. *American Journal of Epidemiology, 149*(1), 41–46.

Melamed, S., Shirom, A., Toker, S., Berliner, S., & Shapira, I. (2006). Burnout and risk of cardiovascular disease: Evidence, possible causal paths, and promising research directions. *Psychological Bulletin, 132*(3), 327–353.

Nelson, D. L., Quick, J. C., & Simmons, B. L. (2001). Preventive management of work stress: Current themes and future challenges. In A. Baum, T. A. Revenson & J. E. Singer (Eds.), *Handbook of health psychology* (pp. 349–364). Mahawah, NJ: Erlbaum.

Neveu, J.-P. (2007). Jailed resources: conservation of resources theory as applied to burnout among prison guards. *Journal of Organizational Behavior, 28*(1), 21–42.

O'Driscoll, M. P., & Schubert, T. (1988). Organizational climate and burnout in a New Zealand social service agency. *Work & Stress, 2*, 199–204.

Penley, J. A., Tomaka, J., & Wiebe, J. S. (2002). The association of coping to physical and psychological health outcomes: A meta-analytic review. *Journal of Behavioral Medicine, 25*(6), 551–603.

Peterson, U., Bergstrom, G., Samuelsson, M., Asberg, M., & Nygren, A. (2008). Reflecting peer-support groups in the prevention of stress and burnout: Randomized controlled trial. *Journal of Advanced Nursing, 63*(5), 506–516.

Pines, A. (1987). Marriage burnout: A new conceptual framework for working with couples. *Psychotherapy in Private Practice, 5*, 31–43.

Pines, A. (1993). Burnout. In L. Goldberger & S. Breznitz (Eds.), *Handbook of stress* (2nd ed., pp. 386–403). New York: The Free Press.

Pines, A., Aronson, E., & Kafry, D. (1981). *Burnout: From tedium to personal growth*. New York: The Free Press.

Prescott, E., Holst, C., Gronbaek, M., Schnohr, P., Jensen, G., & Barefoot, J. (2003). Vital exhaustion as a risk factor for ischaemic heart disease and all-cause mortality in a community sample. A prospective study of 4,084 men and 5,479 women in the Copenhagen City Heart Study. *International Journal of Epidemiology, 32*(6), 990–997.

Rabin, S., Saffer, M., Weisberg, E., Kornitzer-Enav, T., Peled, I., & Ribak, J. (2000). A multifaceted mental health training program in reducing burnout among occupational social workers. *Israel Journal of Psychiatry and Related Science, 37*, 12–19.

Roundtree, B. H. (1984). Psychological burnout in task groups. *Journal of Health and Human Resources Administration, 7*, 235–248.

Rozanski, A., Blumenthal, J. A., Davidson, K. W., Saab, P. G., & Kubzansky, L. D. (2005). The epidemiology, pathophysiology, and management of psychosocial risk factors in cardiac practice: The emerging field of behavioral cardiology. *Journal of the American College of Cardiology, 45*(5), 637–651.

Salmela-Aro, K., Naatanen, P., & Nurmi, J. E. (2004). The role of work-related personal projects during two burnout interventions: A longitudinal study. *Work and Stress, 18*(3), 208–230.

Schaufeli, W. B., & Buunk, B. P. (2003). Burnout: An overview of 25 years of research and theorizing. In M. J. Schabracq, J. A. M. Winnubst & C. L. Cooper (Eds.), *The handbook of work and health psychology* (2nd ed., pp. 383–429). Chichester: Wiley.

Schaufeli, W. B., & Enzmann, D. (1998). *The burnout companion to study and practice: A critical analysis*. Washington, DC: Taylor & Francis.

Schuitemaker, G. E., Dinant, G. J., Van der Pol, G. A., & Appels, A. (2004). Assessment of vital exhaustion and identification of subjects at increased risk of myocardial infarction in general practice. *Psychosomatics, 45*(5), 414–418.

Schuitemaker, G. E., Dinant, G. J., Van Der Pol, G. A., Verhelst, A. F. M., & Appels, A. (2004). Vital exhaustion as a risk indicator for first stroke. *Psychosomatics, 45*(2), 114–118.

Schwartz, S. W., Carlucci, C., Chambless, L. E., & Rosmand, W. D. (2004). Synergism between smoking and vital exhaustion in the risk of ischemic stroke: Evidence from the ARIC Study. *Annals of Epidemiology, 14*, 416–424.

Schwarzer, R., & Fuchs, R. (1995). Changing risk behaviors and adopting health behaviors: The role of self-efficacy beliefs. In A. Bandura (Ed.), *Self-efficacy in changing societies* (pp. 259–288). New York: Cambridge University Press.

Shirom, A. (1989). Burnout in work organizations. In C. L. Cooper & I. Robertson (Eds.), *International review of industrial and organizational psychology* (pp. 25–48). New York: Wiley.

Shirom, A. (2003). Job-related burnout. In J. C. Quick & L. E. Tetrick (Eds.), *Handbook of occupational health psychology* (pp. 245–265). Washington, DC: American Psychological Association.

Shirom, A., & Ezrachi, Y. (2003). On the discriminant validity of burnout, depression, and anxiety: A re-examination of the burnout measure. *Anxiety, Stress and Coping, 16*, 83–99.

Shirom, A., & Melamed, S. (2006). A comparison of the construct validity of two burnout measures in two groups of professionals. *International Journal of Stress Management, 13*(2), 176–200.

Shirom, A., Nirel, N., & Vinokur, A. (2006). Overload, autonomy, and burnout as predictors of physicians' quality of care. *Journal of Occupational Health Psychology, 11*(4), 328–342.

Shirom, A., Vinokur, A. D., & Nirel, N. (in press). Work hours and caseload as predictors of physician burnout: The mediating effects of perceived workload and autonomy. *Applied Psychology: An International Review.* doi: 10.1111/j.1464-0597.2009.00411.x

Singh-Manoux, A., Martikainen, P., Ferrie, J., Zins, M., Marmot, M., & Goldberg, M. (2006). What does self rated health measure? Results from the British Whitehall II and French Gazel cohort studies. *Journal of Epidemiology and Community Health, 60*(4), 364–372.

Soderfeldt, M., Soderfeldt, B., Ohlson, C. G., Theorell, T., & Jones, I. (2000). The impact of sense coherence and high-demand/low-control job environment on self-reported health, burnout, and psychophysiological stress indicators. *Work & Stress, 14*(1), 1–15.

Suls, J., & Bunde, J. (2005). Anger, anxiety, and depression as risk factors for cardiovascular disease: The problems and implications of overlapping affective dispositions. *Psychological Bulletin, 131*(2), 260–300.

Taris, T. W., Le Blanc, P. M., Schaufeli, W. B., & Schreurs, P. J. G. (2005). Are there causal relationships between the dimensions of the Maslach Burnout Inventory? A review and two longitudinal tests. *Work and Stress, 19*(3), 238–256.

Uchino, B. N. (2006). Social support and health: A review of physiological processes potentially underlying links to disease outcomes. *Journal of Behavioral Medicine, 29*(4), 377–387.

Vandenberghe, R., & Huberman, A. M. (1999). *Understanding and preventing teacher burnout: A sourcebook of international research and practice.* New York: Cambridge University Press.

Van Dierendonck, D., Schaufeli, W. B., & Buunk, B. P. (1998). The evaluation of an individual burnout intervention program: The role of inequity and social support. *Journal of Applied Psychology, 83*(4), 392–407.

Vinokur, A., Pierce, P., & Lewandowski-Romps, L. (2009). Disentangling the relationship between job burnout and perceived health in a military sample *Stress and Health, 25*, 355–363.

Worley, J. A., Vassar, M., Wheeler, D. L., & Barnes, L. L. B. (2008). Factor structure of scores from the Maslach Burnout Inventory: A review and meta-analysis of 45 exploratory and confirmatory factor-analytic studies. *Educational and Psychological Measurement, 68*(5), 797–823.

Wright, T. A., & Cropanzano, R. (1998). Emotional exhaustion as a predictor of job performance and voluntary turnover. *Journal of Applied Psychology, 83*(3), 486–493.

Zapf, D., Dormann, C., & Frese, M. (1996). Longitudinal studies in organizational stress research: A review of the literature with reference to methodological issues. *Journal of Occupational Health Psychology, 1*(2), 145–169.

5

Large-Scale Job Stress Interventions
The Dutch Experience

Toon W. Taris
Radboud University Nijmegen and Utrecht University, The Netherlands

Ingrid van der Wal and Michiel A. J. Kompier
Radboud University Nijmegen, The Netherlands

In this chapter we argue that job stress may originate at various levels, ranging from the level of the individual worker or his or her job to that of international socio-economic and legislative developments. Similarly, measures to alleviate job stress may apply at different levels. Although the effectiveness of interventions directed at the individual worker or his or her job has been studied fairly extensively, accounts of the design and effectiveness of higher-level measures to reduce job stress are largely absent. Therefore, in this chapter we discuss the outcomes of a unique experiment conducted in the Netherlands, in which a large-scale concerted effort, involving the Dutch government, trade unions, and employers' organizations and covering many sectors of the labor market, was made to reduce work stress at the national level. The program facilitated the assessment of risk factors for job stress both across organizations and within specific sectors, and provided for the funding of interventions designed to alleviate the condition. Thus, general measures taken at the level of the environment in which organizations operate (opportunities for funding and sector-level assessment of job stress) were presumed to facilitate specific lower-level interventions, i.e., as implemented at the level of the organization, jobs, or workers. In this chapter we provide an evaluation of the findings of this approach. First we examine whether the quality of sector-level approaches affects organizations' actions regarding the reduction of job stress. Then we examine the link between organizational interventions and their effects. We conclude with a short discussion of the lessons to be learned from this approach.

Origins of Job Stress

In recent decades, advanced industrial countries have seen major changes in the organization of work that have been influenced by major economic, technological, legal, political, and other developments (Sauter et al., 2002). The main impetus for these changes was the philosophy of neoliberalism. According to this ideology, the role of the state in all dimensions of social and economic life should be reduced, in order to free up the potential of market forces, by deregulating world trade and increasing the mobility of capital and labor (Navarro, 2007). These transformations in the economic and political spheres have forced organizations to undertake a variety of adaptive strategies, including outsourcing, privatization, mergers and acquisitions, and they often involve reductions in the number of permanent employees through layoffs and the increased utilization of subcontracted and temporary workers (De Cuyper et al., 2008). Further, organizations are implementing flatter management structures that result in a downward transfer of management responsibility and decentralized control, and they are embracing more flexible and lean production technologies, such as just-in-time manufacturing (Sauter et al., 2002).

The adoption and implementation of these *high-performance work systems* has, for many workers, resulted in a variety of potentially stressful circumstances, such as reduced job stability and increased workload. For example, Bluestone and Rose (1998) show that in the U.S. there has been a "clear and nearly unbroken trend toward much greater work effort" (p. 2) since the 1970s, such that the combined total number of hours that American working couples put in has increased by almost 600 hours per year across the 1970–1990 interval. In Europe a reverse trend is visible, with the percentage of employees working more than 41 hours per week decreasing from 32% in 1991 to 25% in 2005 (Parent-Thirion, Fernàndez Macías, Hurley, & Vermeylen, 2007). However, here the *intensity* of work (as defined in terms of the speed at which workers must work and the degree to which they must meet tight deadlines at work) has increased considerably. Whereas in 1991 33% of European workers were confronted with high work intensity, this figure had increased to 45% in 2005. As high job demands (including work intensity) are a major risk factor for worker health (see Belkiç, Landsbergis, Schnall, & Baker, 2004; De Lange, Taris, Kompier, Houtman, & Bongers, 2003, for reviews), it is not surprising that presently the number of workers reporting work-related health complaints is substantial. In 2005, 35% of European workers said that their work negatively affected their health, with psychosocial complaints such as fatigue (23%), stress (22%), and headaches (16%) ranking among the five most prevalent work-related health complaints (Parent-Thirion et al., 2007).

Evidently, job stress is a major health risk in today's industrial society, and as a consequence much research has addressed the effectiveness of interventions that aim to alleviate it. The main emphasis of this research has been on individual-level intervention strategies, such as stress management and health promotion: interventions that seek to improve the capacity of workers to withstand demanding or hazardous job situations (Sauter et al., 2002). A smaller body of research has addressed the reorganization of work, including work rescheduling, workload reduction, role clarification and the redesign of jobs (Semmer, 2003, 2006). However, organizations are complex dynamic systems that often depend on external developments in the socio-economic and political spheres (Kang, Staniford, Dollard, & Kompier, 2008). For example, in many countries state-level legislation obliges organizations to implement family-friendly arrangements. Among these, two main categories can be distinguished: flexible arrangements, which increase employees' flexibility regarding working time and/or working place (e.g., part-time work, and flextime; flexible start and finishing times); and care-related arrangements, which enable employees to perform their care-giving responsibilities (e.g., parental leave and subsidized childcare; cf. Dikkers, Geurts, Den Dulk, Peper, Taris, & Kompier, 2007). Such policies are intended to reduce stress associated with work–family conflict that may otherwise result from the need to combine work and family roles. Similarly, socioeconomic developments may affect levels of job stress and the opportunities to reduce these as well through, for example, the availability of financial resources available for job stress interventions.

The presence and potential effects of such higher-level causes for job stress have been increasingly acknowledged, leading to calls for multilevel models of job stress that link external, organizational, group, and individual levels of job stress (Kang et al., 2008; Sauter et al., 2002). In these approaches, workers are seen as nested in jobs that are themselves nested within organizations; in turn, the possibilities for organizations to address job stress are affected by their external environment, including political and economic developments at state and international levels. This reasoning implies that the origins of job stress may be found at a variety of levels. For example, workers may simply not be qualified for the job (a within-person, individual-level cause); their job may possess particularly stressful features such as unpredictability and confrontation with human suffering (job level); the organizational environment in which they work may be conducive to high levels of stress, e.g., working overtime may be part of the organization's culture (organizational level); new legislation may necessitate changes in the way jobs are performed, e.g., restrictions on the use of herbicides may make it harder for farmers to keep their crop free of weeds (national level); or the increasing number of senior citizens in many Western societies may impinge on the national health care system, leading to an increase in job demands for employees such as nurses (national level).

Whatever the level at which job stress originates, and irrespective of which intervention is chosen to address it, dealing with it successfully requires a tight match between the problem and its solution. This implies that those designing and implementing the intervention should possess thorough insight into the problem. There is no single intervention that will always have a beneficial effect on job stress; for example, although a budget increase may well facilitate the division and implementation of lower-level interventions, *in itself* this will not lead to positive changes with respect to job stress. For such interventions to be effective, they should correspond closely with the problem at hand. This suggests that higher-level interventions may facilitate the design and implementation of lower-level interventions—job stress is often best addressed at the lower (organizational, departmental, job, or individual) levels as only at these levels will the nature of the specific problem as well as possible complications be fully known, meaning that only here can it be addressed effectively.

In summary, we argue that (a) the sources of job stress may originate at various levels, ranging from the individual to the socio-economic and political level; (b) job stress may be addressed at any of these levels, but preferably at the level at which stress originates or lower; (c) higher-level, general interventions may facilitate the implementation of specific lower-level measures to reduce job stress; (d) in order to be successful, there should be a close match between the problem and the intervention; meaning that (e) job stress is usually best addressed at relatively low levels—the organization, the job, or the individual worker.

Although this reasoning may sound compelling, little empirical evidence addresses notions (a) to (c). Intervention research is primarily aimed at the individual or job levels (Sauter et al., 2002), for instance, because stakeholders (such as company management) believe that the sources of job stress are located at these two lowest levels (Kompier, Geurts, Gründemann, Vink, & Smulders, 1998). However, as indicated above, such beliefs are increasingly being challenged by notions that the sources of job stress may lie at a variety of levels, and that higher-level interventions are needed to address job stress, even if the specific interventions needed are implemented at the individual, job or organizational levels. The purpose of the present chapter is to fill this void by describing (and to some degree evaluating) a large-scale approach that was implemented in the Netherlands at the beginning of the present decade.

The Dutch Approach

During the first 5 years of the last decade, the Dutch government, trade unions, and employers' organizations conducted a national program that aimed to reduce job stress in many sectors of the labor market. At that time there were strong indications that job stress was a major problem in the Netherlands (Merllie & Paoli, 2001), resulting in high work incapacity rates (Geurts, Kompier, & Gründemann, 2000; Schaufeli & Kompier, 2001) and associated costs (Gründemann & Van Vuuren, 1997). During this period in many sectors of the Dutch labor market so-called *covenants on health and safety at work* (CHSWs) were established between representatives of the Dutch government, trade unions, and employers' organizations in an attempt to reduce job stress. The labor market sectors included in this approach were so-called *high-risk sectors* (i.e., sectors in which either 40% of the workers or at least 50,000 workers were exposed to primary work risks, including high job demands, high physical demands, and working with health-damaging chemicals). These sectors were explicitly invited by the Dutch Government to join the CHSW approach. Moreover, other sectors could voluntarily participate in this approach. In total about 50 sectors were included.

Within the framework of these CHSWs, within-sector agreements were made concerning the reduction of job stress and burnout, over and above existing policy measures such as working conditions regulations, financial incentives for individual organizations, and public information campaigns. By signing a covenant, trade unions and employers' organizations guaranteed that they would stimulate their members to deal with the work risks in their organizations. Agreements were made on a voluntary basis and were not legally enforceable.

Contents of the covenants on health and safety at work

The CHSWs took the form of large-scale programs conducted within individual sectors. These programs consisted of five phases:

1.   The first phase consisted of a *state-of-the-art study*, in which both the health risks in a particular sector and the knowledge available for dealing with that risk were established. Assessment of these health risks took place in either all or a sub-sample of the organizations in each sector, often in the form of quality-of-employment surveys among workers in the selected organizations. This information was then fed back to the organizations. Moreover, organizations received information about possible interventions that could alleviate the stress-related problems in their own organization. The state-of-the-art studies were usually conducted by external parties.

2.   Based on this information, the second phase involved *signing the respective CHSW*, detailing the role of all parties involved and determining the goals of the covenant (usually involving "a reduction of the number of workers confronted with health risk *x* by 10% in five years"). Based on this covenant, plans were made as to how these goals could be achieved.

3.   In the third phase, *a commission was formed* with representatives of the trade unions, the Dutch Ministry of Social Affairs, and employers' organizations. This commission monitored the progress of the plans developed in phase 2 and made decisions in relation to unforeseen matters.

4.   In the fourth phase, *the plans were executed*. In this phase interventions to deal with particular problems in specific organizations were designed and implemented. On the basis of the information collected in the first phase, organizations could decide which actions they should take (if any) to target problems. The execution of the plans was usually assigned to external parties and organizations, who were supervised and monitored by the commission formed in phase 3, as well as commissions operating at the local (organizational) level.

5.   Finally, in order to assess the effects of this approach, a sectorwide follow-up study was envisaged that, similar to phase 1, assessed the quality of working life (*evaluation*).

The costs of phases 1–3 and 5 were covered by the Dutch Ministry of Social Affairs. Specific interventions (phase 4) were largely paid for by the organizations in which these were implemented. It was expected that this approach would allow organizations in specific sectors of the labor market to effectively address possible work-related health risks such as high work pressure. This, in turn, was expected to result in lower levels of absence due to sickness, work incapacity, and related costs.

The structure of the CHSW program followed the ideas outlined above, namely that higher-level general interventions (provision of funding, coordination of efforts to reduce job stress, making available state-of-the-art knowledge on the reduction of work-related health risks) would facilitate the implementation of specific interventions at a lower level (i.e., the organizational, job, or individual level). In this approach, the Dutch state provided funding and the impetus to deal with job stress; plans were devised and coordinated at the sector level; and specific interventions were chosen and implemented at the organizational and lower levels. In a sense this is both a top-down and bottom-up approach; the higher (top) levels were designed to facilitate interventions at the lower (bottom) levels, but the organizations at the bottom level were expected to know best what the specific problems were and decide whether and how to deal with these. In this way it was expected that job stress could be dealt with efficiently and effectively.

Relations between Sector-Level and Lower-Level Approaches

For the CHSW approach to be successful, actions taken at one (higher) level should facilitate actions taken at another (lower) level. Specifically, the better the quality of the higher-level interventions and actions, the higher the expected quality of lower-level interventions. To examine this issue, we conducted a study of the links between the quality of the sector-level job stress programs (as established in phase 1 of the CHSW approach) and the efforts taken by individual organizations in that sector in reducing job stress (phase 4 of the CHSW approach). In a preliminary qualitative study we first established the quality of the sector-level job stress programs. Then we selected three sectors (offering a low, intermediate and high-quality job stress program) in which we conducted a quantitative survey study among HR professionals employed by the organizations operating in these sectors. Generally, we expected (1) that organizations in the sector offering a high-quality job stress program would be *more active* in taking measures to reduce job stress, (2) that the *quality of these measures would be higher* in terms of the correspondence between the type of problems in these organizations (as established in phase 1 of the sector-level approach) and the type of interventions, and (3) that the effectiveness of these interventions would be higher, relative to organizations in sectors with low and intermediate-quality job stress programs.

Establishing the quality of sector-level job stress approaches

In total about 50 sectors were included in the CHSW approach: job stress was a major risk in 70% of these. The organizations in these sectors operated in a dynamic and quickly changing context that was obviously beyond a researcher's control. Therefore, to minimize the impact of the external environment we decided to focus on not-for-profit organizations that were primarily dependent on governmental funding (i.e., organizations in the educational sector, health care, cultural affairs, defense, and public administration). These organizations shared a set of central characteristics: (1) they were funded through taxes and social contributions; (2) they produced public goods, so that consumption of the good produced by these organizations by one individual did not reduce the availability of the good for consumption by others, and no-one could effectively be excluded from using a good of this kind (e.g., the presence of a police officer during a riot); and (3) they were dependent on political and governmental decisions, both in terms of funding and the regulations that apply to them.

The present study included nine sectors. We aimed to examine (1) the quality of the sector-specific job stress programs in these sectors, (2) the relationship between the quality of these sector programs and the quality of the job stress programs of individual organizations within three of these sectors, and (3) the effects of the sector-level programs on the antecedents and outcomes of job stress. In conjunction, the answers to these three issues provide evidence concerning whether sector-level job stress programs (interventions) affect the quality and effectiveness of lower-level interventions.

Approach

The nine public sector organizations in the qualitative study comprised home care, higher education institutions (universities and colleges), academic hospitals, general hospitals, local government organizations, state government organizations, nursing homes, residential homes for the disabled, and mental health services. All were considered high-risk sectors. In total they covered 1.03 million workers (15% of the Dutch labor force), with the number of workers within these sectors varying from 60,000 (academic hospitals and mental health services) to 200,000 (local government institutions and nursing homes). The programs developed in phase 1 of the CHSW approach for each of these sectors (i.e., a study on the state-of-the-art knowledge regarding the health risks in a particular sector, and a sector-wide quality of employment survey) were judged by the authors of the present chapter on the basis of four main criteria (Table 5.1.). For each criterion a set of specific criteria was delineated; the total score per main criterion reflects the number of specific criteria that was met for each sector. The overall score is simply the number of specific criteria met by the sectors. As the number of specific criteria varied slightly per sector (not all of these applied equally well to all sectors), the overall score provides a rough indication of the quality of the sector-level job stress program.

Criteria. As indicated above, four main criteria were applied to evaluate the quality of the sector-level job stress programs. The first applied to the *quality of the*

Table 5.1. Quality of Sector Programs for Dealing with Job Stress, for Nine Public Sectors

	Scores of sectors on the criteria								
Criteria	General hospitals	Home care institutions	Local government	Mental health services	Nursing homes	Higher education institutions	Homes for the disabled	University hospitals	State government
1. Quality of diagnosis	16	15	17	13	16	10	13	0	1
2. Availability of information on job stress interventions	5	5	4	3	0	5	3	5	1
3. Transfer of information to individual organizations	13	13	12	11	10	12	11	9	5
4. Facilities offered to organizations	10	10	9	8	7	5	8	7	1
Overall score	44	43	42	35	33	32	29	21	8

Note. The number of criteria included in the assessment of the sectors varied slightly across sectors.

diagnosis of job stress in the organizations within the nine sectors, focusing on the following specific questions:

- Was a reliable and valid assessment (i.e., using well-validated psychometric instruments) of possible job stress problems conducted?
- Was this assessment conducted among a representative group of workers, in terms of gender, occupational group, and size of the institutions in the sector?
- Was information available on the risk groups for job stress, the type of job stress risks (e.g., amount of emotional, cognitive, and quantitative job demands), and possible antecedents and consequences of job stress?

Taken together, the scores on these specific criteria reflected the overall quality of the diagnosis of job stress within the nine sectors.

The second criterion pertained to the *availability of information on job stress interventions* within sectors. Specific questions were:

- Did the report on the within-sector job stress assessment include an overview of possible interventions aimed at specific risk groups and risk factors, as well as an example of an organizational-level blueprint of the process for possible organizational-level interventions?
- Were the examples given in this report at least partly based on real-life experiences of managers and employees in this sector?

The third criterion referred to the *transfer of this information to individual organizations*. Specific questions were:

- Did organizations in the sector receive information about possible risk groups for job stress, antecedents and consequences, possible interventions (aimed at specific risks and risk groups), and was this information targeted towards several relevant actors within the organizations in this sector (e.g., the management, work council, employees, human resource officer)?
- Was this information distributed widely, e.g., through written leaflets, symposia and a website?

Finally, the fourth criterion applied to the *facilities offered to organizations for dealing with job stress*. Specific questions were:

- Was a reliable, valid, and useful instrument available that organizations could use to assess job stress in their own organization, e.g., to monitor the effects of interventions implemented in these organizations?
- Were good examples of specific job stress interventions available?
- Could specialists in the area of stress interventions be contacted (e.g., through personal contacts or via a web site)?

Table 5.1. presents an overview of the scores of the nine sectors on the four main criteria listed above. In some cases no points were awarded, e.g., there was no diagnosis phase for the university hospitals and in the nursing homes sector there was no information available on job stress interventions. At one end of the quality distributions of sector-level job stress programs there were the home care sector, the general hospitals and institutions in local government (overall scores ranging from 42 to 44 points); at the other end there was the state government sector with an very low 8 points. The other sectors occupied intermediate positions (scores ranging from 21 to 33 points). In the next phase of our study, we selected one top-tier sector (local government), one bottom-tier sector (state government) and one intermediary sector (nursing homes). In these sectors we conducted an additional empirical study in which we focused on the specific activities of organizations, with an eye to linking these to the quality of the sector programs.

Quality of Sector-Level Job Stress Approaches and Number of Organizational Interventions

To examine the relationship between the quality of the sector-level job stress approach and the quality of the interventions implemented by organizations in that sector, in 2005 (several years after phases 1–3 of the CHSW approach had been completed) we conducted an additional survey among organizations in three sectors that varied in terms of the quality of the sector-level job stress approach. Specifically, we expected (1) that organizations in the sector offering a high-quality job stress program (i.e., the local government organizations) would be more active in taking measures to reduce job stress than organizations in other sectors (i.e., the nursing homes and state government sector, respectively), and (2) that the quality of the interventions implemented by organizations in the sector offering a high-quality job stress program would be higher than that of the interventions implemented by organizations in other sectors.

Approach
The three sectors chosen for the survey study were requested to provide information about the names and addresses of organizations within these sectors, their size, as well as contact information for the human resource officers of these organizations. Where possible, organizations with more than 400 employees were split into units of about 150–200 employees that were contacted separately, as we expected that HR officers in larger organizations would not be fully familiar with developments within specific departments of their organization. Organizations with less than 150 employees were not included in our study. The number of eligible institutions was relatively large in the nursing homes and local government sectors (Ns were 612 and 275, respectively). In order to keep the study manageable we randomly selected 200 organizations in each of these sectors. In total we contacted 107 state governmental organizations, 200 nursing homes and 200 local governmental organizations.

All 507 organizations received a structured questionnaire, to be completed by their HR officer. The questionnaire included items about the number and type of measures taken, implementation procedures and perceived results. The response rates were 50% for the governmental organizations, 33% for the nursing homes, and 40% for the governmental organizations (total overall N was 233). Most respondents were HR officers (73%); other respondents held a supervisory or management position (12%), or any of a wide variety of other jobs (15%). Three-quarters of respondents had held their position for more than three years; hence, it could be expected that they had a good overview of the measures that had been implemented as a result of the sector-level job stress program.

Findings

Table 5.2. presents evidence relevant to the hypothesis that organizations in sectors offering high-quality job stress programs would be *more active* in taking measures to reduce job stress than organizations in sectors offering medium or low-quality job stress programs. As this table shows, 50% of the participating organizations had completed or planned at least one intervention, or were in the process of implementing such an intervention. This figure did not differ significantly across

Table 5.2   Number of Job Stress Interventions as a Function of Sector

| Measures | Total (N = 233) | | Quality of sector-level job stress program | | | | | | |
| | | | Low[1] (N = 43) | | Medium[2] (N = 65) | | High[3] (N = 125) | | |
	M	SD	M	SD	M	SD	M	SD	F
% organizations having implemented at least 1 intervention	50		51		58		45		
Number of interventions per organization	3.6	4.0	3.5	3.8	4.5[a]	4.5	2.9[b]	3.7	4.5*
• Number of work-directed interventions	1.7	1.9	1.5	1.8	2.5[a]	2.2	1.4[b]	1.8	6.4**
• Number of work-person-directed interventions	0.9	1.2	1.0	1.2	1.1[a]	1.3	0.7[b]	1.1	3.4*
• Number of other interventions	1.0	1.3	1.0	1.2	1.3	1.4	0.9	1.2	2.0

Note. *$p < .05$; [1]State government organizations; [2]Nursing homes; [3]Local government organizations. [a,b]means with different superscripts differ significantly from each other, $p < .05$. All F-values have (2,230) degrees of freedom.

organizations, i.e., it was *not* the case that organizations in the sector offering a high-quality job stress program (the local governmental organizations) implemented more interventions than the other organizations. This also applied to the average number of job stress interventions implemented by all participating organizations ($M = 3.6$). Interestingly, the average number of interventions implemented by local government organizations was significantly *lower* than that implemented by the nursing homes. Thus, our findings did not confirm our hypothesis that organizations in sectors with high-quality job stress programs were more active in implementing interventions to reduce job stress than organizations in other sectors.

Types of interventions
Job stress interventions may be classified in terms of their target. For example, DeFrank and Cooper (1987) and Giga, Faragher, and Cooper (2003) have distinguished between work/organization-directed interventions, person/work-directed interventions, and other (mainly person-directed) interventions. Work-directed interventions focus on factual changes in the work content and/or relations at work and are geared towards eliminating, reducing, or altering stressors in the work situation (e.g., through job redesign and restructuring to improve worker decision making and autonomy, ergonomic improvements, or workload reduction). These interventions apply to all members of the organization or all of those in a particular job.

Interventions focusing on the *person/work interface* are usually intended to increase employee resistance to specific job stressors. Such interventions are often targeted towards changing personal characteristics (e.g., broadening one's coping repertoire by giving feedback, training programs), with the explicit aim of improving particular aspects of the employee's functioning at work. Thus, these interventions focus on the individual in the context of the organization, aiming to improve the match between the person and their work environment. Note that this type of intervention may apply to all employees performing a particular task, or only to those who perform poorly or show signs of stress.

Finally, other (*person-directed*) interventions are targeted toward changing personal characteristics without the explicit aim of improving employee functioning at work (e.g., exercise, employee assistance programs, relaxation training). This is not to say that performance at work may not improve as a result of these measures, but rather that no explicit link with particular stressors in the work situation is made. The assumption with respect to these general interventions is that their effects will spill over into the work situation (e.g., stress management programs may focus on increasing employee coping skills in general).

The effectiveness of these different types of intervention has been the subject of extensive debate. Newman and Beehr (1979) presented the first comprehensive and critical review of various strategies for handling job stress. Although their study revealed that many such strategies existed, their main conclusion was that their effectiveness could not be evaluated because methodologically reliable evaluative research was lacking. Since then, many reports on the effects of stress management interventions have appeared, including several reviews (among others, Giardini Murta, Sanderson & Oldenburg, 2007; Giga et al., 2003; Lamontagne, Keegel, Louie,

Ostry & Landsbergis, 2007; Murphy, 1996; Semmer, 2003; Van der Klink, Blonk, Schene & Van Dijk, 2001). The conclusions from this research suggest that there is no simple answer to the question of whether stress interventions really work. As Semmer (2003) stated, "[work-related] interventions do have the potential for positive effects. It is, however, hard to predict specifically which changes are likely to occur" (p. 34). Semmer argued that the question is not so much *whether* organizational stress management programs are effective in reducing job stress but rather *what* can be expected under *which* circumstances. The effectiveness of stress interventions depends on a multitude of factors, including the type of target variables, the match between the intervention and the target variable (ideally the intervention deals directly with the target variable: Kompier, 2002), the severity of the problem, the modifiability of job stressors, and process considerations such as the degree to which workers were involved in the decision-making process concerning interventions (Giardini Murta et al., 2007; Heaney, 2003; Kompier, Cooper & Geurts, 2000; Semmer, 2003).

This inconclusiveness regarding the effectiveness of stress management interventions does not mean that it is impossible to draw some preliminary conclusions. On the basis of their review of 74 intervention studies that met the minimum requirement of presenting an evaluation of the effects of the intervention, Giga et al. (2003) concluded that "there is suggestion that a combination of work-related and worker-related stress prevention and management is likely to be the most effective option" (p. 43). This implies that organizations that do more (i.e., take more measures) to prevent or reduce job stress will generally be more successful in attaining their goal than organizations that do less. Moreover, person-directed measures seem considerably less effective than work- or person-work-related measures. These ideas were confirmed in a large-scale evaluation study in the Dutch home care sector by Taris et al. (2003), who compared the effects of person-directed, person-work-interface-directed, and work-directed interventions, finding that only work-directed interventions were effective in reducing job stress.

Applied to the current study, it may be possible that whereas organizations in sectors offering a high-quality job stress program do not do *more* than other organizations, they may be better in doing the *right* thing—that is, implementing job-directed and person-job-interface-directed interventions. In regard to this proposition, Table 5.2. also presents the number of person-directed, person-job directed and other interventions, as a function of sector. Remarkably, although the differences among the organizations in the three sectors were not always statistically significant, the organizations in the sector offering a high-quality program consistently had the lowest scores on the number of measures implemented in these organizations. Thus, organizations in the sector offering a high-quality job stress program were *not* more likely to take measures that are more effective in reducing job stress than organizations in other sectors.

Quality of sector-level job stress approaches and quality of organizational interventions

Previous research has suggested that if job stress interventions are to be effective, they should closely match the stressor that is responsible for these high levels of stress (Kompier, 2002). Thus, even if organizations in sectors offering high-quality job stress programs do not implement more interventions, or more potentially effective interventions, than do organizations in other sectors, it is still possible that the interventions they implement correspond more closely with the specific problems in their organization. To test this assumption, we asked the HR professionals in our quantitative study what had been the most important reasons in their organizations for implementing job stress interventions since the start of the CHSW approach in 1999. Table 5.3. presents the 10 most frequently mentioned problems. As this table shows, having too much work to do (26% of the organizations), having insufficient

Table 5.3   Number of Job Stress Interventions Fitting Particular Job Stress Problems as a Function of Sector, for the 10 Most Frequently Mentioned Work-related (W), Work/Person-related (W/P) and Other (O) Problems

		Total (N = 233)		Low[1] (N = 43)		Medium[2] (N = 65)		High[3] (N = 125)		
Problems	% Mentioned	M	SD	M	SD	M	SD	M	SD	F
Too much work (W)	26	1.2	2.6	1.7	2.9	1.4	2.9	1.0	2.4	1.3
Internal pressure (colleagues) (W)	20	0.3	0.9	0.5	1.1	0.3	0.8	0.3	0.9	1.2
Insufficient personnel (W)	18	0.2	0.5	0.1[a]	0.5	0.4[b]	0.7	0.1[a]	0.4	4.9**
External pressure (political demands, low budgets) (O)	16	0.1	0.2	0.0	0.2	0.1	0.2	0.1	0.3	0.7
Work interruptions (W)	15	0.3	0.9	0.2	0.8	0.4	0.9	0.3	0.8	0.4
Inefficient procedures (W)	15	0.4	1.2	0.4	1.2	0.3	1.1	0.5	1.2	0.6
Insufficient control (W/P)	15	1.2	1.4	1.2[a]	1.4	1.6[b]	1.5	1.0[a]	1.4	3.7*
Unclear demands/priorities (W)	15	0.2	0.8	0.2	0.8	0.3	0.9	0.2	0.7	0.1
Low quality leadership (W/P)	15	0.5	0.6	0.4 a	0.6	0.6 b	0.6	0.4 a	0.6	3.3*
Insufficient autonomy (W/P)	11	0.3	1.1	0.0	0.0	0.5	1.4	0.4	1.1	2.5

Note. *p < .05; [1]State government organizations; [2]Nursing homes; [3]Local government organizations. [a,b]means with different superscripts differ significantly from each other, p < .05. All F-values have (2,230) degrees of freedom.

personnel (18%) and experiencing internal pressure from colleagues and other departments within the organization (20%) were mentioned most frequently.

Further, we asked the HR professionals about the interventions that had been implemented in their organizations in the five years before our study took place. Completed interventions, interventions in progress as well as planned interventions could be mentioned. The interventions mentioned by the HR professionals were then evaluated by the authors on the basis of their fit with the stress-related problems in their organizations. In this way, we obtained an impression of the degree to which organizations acted in response to their specific problems. Table 5.4. lists the number of interventions associated with the 10 most prevalent stress-related problems, both for all organizations and for the three sectors separately. For example, the problem of having too much work to do was a major impetus for interventions in 26% of the organizations, and on average organizations applied 1.2 interventions for the resolution of this problem (including increasing the number of employees, making time-management programs available, improving work processes, and flexibilizing working times). The average number of interventions that fitted this particular problem varied somewhat across sectors, but not significantly so.

Relevant to the notion that organizations in the sector offering high-quality job stress programs may implement interventions that correspond more closely with organization-specific problems than organizations in sectors offering lower-quality approaches, we found that the number of "fitting" interventions differed significantly across sectors in three instances. However, in all three cases we found that the organizations in the high-quality sector were *less* likely to implement interventions that could address the problems in their organizations than organizations in other sectors. All in all, these analyses provided no evidence that organizations in sectors offering a high-quality job stress program were more likely to implement interventions that could effectively address the problems in their organizations than organizations in other sectors.

Quality of sector-level job stress approaches and intervention effectiveness

The analyses reported above provided no evidence that high-quality sector-level job stress approaches improve the quality of job stress interventions taken at the organizational level. However, it is still possible that, in spite of the fact that such organizations do not implement better or potentially more effective interventions than organizations in other sectors, they are better at implementing these interventions per se. In this way the effectiveness of the measures taken could be higher for organizations in sectors offering high-quality job stress programs than for organizations in other sectors, resulting in better work outcomes for the organizations in the high-quality sector. To examine this issue, we asked the HR professionals in our study to indicate whether they felt the situation had improved, stayed the same, or worsened in the period between 2000 and 2005. Table 5.4. presents the relevant information,

Table 5.4. Changes in Various Stress-related Concepts across Time (2000–2005) as a Function of Sector

	Total (N = 233)		Quality of sector-level job stress program						
			Low[1] (N = 43)		Medium[2] (N = 65)		High[3] (N = 125)		
	M	SD	M	SD	M	SD	M	SD	F
Antecedents of job stress	0.1	0.3	0.0	0.3	0.2	0.2	0.1	0.3	3.1
Job stress	−0.2	0.5	−0.4	0.5	−0.4[a]	0.4	−0.2[b]	0.6	4.6*
Work pleasure	0.1	0.7	0.1	0.8	0.2	0.6	0.0	0.7	1.1
Fatigue	−0.3	0.6	−0.4	0.7	−0.5[a]	0.5	−0.2[b]	0.6	3.8*
Health complaints	−0.1	0.6	0.0 [a]	0.6	−0.5[b]	0.5	0.0[a]	0.6	12.1**
Sickness absence	−0.0	0.8	0.2 [a]	0.8	−0.7[b]	0.5	0.3[a]	0.7	41.2**

Note. *p < .05, **p < .001. [1]State government organizations; [2]Nursing homes; [3]Local government organizations. [a,b]means with different superscripts differ significantly from each other, p < .05. F-values have 2,86 to 2,164 degrees of freedom, depending on the number of valid responses for these items. Scores of .00 indicate no change; positive scores indicate improvement; negative scores indicate deterioration.

with negative scores signifying a deterioration, positive scores, an improvement, and zero scores reflecting an unchanged situation.

Inspection of Table 5.4. shows that, generally speaking, negative changes had occurred for job stress, fatigue, and health complaints (scores ranging from −0.14 to −0.31). Small positive changes were seen for the causes of job stress and job pleasure (scores were 0.11 and 0.09, respectively). For sickness absence there was no change. Four of these scores varied as a function of sector. Interestingly, strong negative changes occurred for the organizations in the sector offering an intermediate-quality job stress program (nursing homes, with scores ranging from −0.42 to −0.67). Conversely, positive changes occurred for the organizations in the sector offering a high-quality job stress program (the local government sector, with scores ranging from −0.17 to 0.34). Thus, although previous analyses provided no evidence that the organizations in the sector offering a high-quality intervention program implemented more or better interventions than organizations in the other sectors, overall the changes occurring in these organizations were *more positive* than those in organizations in the other sectors. This is consistent with our expectations, in that we hypothesized that the interventions implemented in the sector offering a high-quality job stress program would be more effective in improving the quality of working life than the measures taken in other sectors. At the same time, it must be acknowledged that it is difficult to link the findings presented in Table 5.4. to the specific interventions that were discussed previously (or their quality). Apparently, the quality of employment in the sector offering high-quality job stress programs has changed more or less independently of the interventions implemented in that sector, which questions the assumptions guiding the CHSW approach.

Conclusions and Recommendations

The present chapter started from the assumption that job stress could originate at various levels, ranging from the individual level via the job and organizational levels to (inter)national socio-economic and political developments (Kang et al., 2008). We argued that although job stress may originate at any of these levels, the lower (organizational, job and individual) levels are most appropriate for dealing with job stress, because (only) here the nature and context of the problems and the way in which these can be addressed best is fully known. Higher-level interventions may be useful in facilitating specific lower-level interventions to reduce job stress.

These ideas were examined in the context of a large-scale concerted effort to reduce job stress in the Netherlands, which was carried out between 1999 and 2005 in about 50 sectors of the Dutch labor market. In this period Covenants on Health and Safety at Work (CHSWs) were drawn up between representatives of the Dutch government, trade unions and employers' organizations, among others, involving within-sector state-of-the-art studies on the health risks within that sector as well as possible ways to reduce these risks, and the implementation of specific measures to reduce job stress in the organizations within these sectors. This approach meshes well with the notion that higher-level interventions (provision of knowledge to reduce job stress, diagnosis of health risks within a particular occupational sector, and to some degree the provision of funding) may facilitate the implementation of specific lower-level measures. The main questions addressed in this chapter were: was this approach successful?, and what lessons can be learned from this unique social experiment?

To address the issue of the effectiveness of this approach, we conducted two related studies. In the first, qualitative study, we examined the quality of nine sector-level job stress programs. These programs were evaluated in terms of the quality of the diagnosis in that sector and the organizations operating in that sector (i.e., the findings of the state-of-the-art studies on the health risks within specific sectors including an inventory of measures to address these risks), the quality of the transfer of that information to individual organizations, and the facilities offered to organizations. To keep as many confounding variables as possible constant across sectors we focused on public sectors. We found that the quality of the sector-level programs varied strongly across sectors. Some sectors provided the individual organizations with an excellent overview of within-sector health risks and with ways to deal with the latter, while supporting them when they implemented possible interventions; but other sectors performed very poorly in these respects.

If the reasoning is that higher (sector)-level interventions facilitate taking effective lower-level measures to reduce job stress, one would expect organizations in the sectors offering high-quality programs to take more, and more effective, measures than organizations in sectors offering intermediate and low-quality job stress programs. This reasoning was tested in a quantitative survey study among 233 human resource officers of organizations in three of the nine sectors included in the qualitative study, namely one offering a high-quality program, one offering an intermediate-quality program, and one offering a low-quality program. Contrary to our expectations, the results showed that organizations offering a high-quality program did *not* take more measures to reduce job stress than organizations in other sectors did, nor did they take more potentially effective measures. Rather, our findings showed that the organizations in the sector offering an intermediate-quality job stress program were most active in implementing stress interventions. However, our findings did support the idea that the effectiveness of job stress interventions would be higher in organizations in the sector offering a high-quality job stress program. This became evident from ratings of across-time changes in the antecedents and outcomes of job stress.

Lessons to be learned

Based on these findings, it seems fair to conclude that there is modest evidence for the proposition that higher-level interventions may facilitate effective job stress interventions at lower levels. However, the mechanisms linking the quality of the sector-level job stress program, the activity of the organizations in these sectors, and the implications of these activities for the quality of working life, are still far from clear. For example, why were the organizations in the sector providing a high-quality job stress program (i.e., a program that offered a clear diagnosis of possible problems as well as a description and clear examples of suitable interventions to deal with these problems) less active in dealing with stress-related problems than organizations in other sectors? One tentative answer could be that there is a complicated interaction between the quality of a sector-level job stress program and the specific experiences and knowledge that are already present in that sector. As a sector-level program must build upon these experiences and knowledge, it will be difficult to create a high-quality sector program in the absence of relevant knowledge and experiences. Thus, a high-quality job stress program is not only the *start* of a range of successful organizational-level interventions, but also the *result* of such interventions.

This reasoning suggests that organizations in sectors offering a high-quality sector program will often have been relatively active in reducing job stress, meaning that the major job stress problems in these organizations (if there were any) may well already have been dealt with. Thus, these organizations may have had less reason to take measures to reduce job stress than organizations in other sectors. This reasoning was confirmed by a post-hoc inspection of the reasons why organizations had engaged in job stress interventions (cf. Table 5.3.): overall, the two most important stress-related problems were having too much work (26%) and internal pressure (20%), but these problems were most often mentioned by the organizations in the sector offering a low-quality program (37% and 30%, respectively; figures not given in Table 5.3.) and much less often in the sector offering a high-quality program (25% and 20%, respectively). Thus, organizations in the sector offering a high-quality program were indeed considerably less frequently confronted with the two major antecedents of job stress than organizations in the sector offering a low-quality approach, meaning that there was little need for them to engage frantically in all sorts of interventions (cf. Tables 5.2. and 5.3.).

If this reasoning is correct, there are two lessons to be learned. First, *the present sector-level approach (the collection and provision of state-of-the-art knowledge on job stress, as well as ways to deal with this problem) will only be effective if there is sufficient relevant knowledge and experience in the sector.* In its absence, the sector-level approach discussed in this chapter can presumably not guide or facilitate the efforts of individual organizations in reducing job stress, and it would be unrealistic to expect major effects from such a sector-level approach. In such sectors a different approach, involving establishing pilot projects, conducting research into the antecedents of job stress, and providing "good examples" in which job stress was successfully reduced, may be more effective in motivating organizations to reduce job stress. In this way the sector may begin building a body of knowledge on the effects of job stress interventions.

Secondly, *if there is sufficient knowledge and experience available in a particular sector, it is likely that the sector-level approach discussed above will be helpful in reducing job stress even further.* Although organizations in the sector offering a high-quality approach were less active in reducing job stress than organizations in other sectors, the effects of their efforts were larger than those of organizations in other sectors. Apparently the organizations in the high-quality sector were better able to identify the major risk factors for job stress, the measures that could address these issues, or the best way to implement these measures, than organizations in the other sectors.

Taking a more general perspective, the present study underlines Semmer's (2003) statement that the main question to be addressed in intervention research is not *whether* job stress interventions are effective in reducing job stress but rather *what* can be expected under *which* circumstances. The nation-wide approach implemented in the Netherlands has taught us that it is unrealistic to expect job stress interventions to be effective if little knowledge is available on the antecedents of stress in a particular sector (diagnosis) or if it is unclear which interventions could work, given a particular risk factor for job stress. Conversely, it is more likely that stress interventions will have the anticipated effect if organizations are well-informed regarding the nature of their problems as well as possible ways to remedy them. In this sense, we believe that the Dutch approach to addressing job stress has been effective and useful, even if not all organizations in all sectors included in this approach were able to address job stress equally effectively.

References

Belkiç, K., Landsbergis, P. A., Schnall, P. L., & Baker, D. (2004). Is job strain a major source of cardiovascular disease risk? *Scandinavian Journal of Work, Environment and Health, 30,* 85–128.

Bluestone, B., & Rose, S. (1998). *Public policy brief: The unmeasured labor force.* Blithewood, NY: The Jerome Levy Institute of Bard College, Bard Publications Office, No. 39.

De Cuyper, N., De Jong, J., De Witte, H., Isaksson, K., Rigotti, T., & Schalk, R. (2008). Literature review of theory and research on the psychological impact of temporary employment: Towards a conceptual model. *International Journal of Management Reviews, 10*, 25–51.

DeFrank, R. S. & Cooper, C. L. (1987) Work stress management interventions: Their effectiveness and conceptualizations. *Journal of Managerial Psychology, 2*, 4–10.

De Lange, A. H., Taris, T. W., Kompier, M. A. J., Houtman, I. L. D., & Bongers, P. M. (2003). The very best of the millennium: Longitudinal research on the job demands-control model. *Journal of Occupational Health Psychology, 8*, 282–305.

Dikkers, J. S. E., Geurts, S. A. E., Den Dulk, L., Peper, B., Taris, T. W., & Kompier, M. A. J. (2007). Dimensions of work–home culture and their relations with the use of work–home arrangements and work–home interaction. *Work & Stress, 21*, 155–172.

Geurts, S. A. E., Kompier, M. A. J., & Gründemann, R. G. W. (2000). Curing the Dutch disease? Sickness absence and disability in the Netherlands. *International Social Security Review, 53*, 79–103.

Giardini Murta, S., Sanderson, K., & Oldenburg, B. (2007). Process evaluation in occupational stress management programs: A systematic review. *American Journal of Health Promotion, 21*, 248–254.

Giga, S., Faragher, B., & Cooper, C. (2003). Identification of good practice in stress prevention/management. In J. Jordan, E. Gurr, G. Tinline, S. Giga, B. Faragher, & C. Cooper (Eds.), *Beacons of excellence in stress prevention*, HSE Research Report 133 (pp. 1–45). Sudbury, U.K.: HSE Books

Gründemann, R. W. M., & Van Vuuren, C. V. (1997). *Preventing absenteeism at the workplace: European research report*. Dublin: European Foundation for the Improvement of Working and Living Conditions.

Heaney, C. A. (2003). Worksite health interventions: Targets for change and strategies for attaining them. In J.C. Quick and L.E. Tetrick (Eds.), *Handbook of occupational health psychology* (pp. 305–323). Washington, DC: American Psychological Association.

Kang, S. Y., Staniford, A., Dollard, M. F., & Kompier, M. A. J. (2008). Knowledge development and content in occupational health psychology: A systematic analysis of the Journal of Occupational Health Psychology and Work & Stress, 1996–2006. In J. Houdmont and S. Leka (Eds.), *Occupational health psychology: European perspectives on research, education and practice* (vol., 3, pp. 27–63). Maia: ISMAI Publishers.

Kompier, M. A. J. (2002). Job design and well-being. In M. Schabracq, J. Winnubst, & C. Cooper (Eds.), *Handbook of work and health psychology* (pp. 429–454). Chichester, U.K.: Wiley.

Kompier, M. A. J., Cooper, C., & Geurts, S. A. E. (2000). A multiple case study approach to work stress prevention in Europe. *European Journal of Work and Organizational Psychology, 9*, 371–400.

Kompier, M. A. J., Geurts, S. A. E., Gründemann, R. W. M., Vink, P., & Smulders, P. G. W. (1998). Cases in stress prevention: The success of a participative and stepwise approach. *Stress Medicine, 14*, 155–168.

Lamontagne, A. D., Keegel, T., Louie, A. M., Ostry, A., & Landsbergis, P. A. (2007). A systematic review of the job-stress intervention evaluation literature, 1990–2005. *International Journal of Occupational and environmental Health, 13*, 268–280.

Merllie, D., & Paoli, P. (2001). *Ten years of working conditions in the European Union*. Dublin: European Foundation for the Improvement of Working and Living Conditions.

Murphy, L. R. (1996). Stress management in working settings: A critical review of the health effects. *American Journal of Health Promotion, 11*, 112–135.

Navarro, V. (Ed.) (2007). *Neoliberalism, globalization and inequalities.* Amityville, NY: Baywood.

Parent-Thirion, A., Fernàndez Macías, E., Hurley, J., & Vermeylen, G. (2007). *Fourth European Working Conditions Survey.* Dublin: European Foundation for the Improvement of Living and Working Conditions.

Sauter, S. L., Brightwell, W. S., Colligan, M. J., Hurrell, J. J., Jr., Katz, T. M., LeGrande, D. E., Lessin, N., Lippin, R. A., Lipscombe, J. A., & Murphy, L. R. (2002). *The changing organization of work and the safety and health of working people,* DHHS [NIOSH] Publication No. 2002–116. Cincinnati, OH: National Institute for Occupational Safety and Health.

Schaufeli, W. B., & Kompier, M. A. J. (2001). Managing job stress in the Netherlands. *International Journal of Stress Management, 8,* 15–34.

Semmer, N. K. (2003). Job stress interventions and organization of work. In J. C. Quick and L. E. Tetrick (Eds), *Handbook of occupational health psychology* (pp. 325–354). Washington, DC: American Psychological Association.

Semmer, N. K. (2006). Job stress interventions and the organization of work. *Scandinavian Journal of Work, Environment, and Health, 32,* 515–527.

Taris, T. W., Kompier, M. A. J., Geurts, S. A. E., Schreurs, P. J. G., Schaufeli, W. B., de Boer, E.M., & Sepmeijer, K.G. (2003). Stress management interventions in the Dutch domiciliary care sector: Findings from 81 organizations. *International Journal of Stress Management, 10,* 297–325.

Van der Klink, J. J. L., Blonk, R. W. B., Schene, A. H., & Van Dijk, F. J. H. (2001). The benefits of interventions for work-related stress. *American Journal of Public Health, 91,* 270–276.

6

The Neglected Employees
Work–Life Balance and a Stress Management Intervention Program for Low-Qualified Workers

Christine Busch and Henning Staar
University of Hamburg, Germany

Carl Åborg
Karolinska Institutet, Sweden

Susanne Roscher
Verwaltungs-Berufsgenossenschaft, Germany

Antje Ducki
University of Applied Sciences Berlin, Germany

To date, research on work–life balance, occupational health promotion and, in particular, stress management interventions, has largely focused on the individual, qualified employee (Richardson & Rothstein, 2008; Thompson, Smith, & Bybee, 2005). In this chapter, we take a different perspective by studying the work–life balance of low-qualified workers and by presenting a team-based stress and resource management intervention program for this target group. We provide results from the ReSuM project[1], financed by the German Federal Ministry of Education and Research[2], in which the intervention program was developed and is currently being evaluated. We developed the intervention program in close cooperation with prevention providers such as health insurance agencies and company doctors, with a view to integrating the experiences and needs of these key stakeholder groups. This chapter reflects selected contributions from the symposium "Work-Life Balance and a Workplace Health Promotion Program for Low-Qualified Workers", which was convened at the 2008 conference of the European Academy of Occupational Health Psychology, in Valencia, Spain.

In this chapter, therefore, we present a cross-cultural study which investigates the work–family interface of low-qualified workers[3]. It shows that low-qualified German workers, especially women, experience high levels of work–family conflict in comparison to their Swedish counterparts. In contrast to the cross-cultural differences in work–family conflict, however, the same assumed cultural impact on work–family enrichment could not be confirmed for low-qualified workers.

Further, we present a team-based stress and resource management intervention program for low-qualified workers. A team approach has various advantages over conventional stress management training programs focused on individuals. On the one hand, it enables consideration of the work organization and focuses on team resources and collective coping strategies. On the other hand, and this is of paramount importance for low-qualified workers, it facilitates participation, learning processes, and the transfer of acquired skills into everyday practice. The intervention program involves a training intervention for supervisors to secure their support for the program and to strengthen supervisory care of subordinates' health. The program underwent a pilot phase in six companies including an extensive process evaluation. Results from this pilot phase are presented here. On the basis of the results from the process evaluation the whole intervention program was revised. At present the intervention program is going through an evaluation phase with a control-group test design in eight companies ($N = 268$).

The Neglected Employees

Low-qualified workers are at particular risk in terms of their health. Morbidity and mortality statistics from various European countries, such as Germany, indicate that more deaths and illnesses occur among people in low social classes than among those in high social classes (Mackenbach, Kunst, Cavalaars, Groenhof & Geurts, 1997; Robert-Koch-Institut, 2006). Compared with people in higher social classes, people in lower social classes have a higher probability of serious health impairments and chronic illnesses such as back pain, chronic bronchitis, depression, and diabetes mellitus. There are gender differences too; men in low social classes suffer more often from heart attacks, back pain, dizziness and chronic bronchitis than men in high social classes, while women in low social classes suffer more often from heart attacks and diabetes mellitus than women in high social classes. Health-risk behaviors such as smoking and inactivity, are also more prevalent among low-qualified people. Inactivity is the main determinant for the development of chronic illnesses (Robert-Koch-Institut, 2006).

The reason for unhealthy behavior and increased health impairments might be increased psychological stress from a number of circumstances. People in low social classes may experience more critical life events such as migration and periods of unemployment, as well as more daily hassles such as job stress and work–family conflicts. Furthermore, they commonly have insecure jobs. Job insecurity is associated with high morbidity rates (Ferrie, Shipley, Marmot, Stansfeld, & Smith, 1998). On the basis of the job demand-control-support model (Johnson & Hall, 1988; Karasek, 1979) it might be suggested that low-qualified employees are more likely than highly qualified employees to have stressful and/or passive jobs, i.e., jobs with low job control, low social support and low cognitive demands, but high physical and psychosocial demands, as in the case of shift work and monotonous tasks (Björksten, Boquist, Talbäck & Edling, 2001). Social support has been found to be the most important resource for low-qualified people in coping with stressful situations (Gunnarsdottir & Björnsdottir, 2003). At the same time, social support is less available for low-qualified workers than for qualified employees. In the 4th European Working Condition Survey, only 78% of unskilled workers, compared to 92% of senior managers, reported receiving social support from colleagues. Similarly, 69% of unskilled workers and 85% of senior managers reported receiving social support from supervisors; 35% of unskilled workers and 69% of senior managers reported receiving external social support (Parent-Thirion, Macías, Hurley, & Vermeylen, 2007). Low-qualified workers not only have jobs with low cognitive demands, they also tend to have less access to occupational training for professional development and health promotion. There is a strong association between learning opportunities on the job and motivation for training as well as training activities. The level of training is particularly low in qualified, semi-qualified and unqualified industrial and service occupations. In the 4th European Working Condition Survey, only 16% of unqualified workers compared to 50% of senior managers reported receiving training paid for by their employer (Parent-Thirion et al., 2007). Therefore, the opportunities for professional development are limited for these employees. The combination of low job control, high physical and psychosocial demands as well as a lack of opportunities for development on the job, are all associated with increased health risk (Sundquist, Östergren, Sundquist, & Johansson, 2003). Additionally, employers are usually not interested in offering health promotion activities to low-qualified employees. One of the reasons for this lack of interest may be the fact that low-qualified workers are easy to replace if they get ill. The costs of health promotion activities tend to be the major barrier to implementing activities for this target group; a way around this barrier is to utilize the services provided by health and accident insurance agencies. For example, in Germany, health insurance agencies are obliged by law to offer workplace health promotion activities (§ 20 Sozialgesetzbuch, SGB V). They offer preventive services in the areas of stress, physical demands, nutrition, and addictive drugs for employees. They also offer support for professional development, such as the enhancement of leadership skills.

Little is known about the determinants of participation for low-qualified workers in occupational health promotion activities offered by employers. The greater participation shown by high-qualified employees compared with the low-qualified may be due to the former's increased job flexibility, the larger value they place on health, and their higher levels of self-efficacy (Thompson et al., 2005). The perception of one's own state of health as well as the perception of the state of health of significant others are important determinants of participation (Stonecipher & Hyner, 1993). Self-efficacy, attitudes towards health behaviors, and the perception of behavioral control were found to be the main determinants for engagement in healthy behaviors such as exercise (Blue, Black, Conrad, & Gretebeck, 2003; Blue, Wilbur, & Marston-Scott, 2001). Women face unique barriers to participation in workplace health promotion intervention programs, including lack of time due to the requirement to balance multiple roles and responsibilities

(Campbell et al., 2002). Furthermore, traditional workplace health promotion programs tend not to be tailored to the skills, experiences, and needs of low-qualified workers. For example, reading and writing skills are limited among low-qualified people, but traditional intervention programs often require these skills. One exception is the "Health Works for Women" intervention program (Campbell et al., 2002), which is tailored to low-qualified women. It includes two intervention strategies: individualized computer-aided health messages and a natural helpers program at the workplace. Natural helpers are female volunteers drawn from multiple social networks at the workplace for the purpose of enhancing social support among women. Other important issues to consider include legal and ethical concerns, such as data security. For example, if participants complete health risk appraisals and questionnaires, confidentiality of information must be maintained. Participants, particularly low-qualified workers who may experience high job insecurity, may view health risk appraisals and questionnaires as a concrete threat. Increasing employee participation is of paramount importance. The use of modest incentives is often seen as an effective method to increase participation in workplace health promotion programs. These incentives must be in line with the company and employee cultures. Program flexibility can also increase participation. Furthermore, the program should include a variety of activities with differing intensities and commitment levels (Glasgow, McCaul & Fisher, 1993; Thompson et al., 2005). Last, but not least, tailoring interventions based on theoretically sound research to low-qualified workers should increase the likelihood of program effectiveness.

Family and Work: Benefit or Burden for Low-Qualified Workers?

Balancing work and family has become an issue for the vast majority of employees in most countries and cultural contexts. The problem of balancing multiple life domains may be especially true for employees in low-qualified jobs given that they are notably susceptible to strain. However, as of late there has been an intensified recognition of culture as a possible key driver of variations in work–family conflict, suggesting that larger cultural contexts may affect men's and women's perceptions and experiences within the work and family domains (Aycan, 2008; Yang, Chen, Choi, & Zou, 2000). Accordingly, research is required to clarify whether this is also the case for low-qualified workers, and if members of this potential risk-group are equally affected by work and family problems across cultures. The intention of this cross-cultural study within the ReSuM project was, firstly, to empirically confirm suggested differences in the work-related and family-related cultural values and attitudes of low-qualified workers of two different national cultures and, building on that, to secondly assess how these differences in cultural values may influence individuals' perceptions and experiences of the work–family interface.

Work, Family, and Culture

Perhaps due to the fact that expectations underpinning role performance in work and family domains have been shown to be different and frequently incompatible, much of the extant research has primarily focused on *work–family conflict* (WFC) that individuals experience as they simultaneously attempt to balance these two areas of life (Aryee, Luk, Leung, & Lo, 1999). According to Greenhaus and Beutell (1985), WFC can be defined as a specific "form of interrole conflict in which the role from the work and family domains are mutually incompatible in some respect" (p. 77). Most researchers agree that the work–family interface contains two separate but related components: work-to-family and family-to-work. Consequently, WFC can arise from two directions: work interferes with family (WIF) or family interferes with work (FIW; e.g., Frone, Russell, & Cooper, 1992; Gutek, Searle, & Klepa, 1991).

Although the conflict perspective, with its emphasis on resource drain, has dominated the work family literature to date (Frone et al., 1992; Greenhaus & Beutell, 1985), an emerging trend toward more positive conceptualizations of the work–family interface can be discerned (e.g., Frone, 2003; Grzywacz & Marks, 2000; Rothbard, 2001;). Following Frone (2003), *work–family enrichment* (WFE) can be defined as the extent to which participation at work (or home) is made easier by virtue of the experiences, skills, and opportunities gained or developed at home (or work). Analogously for the negative side of the interface, a bi-directional relationship between life domains is assumed: work can enrich family life and vice versa (WEF, FEW; e.g., Greenhaus & Powell, 2006).

With his taxonomy of *work-family balance* (WFB), Frone incorporates both constructs into a common model, thereby providing a conceptual lens through which to examine work and family not only as mutually constraining, but also as mutually reinforcing. He argues that WFB results from low levels of WFC and high levels of WFE, suggesting that WFB may be a formative rather than reflective latent construct (Edwards & Bagozzi, 2000, in Carlson & Grzywacz, 2007). In accordance with Frone's model, the present study aims to operate within the WFB perspective with both components, WFC and WFE, integrated.

The current literature indicates a growing recognition that larger cultural, social, and political contexts may affect individuals' perceptions and experiences within the work–family domains (Westman, 2002). In this work, the word culture corresponds to the definition given by Hofstede (1997), that culture is "the collective programming of the mind which distinguishes the members of one group category of people from another" (p. 5). Based on his influential study of cross-cultural differences in work-related values, Hofstede (2001) and Hofstede and Bond (1984, 1988) concluded that the values of different societies would vary substantially along five cultural dimensions: individualism/collectivism, power distance, uncertainty avoidance, masculinity/femininity, and long-term orientation. However, when taking these cultural dimensions into account, a special emphasis has been placed on geographically distant national cultures such as the U.S. and Asia, where cultural differences on

Table 6.1   Descriptions of Masculine/Feminine Cultures (Hofstede, 1998, 2001)

Masculine societies		Feminine societies
Higher work centrality	↔	Lower work centrality
Higher job stress	↔	Lower job stress
Employer may invade employees' private lives	↔	Private life is protected from the employer
Distinct gender roles	↔	Overlapping gender roles

individualism/collectivism have been assessed (e.g., Yang et al., 2000). However, as suggested by Bartusch and Lindgren (1999), noteworthy cultural differences are likely to exist even between neighbouring European national cultures such as Sweden and Germany: "The fact that Swedes and Germans are relatively alike on the surface implies that the existing cultural distinctions between these two countries are particularly critical" (p. 2). Nevertheless, no cross-cultural comparison between these two countries has been conducted. Moreover, the extant body of research has neglected to include the masculinity/femininity dimension in examinations of individuals' work–family experiences. This is quite surprising given researchers' assertion that this cultural dimension may be of great importance in understanding cross-cultural differences and similarities in work–family issues (Shafiro & Hammer, 2004; Westman, 2002). Moreover, as can be seen from Table 6.1, the descriptions of masculine and feminine cultures regarding their importance in understanding the role that work plays, and different attitudes towards men and women, etc., give reason to assume that this cultural dimension may greatly contribute to explaining cross-cultural differences in the work–family interface.

However, extant research has largely refrained from making concrete theoretical assumptions on how to translate masculine/feminine cultural values into work–family matters. Recently, Aycan (2008) has started to address this theoretical gap in cross-cultural research, arguing that in cultures that value high work-centrality, which may be regarded as the central characteristic of masculine societies, employees might be expected to experience more demands in their work role compared to those in cultures that place less emphasis on competition and achievement. Further indication can be drawn from Carlson and Kacmar (2000) who found that high work centrality in people's lives was associated with greater levels of WFC and less family satisfaction from family antecedents. The authors argue that when work is the central feature in life, sources of conflict in the family domain may cause them to spend effort and time in an area where they are not as focused, diminishing satisfaction in that domain. Accordingly, double engagement in work and family may be experienced as more burdensome and less beneficial. Similarly, Greenhaus and Powell (2006) argue that individuals who place high psychological importance on their work are more likely to "allow" their work responsibilities to interfere with their family life (Greenhaus & Powell, 2006; Parasuraman, Purohit, Godshalk, & Beutell, 1996).

Given this, masculinity/femininity can be suggested to have high explanatory power with respect to cross-cultural differences in the work–family interface. Consequently, this cultural dimension became the criterion for selecting the countries that were included in the research design. Sweden and Germany provide representative examples of feminine and masculine countries, respectively. Hofstede's research classified Sweden as the most feminine country in the world, and one with less differentiated gender roles. In contrast, Germany has been assessed as having a strong masculine culture where gender role expectations in work and family are highly differentiated (see, e.g., Hofstede, 1998, 2001). Taking these cultural work and family related differences into consideration the following hypotheses were devised:

H1:   The German sample is likely to rank higher on masculinity than the Swedish sample.

H2:   Swedish workers are likely to report a better work–family balance than German workers (lower levels of conflict, higher levels of enrichment).

H3 (a): The distribution of household chores is likely to differ between male and female workers in the German sample.

H3 (b): The distribution of household chores will not significantly differ between male and female workers in the Swedish sample.

H4:   In the German sample there will be greater gender differences in the reported levels of work–family conflict compared to the Swedish sample.

Method

To empirically verify the *masculine/feminine values* of respondents from both cultures, four items from the Value Survey Module 94 were taken (Hofstede, 1994) which allows calculation of the countries' index scores. WFC was assessed using an eight-item inventory based on Gutek et al. (1991) and Stephens and Sommer (1996). The items belong to two subscales which estimate both directions of WFC. The assessment of WFE was conducted with a four-item inventory, based on the work of Greenhaus and Powell (2006). Again, the items belong to two subscales which examine both directions of work–family enrichment. The distribution of family-related demands was measured via a single item with three response options: (1) having to do most of the work on one's own, (2) sharing household chores with a spouse or other people, and (3) leaving most of the chores to one's spouse. Additionally, sociodemographic data such as gender, age, nationality, occupational activity, and number of hours worked per week were assessed.

All items of interest were slightly adjusted and translated into German and Swedish, respectively. Cronbach's alphas for the translated versions ranged from $\alpha = .63$ to $\alpha = .90$. The assessment of the German sample took place within the ReSuM project at the University of Hamburg. Equivalent Swedish employees were simultaneously recruited through partners at the University of Örebro. The total sample consisted of 203 participants: 98 German and 105 Swedish employees. The German sample consisted of low-qualified workers (production workers, cleaners), while the Swedish sample was made up of 50 low-qualified and 55 higher-qualified production workers. Overall, 79 women and 123 men participated. This meant that in both the Swedish and the German samples, men and women were not equally distributed: male respondents outnumbered female respondents. The chi-square test ($\chi^2 = 0.038$; $df = 1$; $p = .846$) showed no significant differences between the two national groups regarding gender distribution. The majority of the respondents were in their middle years, with 123 participants (62.1%) between 31 and 50 years of age. No significant differences ($\chi^2 = 7.454$; $df = 4$; $p = .114$) were found between the German and Swedish samples in relation to age. The vast majority of respondents were committed to full-time employment with a mean value of approximately 39 working hours per week. t-tests revealed that Swedish and German participants did not significantly differ in their mean working hours ($t = -.35$; $df = 178$; $p = .730$).

Results

Cultural differences between German and Swedish employees

The German sample of low-qualified employees showed higher scores on masculinity than the Swedish sample, with scores of 70 compared to 27, hence supporting the first hypothesis. A comparison between these results and the scores from Hofstede's (2001) study indicated that the average score of the German sample exceeded that of Hofstede's German sample with the latter showing an index score of 66. The same tendency was discovered for Swedish samples: The average scores on the masculinity/femininity dimension for Swedish workers in this study greatly exceeded those of the Hofstede study in which Sweden was listed as the least masculine country with a score of 5. Given these results, it can be stated that both countries' masculinity scores are higher in the present sample, but a similar difference between both countries' scores still prevails.

Differences in experienced levels of WFB between German and Swedish employees

As noted above, WFB was assessed via its components, WFC and WFE. The two Swedish subsamples differed in their demographic characteristics. Due to the fact that half of the Swedish sample consisted of workers holding an occupational status other than that of low-qualified worker, t-tests were used to determine whether the Swedish subsamples significantly differed from each other with regard to the dependent work–family variables. The results showed no significant differences for both WFC variables indicating that, for this sample, the professional status of Swedish workers was unrelated to conflict experiences. With regard to WFE, however, the Swedish subgroups demonstrated significant differences across all measured forms of

Table 6.2   t-tests for WFC and WFE between Germans and Swedes

Variables	German (n=95) M (SD)	Swedish (n=103) M (SD)	t	df	p	d
WIF	3.5 (0.9)	2.4 (0.8)	8.73	196	.000***	1.25
FIW	2.7 (1.1)	1.8 (0.6)	6.88	196	.000***	1.04
Variables	German (n=94) M (SD)	Swedish (n=49) M (SD)	t	df	p	d
WEF	2.6 (0.9)	2.5 (1.0)	0.75	141	.456	0.13
FEW	2.7 (0.9)	2.9 (1.1)	−0.94	141	.351	0.16

***p<.001

enrichment. The professionals' ratings were consistently higher than those of their low-qualified associates. To eliminate the influence of occupation level with respect to H2, only the subgroup of low-qualified workers was considered for the analysis of WFE presented in Table 6.2. Accordingly, in considering the proposed hypotheses, any significant differences between the Swedish subgroups on dependent variables was described and taken into account in the analysis. The comparability of the German sample and the Swedish sample in respect of sociodemographic variables was estimated before testing. There were no significant differences between groups. Accordingly, differences cannot to be traced to sociodemographic variables.

As regards WFC, results revealed that German employees experienced significantly more conflict in both directional forms than Swedish employees, WIF (t = 8.73; p = .000***) and FIW (t = 6.88; p = .000***). Thus, strong evidence to support H2 was found. As regards experiences of WFE, t-tests were again performed to determine whether group differences existed between the two cultural samples. Contrary to expectations, no significant differences between Swedish and German workers were found for WEF or FEW when occupational level was controlled. Accordingly, results failed to provide evidence to support the WFE component of H2.

Differences in the distribution of household chores

It was hypothesized that, given more traditional gender roles at home, the distribution of household chores was likely to differ between German male and female low-qualified workers. Furthermore, it was assumed that this should not be true for Swedish working men and women whose cultural background is considered to promote fairly equal gender roles. The majority of German women (54.3%) were responsible for household duties, and only a small percentage of them (8.6%) left household responsibilities to their partners. In contrast, almost half of the German men (49.1%) abstained from family-related demands. Accordingly, men and women in the German sample significantly differed in the distribution of household labour (χ^2 = 18.33; df = 2; p = .000***). Also, in accordance with H3, the chi-square test for the Swedish sample revealed no significant results. Swedish respondents showed a similar distribution across gender. In addition, Swedish women were more likely than Swedish men to manage household responsibilities without spousal support. Nevertheless, as depicted in Table 6.3, the majority of both Swedish male and female employees reported that they shared household chores.

Table 6.3   Distributions of Household Demands

Responsibility for household duties	German women n (%)	German men n (%)	Statistical significance χ^2	p
respondent alone	19 (54)	11 (20)		
together with partner	13 (37)	17 (31)	18.33	.000***
other than respondent	3 (9)	27 (49)		
Total	35 (100)	55 (100)		

***p<.001

Responsibility for household duties	Swedish women n (%)	Swedish men n (%)	Statistical significance χ^2	p
respondent alone	15 (43)	14 (26)		
together with partner	20 (57)	34 (63)	5.88	.053
other than respondent	0 (0)	6 (11)		
Total	35 (100)	54 (100)		

Table 6.4   Results of ANOVA on FIW

Variable	n	M (SD)	Factor	F(df)	p	Eta²
FIW						
German						
women	36	3.2 (1.1)				
men	57	2.4 (1.1)				
Swedish			Gender	15.64 (1,191)	.000***	.07
women	39	1.9 (0.8)	Culture	62.70 (1,191)	.000***	.25
men	63	1.7 (0.5)	Gender x Culture	5.01 (1,191)	.026*	.03

*p<.05; ***p<.001

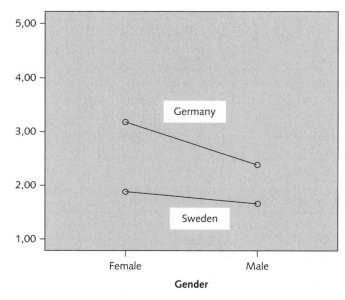

Figure 6.1   Interaction of FIW

Cross-cultural investigation of work–family conflict and gender

It was hypothesized that there would be greater gender differences in the reported levels of WFC in the German sample than in the Swedish. With regard to FIW there was a significant main effect for cultural background ($F(1,191) = 62.70$; $p = <.001$; $\eta^2 = .25$). Furthermore, a significant main effect for gender was found ($F(1,191) = 15.64$; $p = <.001$; $\eta^2 = .08$) showing strong and medium effects for culture and for gender, respectively. The ANOVA revealed a significant ordinal interaction ($F(1,191) = 5.01$; $p = <.05$; $\eta^2 = .03$) of medium effect size. As can be seen in Figure 6.1, German women revealed the highest level of FIW, followed by German men. Swedish women experienced lower FIW on this factor than German men. Again, Swedish men experienced the least FIW. The profile plot clearly shows a substantial difference between FIW experiences reported by German women and men. Despite this gender divide in the German sample, German men revealed higher levels of FIW than Swedish women and men.

Stress and Resource Management for Low-Qualified Workers: A Team-Based Intervention Program

Occupational stress theories, including the influential demand-control-support model (Johnson & Hall, 1988; Karasek, 1979), emphasize the importance of resources in the stress process. Low-qualified workers often have few resources and experience poor work–life balance, as we have mentioned in the sections above. Therefore an intervention program was developed that was designed to strengthen resources and improve work–life balance.

We chose a team-based intervention program for several reasons. A team approach has various advantages over conventional stress management training programs focused on the individual. On the one hand, it enables a consideration of the organization of teamwork. In European countries, 50% of unskilled employees do part or all of their work in teams, even if the quality of teamwork seems to be limited (Parent-Thirion et al., 2007). Occupational stress models do not refer to teamwork, but the socio-technical system approach does (Emery & Trist, 1960). It is not a stress theory, but a theory of the organization of production processes that has important implications for the quality of work. According to the sociotechnical system approach, technical and social systems can be distinguished in teamwork. The fit between these two systems is essential for the quality of work. Stress emerges when team workers meet demands without having suitable latitude for self-regulation in the system and without having suitable competencies for successful self-regulation. Latitude and competencies for self-regulation can be conceptualized as resources in teamwork. The few empirical studies on teamwork and well-being show that the presence of a system of job rotation is positively related to health factors. At the same time, line-paced assembly work with limited regulation latitude is negatively related to health factors (Delarue, 2007). In a longitudinal study, processes of internal self-regulation such as social support, conflict management, taking responsibility, continuous improvements, and relations to others (Kuipers, 2005) were found to be positively related to health outcomes. Furthermore open group processes, group cohesiveness (Carayon, Haims, Hoonakker, & Swanson, 2006), participation (Campion, Medsker, & Higgs, 1993) and task orientation (Carter & West, 1998) have been shown to be positively related to health or well-being factors. Team-based intervention programs provide an excellent opportunity for strengthening resources in teamwork. Additionally, team-based intervention programs may also support collective coping strategies such as mutual social support and collective problem-solving activities.

On the other hand, and this is of particular importance for low-qualified people, a team approach facilitates participation among low-qualified workers by providing a perception of psychological safety. The personal decision to participate will be easier if teammates participate. A team approach also makes behavior change easier. It facilitates cognitive-affective intervention strategies such as reflection and communication with significant others. It also supports behavioral intervention strategies such as public statements of the intention of change, the development of action plans, or exercises in social support. According to the influential transtheoretical theory of behavior change, these intervention strategies are important ones for behavior change (Prochaska & DiClemente, 1983). Furthermore, team-based intervention programs facilitate learning processes and transfer due to the presence of stable social relations during the intervention (Edmondson, Bohmer, & Pisano, 2001).

As has been shown, low-qualified German workers, particularly German women, experience low levels of work–life balance. Participants in this intervention program were therefore encouraged to reflect on their life domains and learn about goal-setting to strengthen work–life balance. Individual action plans were developed within the intervention program. We also mentioned above that low-qualified workers are at highest risk of chronic illnesses due to relatively high levels of inactivity. The intervention program therefore also focused on increasing physical exercise in work and leisure time.

The success of intervention programs, particularly for low-qualified workers, depends heavily on the support that is received from supervisors. Supervisors influence subordinates' health because they play a major role in work design (Kuoppala, Lamminpää, Liira, & Vainio, 2008). They strongly influence participation and transfer of acquired skills into everyday practice. Without support from supervisors, activities such as regular team meetings are unlikely to take place, yet these are fundamental to facilitating reflection on stressful situations and to the generation of solutions. Low-qualified workers need support to implement activities for stress reduction. Therefore, this intervention program integrates a training for the supervisor to secure their support for the program and to strengthen supervisory care for subordinates' health.

Last but not least, participation among employers was taken into account by developing the intervention in close cooperation with various prevention providers in Germany such as health insurance agencies. Workplace health promotion activities offered by prevention providers are cost-effective and therefore attractive for employers.

The Intervention

The intervention in the pilot phase consisted of five self-contained sessions. Four were designed for team workers of one or more teams with a maximum of twenty participants. Each session lasted four hours. Two trainers were involved; this was found to be especially necessary when more than one team was trained. The first session treated the stress process through the provision of information and the encouragement of reflection on stress, resources, and coping behavior. Physical exercises that might be used in leisure time, and short preventive physical exercises at work, were practiced. In addition, action plans were developed and supported by modest incentives at the team and individual levels. The second session started with a reflection on cooperation. Mutual social support, appreciation, and conflict management were dealt with. In session three, information about problem-focused coping was given, and practical exercises were conducted to develop collective, problem-focused coping skills in teamwork. Training for supervisors was carried out after session three with a focus on the support that they might give to subordinates in respect of problem-solving activities and the strengthening of supervisory care for subordinates' health. The last team session dealt with work–life balance. Different life domains were reflected upon, information concerning goal-setting was given, and individual action plans were developed. The program also involved an information session for all participants that was held three to four weeks before commencement of the intervention, and an on-site inspection by the trainers with a screening instrument. The transfer session took place three months later.

Process Evaluation

The pilot phase was exposed to extensive process evaluation. Low-qualified team workers from various industries participated. In the following sections we report on the participants in the pilot phase, the quality of their teamwork, trainers' adherence to the manual and session evaluation by participants. Last but not least we report on the participation of employers and health prevention providers.

Method

Participants and quality of teamwork

Quality of teamwork was separately assessed for the technical and social systems. Resources in the technical system were assessed on the basis of the following four teamwork characteristics through interviews and observation during the on-site inspection (1 = none of the four teamwork characteristics exist; 5 = all four teamwork characteristics exist). *Job rotation*: As already mentioned, the presence of a system of job rotation is positively related to health factors (Delarue, 2007). *Self-nominated team speaker*: It is assumed that workers have less stress and feel better with a self-nominated team speaker. Workers trust their self-nominated team speaker to obtain appropriate external support for work-related stress. Team workers nominated a colleague, who had good relationships with others. This was considered important given that relationship to others is positively related to health factors (Kuipers, 2005). *Payment on team level*: If payment also depends on the extent to which performance targets are attained by the whole team, team members will cooperate in a better way. *Regular team meetings*: Regular team meetings are necessary to reflect collectively on stressful situations and to solve problems. Resources in the social system were measured by a 12-item scale. The respondent was required to indicate the extent to which the statements were true (ranging from 1 = that is not the case at all, to 5 = that is completely the case). The items covered task reflexivity, collective self-efficacy, goal orientation, taking responsibility, participation in decision-making situations, and collective task management. The items were developed on the basis of team process research and team process instruments (Kauffeld, 2001; West, 1996).

Trainers' adherence to the manual

Trainers' adherence to the training manual was assessed by observation with a structured observation sheet.

Session evaluation by participants

Participants were asked to fill out a questionnaire after each session. This concerned their post-session mood, activity and perceived relationship with the trainer. In addition, insight into self or the team and the experienced support for stress management was measured. Post-session positive mood and activity was measured by adjectives (Becker, 1988; ranging from 1= that is not the case at all, to 4 = that is completely the case). The relationship to the trainer, insight into self or the team, and post-session experienced help for stress management were assessed by adapted items from validated scales that were developed to evaluate psychotherapy sessions (Krampen & Wald, 2001).

Organizational decision and implementation process

The organizational decision and implementation process was studied through an interview study using a semi-structured format. For each intervention program, two interviews were carried out; one with the contact person in the company and another with one of the trainers. The interviews were recorded, transcribed and analysed according to qualitative content analysis (Miles & Huberman, 1994).

Results

Participants and quality of teamwork

Missing data were imputed using IVEware (Raghunathan, Solenberger, & Van Hoewyk, 2002). Three data sets were generated (Schafer & Olsen, 1998). Seventy-three low-qualified workers from six companies from various industries took part in the intervention program. 50.7% were women. The participants worked in manufacturing, cleaning, kitchen work, and in the waste disposal industry. The intervention program ran five times; teams of two companies (D) were trained together. A high percentage of migrant-workers participated (34.2 %). A further striking feature was the low average monthly household income (500 to 1000 Euro); both features differed significantly between the companies. Working hours per week differed significantly between the companies as did the percentage of participants who had been unemployed in the last five years (see Table 6.5).

Exploratory factor analysis was conducted on the newly developed items concerning resources in teamwork. The mean values of factor loadings in the explorative

Table 6.5 Sample Description—Pilot Phase

	Total	A Manu.	B City cleaning	C School cleaning	D Kindergarten cleaning and kitchen work	E Waste disposal
% of women	50.7	100	0	92.9	100	0
Working hours per week	31.6	23.3	39	21.7	24.6	44
% of participants, who were unemployed in the last 5 years	22.8	0	27.8	35.7	0	45.5

Table 6.6   Regression Analyses for Resources in Teamwork and Health Factors

	GHQ ß/ Δ R²	Strain ß/ Δ R²	Well-being ß/ Δ R²
1st step	.14	.00	.10
sex	−.33*	−.12	.26*
age	.26	.14	−.06
working hours	−.10	−.01	.18
job tenure	−.13	.14	.17
2nd step	.00	.04	.04
Resources in teamwork (social system)	−.13	−.26*	.24*
R²	.14	.04	.14

*p<.05

factor analyses over three imputations were all above .4. Cronbach's alpha over three imputations for the scale was .89.

The newly developed scale for resources in teamwork should predict well-being and strain. Hierarchical regression analysis with health parameters such as the general health questionnaire (GHQ – 12, Goldberg, 1972), job-related strain (Mohr, Rigotti, & Müller, 2005), and well-being (Herda, Scharfenstein, & Basler, 1998) showed that the scale was negatively related to the GHQ (nonsignificant) and job-related strain, as hypothesized. It was positively related to well-being (see Table 6.6).

Resources in teamwork (social system) differed significantly between companies and the sexes. Women rated the resources in teamwork (social system) significantly higher than men. Resources in the technical system and in the social system did not fit in companies A, C and D (nonfit > |1|). Cleaning staff in schools and kindergarten had little teamwork according to the teamwork criteria (technical system), but the mostly female participants rated the resources in teamwork (social system) as quite high (see Table 6.7).

Trainers' adherence to the manual

Trainers' adherence was highest in Company C at 61 %; in Company B only 40% of the manual was implemented. Trainers stuck strongly to the manual for session three, implementing 64% of its content, as can be seen from Table 6.8.

Session evaluation by participants

Forty percent of the data was missing for the session evaluation, thus precluding multiple imputations. Participants in the waste disposal company were not able to fill out the questionnaires due to the literacy skills demanded for completion. Only those participants who filled out the questionnaires after each session were integrated in the

Table 6.7   Quality of Teamwork

	Total	A Manuf.	B City cleaning	C School cleaning	D Kindergarten cleaning and kitchen work	E Waste disposal
Resources in teamwork (technical system) (1–5)	2.6	5	3	1	2	2
Resources in teamwork (social system) (1–5) over three imputations	3.13(0.96)	3.86(0.49)	2.74(0.56)	3.49(0.9)	3.37(0.98)	2.62(1.31)
Fit	−.53	1.14	.26	−2.49	−1.37	−.62

Table 6.8   Trainers' Adherence to the Manual

% of adherence	Total	A Manuf.	B City cleaning	C School cleaning	D Kindergarten cleaning and kitchen work	E Waste disposal
Session 1	50	44	33	78	39	56
Session 2	50	67	42	58	33	50
Session 3	64	64	50	71	71	64
Session 4	56	56	33	67	56	67
Session 5	37	31	*	31	38	46
Intervention	51	52	40	61	47	57

* = adherence was not assessed

analyses ($n = 28$). Reliabilities for post-session mood (4 items) were between .82 and .92, for relation to trainer (3 items) between .58 and .78, for post-session activity (10 items) between .91 and .94, for insight into self or team (5 items) between .80 and .89, and for experienced support for stress management (5 items) between .70 and .82. Means and standard deviations of session evaluation variables are depicted in Table 6.9. Thus, relation to trainer and post-session positive mood were higher rated than post-session activity and insight into self or team. Session two was rated highest.

Two-factorial univariate ANOVAs (Sessions 1 to 4; Companies A to D) were performed. In contrast to trainers' adherence to the manual, participants in Company C rated the relation to trainer significantly worse than participants in Company B. Session two was evaluated significantly better than session three concerning post-session

Table 6.9   Means and Standard Deviations of Session Evaluation Variables

Variables	n	Intervention	Session 1	Session 2	Session 3	Session 4
			M(SD)	M(SD)	M(SD)	M(SD)
Post-session pos. mood	27	3,00(.73)	2,91(.68)	3,15(.62)	2,86(.83)	3,08(.78)
Relation to trainer	28	3,17(.54)	3,29(.49)	3,30(.58)	3,02(.63)	3,08(.45)
Post-session activity	27	2,73(.63)	2,68(.54)	2,82(.65)	2,66(.67)	2,75(.65)
Insight into self/team	28	2,75(.52)	2,62(.56)	2,82(.53)	2,74(.51)	2,81(.49)
Experienced support for stress man.	28	2,87(.54)	2,71(.60)	3,04(.50)	2,84(.45)	2,88(.60)
Total		2,90(.59)	2,84(.57)	3,02 (.58)	2,82(.62)	2,92(.59)

Table 6.10   Two-factorial Univariate ANOVA (Session 1 to 4; Company A to D), $* = p < .05$

Variables	Session F (df)	Company F (df)	Interaction F(df)
Post-session positive mood	3.23* (3,69) (2 vs. 3)	0.84 (3,23)	2,01 * (3,69)
Relation to trainer	4.08* (3,72) (2 vs. 3)	3.70*(3,24) (B vs. C)	2,76* (3,72)
Post-session acitivity	1.15 (3,69)	1.19 (3,23)	2,31* (3,69)
Insight into self/team	2.49 (3,72)	0.87 (3,24)	2,19* (3,72)
Experienced support for stress management	3.93* (3,72) (2 vs. 1)	0.73 (3,24)	1,35 (3,72)

mood and relation to trainer. Experienced support for stress management was rated significantly higher after session two than after session one.

Organizational decision and implementation process

Participation: Prevention providers mainly participated because the intervention program was tailored for low-qualified workers who are at risk in terms of their health and difficult to reach by conventional health promotion activities. The companies participated to show appreciation to low-qualified employees by offering a qualification and health intervention program. Another driver to involvement was that the intervention program was developed and evaluated by university staff, which promised high public visibility.

People involved: In three of the six participating companies, representatives of the human resource department were heavily involved. In one company, the company physician showed a high level of commitment. In the waste disposal company the managing director chaired the project.

Implementation process: Representatives of the human resource department reported that it was difficult to take whole teams out of the work process and to

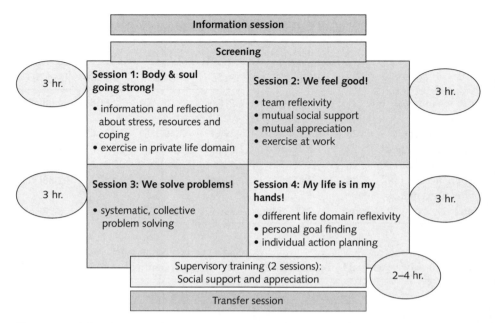

Figure 6.2   The Team-Based Intervention Program for Low-Qualified Employees: ReSuM

organize stand-ins. Lack of support from direct supervisors hindered the implementation process in Company C.

Evaluation: Trainers found the intervention program too dense. The contact person in each of the companies suggested shortening the intervention to reduce costs. Interviewees further pointed to the importance of the pre-session information and the transfer session three months after the intervention. It was suggested that the training for supervisors should be lengthened and split into two sessions; one should be carried out before the team-based intervention starts to inform supervisors about the intervention and their role in the process of generating stress for subordinates, while the other should take place after session three to support team workers' collective problem-solving activities.

On the basis of the results of the process evaluation the whole program was revised (Figure 6.2). The intervention for team workers was shortened to 12 hours; the training for supervisors was lengthened and split into two sessions. At the time of writing, the revised intervention program is going through a process of summative evaluation in eight German companies ($N = 268$).

Conclusions

Very few studies have focused on the situation of low-qualified workers. Moreover, research has refrained from exploring cross-cultural differences in how individuals from the low social classes respond to multiple demands. Therefore, the present study within the ReSuM project makes a significant contribution to bridging the knowledge gap about work–family issues from a cross-cultural perspective. Moreover, as the theoretical explanations for cross-cultural differences in this study relied on the core values of masculinity/femininity, a cultural dimension has been brought into play that was widely neglected in previous research.

The present work has followed Frone's approach whereby WFB is considered to have two constitutive components that contribute to feelings of balance between life domains: the degree of conflict and the degree of enrichment. In this vein it was assumed that Swedish employees would balance work and family life better than German employees. Based on Frone's model, this should be reflected both in lower levels of conflict and higher levels of enrichment in the Swedish sample.

The study has sharpened our assumptions regarding work- and family-related values and, indeed, there is impressive support for the view that Swedish employees, embedded in their feminine culture in which both domains are highly valued and protected from interference, perceive multiple demands as less burdensome and thus experience lower levels of conflict. On the other hand, due to the high value of work and achievement that exists in cultures such as the German, this country's employees could feel more pressured to live up to expectations provided by the working environment. On this note, perhaps the most important implication of the study is that low-qualified employees from a culture with high work centrality, e.g., Germany, are likely to face severe difficulties in balancing both life domains. A society in which work and achievement are central features may be more likely to permit interference from one domain to another. As a result, engagement with multiple demands is perceived as burdensome and as a waste of resources. In contrast, a culture's feminine value orientation may buffer work–family demands on individuals' WFC experiences, which may be essential, especially for at-risk groups such as low-qualified workers. In other words, Swedish employees' lower levels of WIF and FIW could be traced back to values that consider work and family as mutually complementary life domains that are equally valued and largely protected from mutual interference.

With respect to WFE, however, the findings are not as clear: When comparing Swedish and German low-qualified workers, no significant differences emerged on any of the assessed forms of enrichment. However, both the German and the Swedish samples of low-qualified workers showed significantly lower levels of enrichment compared with Swedish professionals. Therefore, regardless of cultural background, a lower occupational level was related to lower levels of enrichment in the study samples. Accordingly, these results lead to the conclusion that aspects related to occupational level may play a more decisive part in enrichment processes than cultural factors. For instance, higher occupational levels are likely to be related to higher income which has been found to be an antecedent factor for WFE (Greenhaus & Powell, 2006). Additionally, professionals are expected to be engaged in more complex tasks at work and to benefit from a comparatively greater freedom of action and accountability for work-related tasks. These characteristics may provide employees with better opportunities to transfer their skills to other skill or life domains, or they may lead to increased feelings of self-esteem, therewith promoting higher levels of

WFE (Barnett & Hyde, 2001; Marks, 1977). In sum, these results indicate that the assumed cultural impact of masculinity/femininity on WFB needs to be divided. On the one hand, Swedish employees experienced the work–family interface as less burdensome, as represented by lower levels of WFC. However, this did not go along with a similar impact on WFE. Thus, it can be concluded that feminine values may be appropriate to ease the burden of multiple demands, but they are less likely to promote enrichment processes between life domains. For the latter, other factors such as occupational level appear to have more predictive value. Given the fact that until now little conceptual and empirical attention has been devoted to exploring and understanding the antecedents of WFE (Frone, 2003), subsequent research may help to shed more light on these findings.

Health promotion intervention programs for low-qualified workers are lacking. In this chapter we have presented a stress and resource management intervention program for low-qualified workers. The intervention program is innovative in that it is a team-based intervention program combined with an intervention program for supervisors. The team-based intervention program focuses on physical exercise, teamwork resources, and collective coping in teamwork, and on work–life balance. The training intervention for supervisors concentrates on securing their support for the program and on strengthening supervisory care for subordinates' health.

Special attention was given to participation because participation in workplace health promotion intervention programs for low-qualified workers is problematic among employers and employees.

For employers, the costs of health promotion activities tend to be the major barrier to their implementation for this target group. A solution to this barrier is to utilize the services provided by health and accident insurance agencies. They are the main multipliers of workplace health promotion programs. For this reason, the intervention program was developed in close cooperation with prevention providers.

In order to improve participation among low-qualified workers, a team approach was chosen. The team approach enhances participation, behavior change, learning processes, and transfer among low-qualified workers because of the psychological safety and stable social relations that are evident during the intervention. Furthermore, the team-based intervention program gives the opportunity to strengthen teamwork resources such as collective self-efficacy and collective coping measures such as collective problem solving. Resources in teamwork were conceptualized on the basis of the socio-technical system approach and team process research. An instrument to assess resources in cooperation, i.e., in the social system of teamwork, was developed. It proved to be a useful in assessing resources possessed by low-qualified workers working in teams. The quality of teamwork varied strongly. In manufacturing industry teamwork was characterized by regular team meetings, job rotation, nominated team-speakers, and payment on the team level; for cleaning staff in schools and kindergartens no real teamwork could be found, but resources in cooperation were rated highly by participants. Resources in cooperation were rated significantly higher by female than by male participants, but gender is confounded with the industry in which participants worked; for example, cleaning staff in schools and in kindergarten were mainly women; workers in the waste disposal industry and in the street cleaning industry were male. The observed misfit between resources in the technical and social systems of teamwork provided direction on how to intervene— with a work design intervention or training intervention.

Trainers' adherence to the manual was observed and showed interesting results in combination with the session evaluation by participants. There seemed to be a negative relationship between trainers' adherence to the manual and participants' relationship with the trainer. The trainers' adherence to the manual was highest in company C, in which the relationship to the trainer during the intervention program was assessed as worst by participants. The trainers' adherence to the manual was highest for session three, which addressed collective problem-solving, but the session evaluation by participants showed that this session was evaluated significantly worse than session two that concerned relation to the trainer. The low values on post-session positive mood are not surprising as problem-solving is an exhausting procedure, especially for participants who are not used to problem-solving processes. The unsatisfying relationship with the trainer can be explained by the trainers' adherence to manual: trainers appeared to lose contact with participants when they stuck to the manual. They probably stuck to the manual because they felt uneasy with the training. It is possible that session three was not designed well enough and that trainers in company C were not sufficiently experienced to perform a team-based intervention program. Therefore, session three was revised and improved. Multilevel analyses in the evaluation phase of the ReSuM-project with more intervention programs carried out will be necessary to test the assumed relationship between trainers' adherence to the manual and session evaluation, as well as the association between participants' relationship with the trainer and training effectiveness. The experienced support for stress management was rated significantly higher after session two, which addressed social relations in teamwork. This was in contrast to session one, which dealt with an introduction to stress management and physical exercise. Therefore session one had to be revised by giving participants more information about stress management and the enhancement of the physical exercise dimension.

Organizational decision and implementation processes were largely the responsibility of representatives from the human resource departments. The team-based intervention program was not only seen as a health promotion intervention but also as a qualification scheme. Lack of support from supervisors was a major hindrance in the intervention implementation process.

Taken together, these results suggest that the team-based intervention program, focusing on physical exercise, teamwork resources, and collective coping in teamwork, as well as work-life balance, seems to be appropriate for low-skilled workers, as well as other stakeholders such as health promotion providers and employers. Prevention providers mainly participated because the intervention program was tailored for low-qualified workers, who are at risk in terms of their health and difficult to reach via conventional health promotion activities. Employers participated to show appreciation to low-qualified employees. The revised intervention program may show promising effects within the summative evaluation.

Notes

1. ReSuM stands for "Stress- und Ressourcenmanagement für un- und angelernte Beschäftigte: Entwicklung eines Multiplikatorenkonzepts" [Stress and Resource Management for Low-Qualified Workers: The Development of a Multiplier Concept].
2. Project registration number 01EL0412, Duration: 2006–2009; Project leader: C. Busch; Co-project: Multiplikatorenkonzept für Betriebsärzte [A Mulitplier Concept for Company Doctors], Project leader: A. Ducki, registration number 01EL0417. Project applicants: C. Busch, E. Bamberg & A. Ducki.
3. The study is the diploma thesis of Henning Staar, University of Hamburg (2008) and was carried out in co-operation with C. Åborg, Sweden (international cooperation partner of the ReSuM-project).

References

Aryee, S., Luk, V., Leung, A., & Lo, S. (1999). Role stressors, interrole conflict, and well-being: The moderating influence of spousal support and coping behaviors among employed parents in Hong Kong. *Journal of Vocational Behavior, 54*, 259–278.

Aycan, Z. (2008). Cross-cultural approaches to work–family conflict. In K. Korabik, D. Lero, & D.S. Whitehead (Eds.), *Handbook of work–family integration: Research, theory and best practices* (pp. 353–370). San Diego, CA: Elsevier.

Barnett, R. C., & Hyde, J. S. (2001). Women, men, work, and family: An expansionist theory. *American Psychologist, 56*, 781–796.

Bartusch, C., & Lindgren, K. (1999). A grounded theory of national cultures' impact on Swedish–German business relationships. *Studies in Business Administration and Informatics, 2*, 1–21.

Becker, P. (1988). Ein Strukturmodell der emotionalen Befindlichkeit [A structural model of a person's emotional state]. *Psychologische Beiträge, 30*, 514–536.

Björksten, M. G., Boquist, B., Talbäck, M., & Edling, C. (2001). Reported neck and shoulder problems in female industrial workers: The importance of factors at work and at home. *International Journal of Industrial Ergonomics, 27*, 159–170.

Blue, C. L., Black, D. R., Conrad, K., & Gretebeck, K. A. (2003). Beliefs of blue-collar workers: Stage of readiness for exercise. *American Journal of Health Behavior, 27*, 408–420.

Blue, C. L., Wilbur, J. E., & Marston-Scott, M. V. (2001). Exercise among blue-collar workers: Application of the theory of planned behavior. *Research in Nursing & Health, 24*, 481–493.

Campbell, M. K., Tessaro, I., Devillis, B., Benedict, S., Kelsey, K., Belton, L., & Sanhueza, A. (2002). Effects of a tailored health promotion program for female blue-collar workers: Health Works for Women. *Preventive Medicine, 34*, 313–323.

Campion, M. A., Medsker, G. J., & Higgs, A. C. (1993). Relations between work group characteristics and effectiveness: Implications for designing effective work groups. *Personnel Psychology, 46*, 823–847.

Carayon, P., Haims, M., Hoonakker, P., & Swanson, N. (2006). Teamwork and musculoskeletal health in the context of work organization interventions in office and computer work. *Theoretical Issues in Ergonomics Science, 7*, 39–69.

Carlson, D. S. & Kacmar, K. M. (2000). Work–family conflict in the organization: Do life role values make a difference? *Journal of Management, 26*,1031–54.

Carlson, D. S. & Grzywacz, J. (2007). Conceptualizing work–family balance: Implications for practice and research. *Advances in Developing Human Resources, 9,* 455–471.

Carter, A. J. & West, M. A. (1998). Reflexivity, effectiveness and mental health in BBC-TV production teams. *Small Group Research, 29,* 583–601.

Delarue, A. (2007). *The impact of structural features of teams on the stress level of the team members: A multilevel analysis.* Paper presented at the 13th EAWOP congress, Stockholm.

Edmondson, A. C., Bohmer, R., & Pisano, G. P. (2001). Disrupted routines: Team learning and new technology adaptation. *Administrative Science Quarterly, 46,* 685–716.

Emery, F. E. & Trist, E. L. (1960). Socio-technical systems. In C.W. Churchman & M. Verhulst (Eds.), *Management, science, models and techniques 2* (pp. 83–97). Oxford: Pergamon Press.

Ferrie, J. E., Shipley, M. J., Marmot, M. G., Stansfeld, S. A., & Smith, G. D. (1998). An uncertain future: The health effects of threats to employment security in white-collar men and women. *American Journal of Public Health, 88,* 1030–1036.

Frone, M. R. (2003). Work–family balance. In J. C. Quick & L. E. Tetrick (Eds.). *Handbook of occupational health psychology* (pp. 143–162). Washington, DC: American Psychological Association.

Frone, M. R. Russell, M., & Cooper, M. L. (1992). Antecedents and outcomes of work–family conflict: Testing a model of work–family interface. *Journal of Applied Psychology, 77,* 65–78.

Glasgow, R. E., McCaul, K. D., & Fisher, K. J. (1993). Participation in worksite health promotion: A critique of the literature and recommendations for future practice. *Health Education Quarterly, 20,* 391–408.

Goldberg, D. P. (1972). *The detection of psychiatric illness by questionnaire. A technique for the identification and assessment of non-psychotic psychiatric illness (GHQ).* London: Oxford University Press.

Greenhaus, J. H., & Beutell, N. J. (1985). Sources of conflict between work and family roles. *Academy of Management Review, 10,* 76–88.

Greenhaus, J. H., & Powell, G. N. (2006). When work and family are allies: A theory of work–family enrichment. *Academy of Management Review, 31,* 72–92.

Grzywacz, J. G., & Marks, N. F. (2000). Reconceptualizing the work–family interface: An ecological perspective on the correlates of positive and negative spillover between work and family. *Journal of Occupational Health Psychology, 5,* 111–126.

Gunnarsdottir, S., & Björnsdottir, K. (2003). Health promotion in the workplace: The perspective of unskilled workers in a hospital setting. *Scandinavian Journal of Caring Sciences, 17,* 66–73.

Gutek, B. A., Searle, S., & Klepa, L. (1991). Rational versus gender role explanations for work–family conflict. *Journal of Applied Psychology, 76,* 560–568.

Herda, C., Scharfenstein, A., & Basler, H.D. (1998). *Marburger Fragebogen zum habituellen Wohlbefinden* [Marburg questionnaire on habitual well-being]. Schriftenreihe des Zentrums für Methodenwissenschaften und Gesundheitsforschung, Arbeitspapier, 98–1. Marburg: Philipps-Universität.

Hofstede, G. (1994). VSM 94 – *Modul für Werterhaltungsumfrage* 1994 Fragebogen (Deutsche Version) [Module of a value preservation survey 1994 Questionnaire (German version)]. Retrieved from http://feweb.uvt.nl/center/hofstede/ deutsche.html

Hofstede, G. (1997). *Cultures and organizations: Software of the mind, 2.* New York: McGraw-Hill.

Hofstede, G. (1998). *Masculinity and femininity: The taboo dimension of national cultures.* Thousand Oaks, CA: Sage Publications.

Hofstede, G. (2001). *Culture's consequences: Comparing values, behaviors, institutions and organizations across nations.* Beverly Hills, CA: Sage Publications.

Hofstede, G. & Bond, M. H. (1984). Cultural dimensions: An independent validation using Rokeach's value survey. *Journal of Cross-Cultural Psychology, 15,* 417–433.

Hofstede, G. & Bond, M. H. (1988). The Confucius connection: From cultural roots to economic growth, *Organizational Dynamics, 16,* 4–22.

Johnson, J. & Hall, E. M. (1988). Job strain, work place social support and cardiovascular disease: A cross-sectional study of random sample of the Swedish working population. *American Journal of Public Health, 78,* 1336–1342.

Karasek, R. A. (1979). Job demands, job decision latitude and mental strain: Implications for job redesign. *Administrative Science Quarterly, 24,* 285–308.

Kauffeld, S. (2001). *Teamdiagnose* [Team diagnosis]. Göttingen: Verlag für Angewandte Psychologie.

Krampen, G., & Wald, B. (2001). Instruments for formative evaluation and indication in general and differential psychotherapy and counseling: Short inventories for single psychotherapy and counseling. *Diagnostica, 47,* 43–50.

Kuipers, B. S. (2005). *Team development and team performance. responsibilities, responsiveness and results: A longitudinal study of teamwork at Volvo Trucks Umea,* PhD, University of Groningen.

Kuoppala, J., Lamminpää, A., Liira, J., & Vainio, H. (2008). Leadership, job well-being, and health effects – A systematic review and a meta-analysis. *Journal of Occupational & Environmental Medicine, 50,* 904–915.

Mackenbach, J. P., Kunst, A., Cavalaars, A. E., Groenhof, F. & Geurts, J. J. (1997). Socioeconomic inequalities in morbidity and mortality in Western Europe. *The Lancet, 349,* 1655–1659.

Marks, S. R. (1977). Multiple roles and role strain: Some notes on human energy, time and commitment. *American Sociological Review, 42,* 921–936.

Miles, M. B., & Huberman, A. M. (1994). *Qualitative data analysis. An expanded sourcebook.* Thousand Oaks, CA: Sage.

Mohr, G., Rigotti, T., & Müller, A. (2005). Irritation—Ein Instrument zur Erfassung psychischer Beanspruchung im Arbeitskontext. Skalen- und Itemparameter aus 15 Studien [Irritation—An instrument for assessing mental stress in the work context. Scales and item parameters from 15 studies]. *Zeitschrift für Arbeits- und Organisationspsychologie, 49,* 44–48.

Parasuraman, S., Purohit, Y. S., Godshalk, V. M., & Beutell, N. J. (1996). Work and family variables, entrepreneurial career success, and psychological well-being. *Journal of Vocational Behavior, 48,* 275–300.

Parent-Thirion, A., Macías, E., Hurley, J., & Vermeylen, G. (2007). *Fourth European Working Conditions Survey.* Luxembourg: Office for Official Publications of the European Communities.

Prochaska J. O., & DiClemente, C. C. (1983). Stages and processes of self-change of smoking: Toward an integrative model of change. *Journal of Consulting and Clinical Psychology, 51,* 390–395.

Raghunathan, T. E., Solenberger P. W., & Van Hoewyk, J. (2002). *IVEware: Imputation and Variance Estimation Software. User Guide.* University of Michigan.

Richardson, K. M. & Rothstein, H. R. (2008). Effects of occupational stress management intervention programs: A meta-analysis. *Journal of Occupational Health Psychology, 13,* 69–93.

Robert-Koch-Institut (Ed.) (2006). *Gesundheit in Deutschland. Gesundheitsberichterstattung des Bundes* [Health in Germany. Health report on the Federal Republic]. Berlin: Robert-Koch-Institut.

Rothbard, N. P. (2001). Enriching or depleting? The dynamics of engagement in work and family roles. *Administrative Science Quarterly, 46,* 655–684.

Schafer, J. L. & Olsen, M. K. (1998). Multiple imputation for multivariate missing-data problems: A data analyst's perspective. *Multivariate Behavioral Research, 33,* 545–571.

Shafiro, M. & Hammer, L. (2004). *Work and family: A cross-cultural psychological perspective.* Retrieved from http://wfnetwork.bc.edu/encyclopedia_entry.php?id=226.

Stephens, G. K., & Sommer, S. M. (1996). The measurement of work to family conflict. *Educational and Psychological Measurement, 56,* 475–486.

Stonecipher L., & Hyner G. C. (1993). Health practices before and after a work-site health screening. *Journal of Occupational Medicine, 35,* 297–306.

Sundquist, J., Östergren, P. O., Sundquist, K., & Johansson, S. E. (2003). Psychological working conditions and self-reported long-term illness: A population-based study of Swedish-born and foreign-born employed persons. *Ethnicity and Health, 8,* 307–317.

Thompson, S. E., Smith, B. A., & Bybee, R. F. (2005). Factors influencing participation in worksite wellness programs among minority and underserved populations. *Family & Community Health, 28,* 267–273.

West, M. A. (Ed.) (1996). *Handbook of work group psychology.* New York: Wiley.

Westman, M. (2002). *Work–family conflict: A cross-cultural perspective.* Paper presented as part of at the annual meeting of the Society for Industrial and Organizational Psychology, Toronto, Canada.

Yang, N., Chen, C. C., Choi, J., & Zou, Y. (2000). Sources of work–family conflict: A Sino-U.S. comparison of the effects of work and family demands. *Academy of Management Journal, 43,* 113–123.

7

Personal Resources and Work Engagement in the Face of Change

Machteld van den Heuvel, Evangelia Demerouti, and Wilmar B. Schaufeli
Utrecht University, The Netherlands

Arnold B. Bakker
Erasmus University Rotterdam, The Netherlands

Introduction

Organizations are continuously changing. Developments in society such as the current financial crisis and ongoing technological innovation increase pressure on employees to show change-ability and resilience. Most planned change initiatives, whether they concern a restructuring, cultural change, or policy innovation, share the aim of maximizing organizational performance. Recently, organizations have begun to refer to the "new world of work" indicating a digital work style characterized by flexible hours and no fixed locations (Microsoft, 2005). The ideal "new" employee is a self-directed, proactive, networking entrepreneur, taking responsibility for his or her own performance and development. Innovative IT systems aim to make working life easier and support employee productivity. However, the pace of change is high and multiple change efforts often coincide and overlap, adding to the demands on employees' adaptive capacities (Herold, Fedor, & Caldwell, 2007). Change *processes* have become a stressor irrespective of the *content* of the change (Korunka, Weiss, & Karetta, 1993).

In order to successfully implement change, many factors at many levels (societal, organizational, departmental, individual) need to be managed simultaneously (Armenakis, Harris, & Mossholder, 1993; Fernandez & Rainey, 2006). However, considering that ultimately work is carried out by employees, individual knowledge, attitudes and behavior are crucial aspects of any change endeavor (Woodman & Dewett, 2004). In spite of this, most empirical organizational change studies have focused on macrolevel factors. Empirical studies that do include employee-level variables tend to focus on the influence of organizational factors on attitudinal outcome variables (e.g., resistance to change). Organizational change research has not sufficiently included the role of individual resources in successful change implementation (Armenakis & Bedeian, 1999; Judge, Thoresen, Pucik, & Welbourne, 1999).

Therefore, in line with the positive approach to studying employee development and performance in organizations (Bakker & Schaufeli, 2008; Luthans, Youssef, & Avolio, 2007), we focus in this chapter on the sustainability of work engagement during change. We aim to advance the knowledge of antecedents of healthy organizational change, both from an organizational and employee perspective. This chapter provides an overview of the role of personal resources in the process of positive adaptation to change. Also, we present a research model that offers a micro-level framework for studying how personal resources are related to work engagement and performance during change.

Healthy Organizational Change

Three themes can be distinguished in change research, reflecting the multiple processes involved in organizational change (Armenakis & Bedeian, 1999). First, research on organizational *context* variables examines the work environment (internal context) or broader societal (external) contexts. Internal context (e.g., working conditions, support, or culture) is relevant to our focus on the employee level. Secondly, *process* variables refer to how the change is implemented, for example, in terms of employee participation and information provided. Thirdly, the *content* theme reflects studies on the substance of change (e.g., strategic change, performance-incentives, etc.) and its relationship with organizational effectiveness. In line with Holt, Armenakis, Field, and Harris (2007), we include a fourth theme – namely, individual characteristics and, specifically, personal resources. We will first focus on how work environments influence well-being and performance at work, before turning to the individual factors that are important for healthy organizational change.

Effects of change on employees

Many change initiatives do not reach their objectives within the given timeframe, partly due to individual reactions to change (Sorge & Van Witteloostuijn, 2004). How does change affect employees? First, organizational change has an impact on the working environment and subsequently it may affect employee well-being, motivation, and performance. Studies have focused on the mediating role of psychosocial working conditions, and their subsequent impact on health and well-being. For example, it was shown that when employees perceived a reduction in decision latitude and an increase in job demands, they were more likely to go on long term sickness absence. In contrast, an increase in support at work led employees to have fewer long spells of sickness absence (Head et al., 2006; Vahtera, Kivimaki, Pentti, & Theorell, 2000). Amabile & Conti (1999) showed that changes due to downsizing negatively impacted creativity-enhancing aspects of the work environment, i.e., freedom, challenge, resources, encouragement, and support. Individual characteristics may explain or buffer the effects of organizational change (Judge et al.,1999; Wanberg & Banas, 2000).

Secondly, *how* change is implemented can affect employee health. This has been studied by focusing on change process characteristics, often leading to practitioner guidelines (Armenakis & Bedeian, 1999). For example, in a recent study by Saksvik et al. (2007), five implementation criteria for healthy organizational change were identified. The criteria were: (1) awareness of norms and how imposed change may conflict with unwritten rules, (2) awareness of diversity, or how different departments may respond differently to change, (3) manager availability, for support and information, 4) constructive conflict, whereby resistance is welcomed and dealt with rather than avoided, emphasizing dialogue regarding the change, and 5) role clarification, similar to role clarity, a job resource (e.g., Abramis, 1994) that becomes even more important in times of transition. Organizational change will nearly always include new ways of working, new roles and new ways of relating to others. These points are linked to our focus on the interplay of the changing work environment and the individual. First, the diversity in change reactions and use of constructive conflict underlines the importance of taking into account individual factors. Secondly, awareness of norms, role clarification and manager availability underline the importance of job demands and resources.

Job demands–resources model

Our approach is based on the assumptions of the job demands–resources model (JD–R) model (Bakker & Demerouti, 2007; Demerouti, Bakker, Nachreiner, & Schaufeli, 2001). This model (see Figure 7.1) provides a framework for studying the

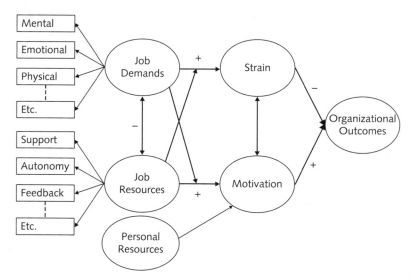

Figure 7.1   Job Demands–Resources model (adapted from Bakker & Demerouti, 2007, 2008)

processes by which work environment factors determine well-being and motivation, often operationalized as burnout and engagement. The JD–R model proposes that each workplace has its own unique demands and resources. *Job demands* refer to those physical, psychological, social, or organizational aspects of the job that require sustained physical and/or psychological (cognitive and emotional) effort or skill and are therefore associated with physiological and/or psychological costs. Examples are high work pressure, unfavourable physical environments, or emotionally demanding client interactions. Job demands are not necessarily negative; however, they may turn into job stressors when meeting those demands requires high effort from which the employee cannot adequately recover (Meijman & Mulder, 1998). *Job resources* are defined as those physical, psychological, social or organizational aspects of the job that may do any of the following: (1) are functional in achieving work related goals, (2) reduce job demands and the associated physiological and psychological costs, and (3) stimulate personal growth and development. Studies using the JD–R model have shown the positive impact of job resources on work engagement and subsequent performance (Bakker & Demerouti, 2007, 2008; Bakker, Schaufeli, Leiter, & Taris, 2008; Schaufeli & Salanova, 2007).

The JD–R model was recently expanded to include personal resources (Xanthopoulou, Bakker, Demerouti, & Schaufeli, 2007). Recent studies show the important role of personal resources in explaining why job resources are translated into engagement and in turn, job performance (Xanthopoulou, Bakker, Heuven, Demerouti, & Schaufeli, 2008; Xanthopoulou, Bakker, Demerouti, & Schaufeli, 2009a, 2009b). Personal resources mediated the relationship between job resources and work engagement/exhaustion. Moreover, personal resources influenced the perception of job resources over time and predicted objective financial turnover via work engagement.

As of yet, the JD–R model has not been tested in dynamic work environments. In this chapter we propose a framework that allows us to test the JD–R model in changing work environments. First, we outline the nature of personal resources.

What Are Personal Resources?

Interest in personal resources originates in stress and coping research. As research showed that there were no fixed associations between stressful life events and distress, attention shifted to mediators in the stress process, e.g., personal resources (Rabkin & Streuning, 1976). Personal resources have been described as "aspects of the self that are generally linked to resiliency" (Hobfoll, Johnson, Ennis, & Jackson, 2003, p. 632). Many researchers use similar concepts, for example, psychological resources (Taylor, Kemeny, Reed, Bower, & Gruenewald, 2000), psychological capital (Luthans & Youssef, 2004), personal coping resources (Aldwin, Sutton, & Lachman, 1996; Wheaton, 1983), and general resistance resources (Antonovsky, 1979). What is less clear in the broad definition is the ontological status of the umbrella-term "resources". What are the defining attributes of a personal resource and how do they relate to personality traits, states and coping styles? In order to add to the conceptualization of the term "personal resources" we propose a more detailed definition.

Key attributes of personal resources

Inherent in the term "resource" is a reference to it being a means of supplying a want or deficiency. What value the resource has is closely linked to the value of the outcome that it will produce or contribute towards (Ashford, 1986). "Personal" in personal resources refers to the idea that individual characteristics can function as a means of dealing with the outside world (Hobfoll, 1986). Personal resources refer to a person-environment interplay and can pertain to a specific domain, e.g., work-related self-efficacy. In personality research and occupational health psychology the importance of this interplay of person and (work) environment is widely accepted. Mischel (2004) states that in order to advance our knowledge of human behavior, the focus should be on patterns that can be found when studying the person–situation interaction.

Semantic definitions of the word "resource" include that resources (1) are useful in coping with (adverse) situations, and (2) add to the creation of a more favorable situation or goal attainment. Pearlin and Schooler (1978) defined psychological resources as "the personality characteristics that people draw upon to help them withstand threats posed by events and objects in their environment" (p.5). In occupational health psychology, studies have shown that the positive influence of personal resources is particularly salient at times when resources are needed, for example, during stressful events (Bakker, Hakanen, Demerouti, & Xanthopoulou, 2007; Callan, Terry, & Schweitzer, 1994; Hakanen, Bakker, & Demerouti, 2005; Hobfoll, 2002). Therefore a key attribute of personal resources is that they facilitate goal attainment in the face of adversity.

Personal resources can be measured both as traits and states; however, most studies take a state-perspective. In order to develop interventions, it is relevant to focus on characteristics that are malleable. Personal resources can be developed over time, influenced by significant life experiences and specific personal development interventions or coaching (Luthans, Avey, Avolio, Norman, & Combs, 2006; Lyubomirsky, Sousa, & Dickerhoof, 2006). Jerusalem (1993) refers to personal resources as self-beliefs and commitments. Personal resources can have both affective and cognitive components and are often valued in their own right (e.g., self-esteem: a combination of positive beliefs about intrinsic self-worth accompanied by positive affect). Personal resources can be considered as lower-order, malleable elements of personality (Gist & Mitchell, 1992).

Personality traits may influence the ease with which personal resources are developed. For example, people who are high on extraversion may be more likely to think optimistically than people who are low on extraversion. However, regardless of traits, it is possible to develop optimistic explanatory styles (Seligman, 1991). In our view, the mobilization of personal resources takes place as follows: when confronted with adversity or ambiguous events, underlying traits influence the presence of lower-order cognitive/affective states. In a stressful situation, these states either function as personal resources or as vulnerability factors (characteristics that increase a person's vulnerability to the adverse impact of stressors). These states influence the perception of the situation and, in turn, how a person will manage the situation (strategies).

We propose the following working definition for the concept of personal resources in organizational settings:

> Personal resources are lower-order, cognitive-affective aspects of personality; developable systems of positive beliefs about one's "self" (e.g., self-esteem, self-efficacy, mastery) and the world (e.g., optimism, faith) which motivate and facilitate goal-attainment, even in the face of adversity or challenge.

Personal Resources at Work

There is a growing tendency in occupational health psychology to focus on personal resources. Personal resources have been studied in relation to the work environment and in relation to outcomes such as performance, job satisfaction, commitment and work engagement. A number of theories have included personal resources and their influence on well-being and performance.

First, *cognitive adaptation theory* states that individuals who are able to adjust well to stressful life events are those who are high on optimism, self-esteem and personal control (Taylor, 1983). The theory proposes that the process of adjustment to threatening events is structured around the processes of (1) searching for meaning in the experience, (2) attempting to gain control of the situation in order to restore a general sense of mastery over one's life and (3) restoring self-esteem through self-enhancing evaluations (Taylor, 1983). This theory is mostly used in health psychology studies (e.g., Helgeson, 1999, 2003). However, it has also been applied to the study of organizational change, where it was found that personal resources predicted openness to change (Wanberg & Banas, 2000).

Another approach to personal resources in the workplace is Positive Organizational Behavior (POB), which focuses on positive attributes of people and organizations (Bakker & Schaufeli, 2008; Luthans, 2002). POB was introduced as "the study and application of positively oriented human resource strengths and psychological capacities that can be measured, developed and effectively managed for performance improvement in today's workplace" (Luthans, Youssef, & Avolio, 2007, p.10). *Psychological Capital* or "PsyCap" was introduced as a higher order construct that operationalizes the individual component of POB, including self-efficacy, hope, optimism and resilience (Luthans & Youssef, 2004). In contrast with signature strengths and virtues (Peterson & Seligman, 2004), PsyCap constructs are operationalized as developable states (Luthans, Avolio, Avey, & Norman, 2007). Even though some concerns have been raised about PsyCap's discriminant validity (Little, Gooty, & Nelson, 2007), PsyCap has been found to predict work-related performance and job satisfaction, both as a higher-order construct and the components individually (Luthans, Avolio, Walumbwa, & Li, 2005; Luthans, Norman, Avolio, & Avey, 2008). Below we describe the four personal resources used in the PsyCap construct. In addition, two other relevant resources (meaning-making and regulatory focus) are briefly described.

Optimism

Optimism has been defined as generalized, positive outcome expectancies (Scheier & Carver 1985). Optimism has also been approached as an explanatory style, which indicates a tendency to attribute causes of negative events to external, transient circumstances, rather than personal factors (Seligman, 1991). Optimism can be measured either state-like or trait-like, and in general or work-related terms, depending on the research question. Optimism has been shown to predict academic performance (Peterson & Barrett, 1987), effective coping with life stressors (Nolen-Hoeksema, 2000), successful management of stressors (Aspinwall & Taylor, 1997), physical health (Peterson, 2000), and work productivity (Seligman & Schulman, 1986). The PsyCap measure reflects work-related optimism. In a recent study, optimism was found to (partially) mediate the relationship between job resources and work engagement, and indirectly influenced organizational performance (Xanthopoulou et al., 2009b).

Hope

Related to optimism, the concept of hope has been defined as the ability to plan pathways to desired goals despite obstacles, and the agency or motivation to use these pathways (Snyder, 2000). Hope is viewed as a result of these two components, and as such differs from the lay person's meaning of "hope". This definition has an active nature, in that it speaks of motivation to the ability to plan. This motivational and agency component of hope suggests some overlap with self-efficacy. Peterson & Luthans (2003) showed that hope can influence financial performance. In order to build hope, the focus needs to be both on goal setting and building pathways towards these goals. Empowerment and mental rehearsal are ways of enhancing sense of control and finding pathways to attain goals (Snyder, 2000).

Resilience

Resilience refers to the ability to bounce back from adverse events, or cope successfully (Rutter, 1985). The interest in resilience originates from the field of developmental psychology (Masten, 2001). Resilience is related to processes of adaptation under stress, or the capacity to maintain positive outcomes in the face of negative life events (Ryff & Singer, 1996). Resilience can be measured as a trait, for example, ego-resiliency (Block & Kremen, 1996), indicating general resourcefulness regardless of the situation (Earvolino-Ramirez, 2007). Over the past two decades, resilience has also been used to indicate a dynamic, modifiable process that occurs during exposure to adversity (Luthar, Cicchetti, & Becker, 2000). Positive relationships, assertiveness, self-worth, sense of humor, and decision-making abilities have been identified as protective factors within the resilience process (Earvolino-Ramirez, 2007). The process of resilience can be built using cognitive coaching interventions (Luthans, et al., 2006). Resilience is slightly different from the other PsyCap constructs in that it always has an object, i.e., resilience is a response to a situation.

Self-efficacy

Self-efficacy is one of the most studied personal resources and has been extensively used in research in educational, clinical, and organizational settings (Hodgkinson & Healey, 2007). Derived from Bandura's social learning theory, the construct is concerned with how knowledge influences action. Perceived self-efficacy is defined as judgments about how capable one is of organizing different skills in order to execute appropriate courses of action to deal effectively with the environment (Bandura, 1989, 1997), or beliefs about one's ability to mobilize the relevant resources to meet situational demands (Gist & Mitchell, 1992). It is a dynamic construct, i.e., the beliefs or judgments can change over time. Self-efficacy influences thought-patterns, emotions, and actions, and as such it is a motivational construct. In work settings, significant correlations have been found between self-efficacy and work performance (Stajkovic & Luthans, 1998).

Meaning-making

Many influential theorists have acknowledged the importance of being able to experience meaning for optimal human functioning (Baumeister & Vohs, 2002; Frankl, 1963; Jahoda, 1958; Maslow, 1968; Rogers, 1961). Research has shown that an ability to make meaning, (i.e., to understand why an event has occurred and what its impact is) when faced with adversity can be beneficial to both mental and physical health (Frankl, 1963; Taylor et al., 2000).

Recently, interest in the study of meaning at work has increased. Many studies focus on the importance of meaningful work for organizational outcomes (e.g., Chalofsky, 2003; Cartwright & Holmes, 2006; May, Gilson, & Harter, 2004; Wrzesniewski, Dutton, & Debebe, 2003). What personal resource or strategy leads to the experience of meaningful work? Our view is that deliberate efforts to reflect on what happens at work and the ability to link this to broader values and life goals is a form of meaning-making that can help employees deal with ongoing change. In line with other theories, we view employees as self-regulating, active agents (Bandura, 1989; Bell & Staw, 1989; Wrzesniewski & Dutton, 2001). In deliberate meaning-making, ambiguous or challenging events are integrated into a framework of personal meaning, values and goals, which results in a sense of meaningfulness. Meaning-making is viewed as a cognitive/affective resource that one can develop. Recently, we developed a scale to capture the degree to which people engage in meaning-making (Van den Heuvel, Demerouti, Schreurs, Bakker, & Schaufeli, 2009). Meaning-making was shown to be related to willingness to change and in-role performance. We expect that meaning-making will facilitate positive attitudes to change and motivation to engage with the changed situation, resulting in more work engagement and enhanced performance.

Self-regulatory focus

Regulatory focus theory (Brockner & Higgins, 2001) states that people can operate in two distinct self-regulatory foci. A *promotion focus* indicates a tendency to perceive the environment in terms of growth and development opportunities (approach), while *prevention-focused* individuals are motivated by security needs and focus on avoiding risks and threats (avoidance). These tendencies may influence appraisal in change situations. Regulatory focus can be studied both as state or trait; chronic regulatory focus pertains to a dispositional focus, while situational regulatory focus is influenced by situational factors (Brockner & Higgins, 2001). The regulatory fit between the type of regulatory cues in the situation and the regulatory focus of the person is central to the theory. Both promotion and prevention are associated with positive outcomes, although some negative correlates of prevention focus have been noted, while for promotion focus, mainly beneficial impacts are emphasized (Brockner & Higgins, 2001; Dewett & Denisi, 2007; Kark & Van Dijk, 2007). Therefore, we propose that a promotion focus may function as a personal resource during change. The different foci will influence how employees perceive changes in work processes. In turn, this may influence how change demands and resources are dealt with.

Personal Resources and Organizational Change

As described above, and recognized by many authors in the management literature (Kotter, 1996, 2005; Stewart-Black & Gregersen, 2008), ultimately it is not organizations as entities that change, it is the people who are part of the organizations who change (Bovey & Hede, 2001, Woodman & Dewett, 2004). Obviously, employees need the right knowledge, skills and tools in order to work in the new ways that the organizational change imposes. However, in addition to this, the role of personal resources in change contexts should be explored. Individual characteristics have been included in the study of organizational change in different ways. Besides the studies that included attitudes, personal resources have also been included, either as predictors, mediators, or moderators.

Self-efficacy is often included as a *predictor* in studies on the adoption of technological innovations (e.g., Lam, Cho, & Qu, 2007). For example, Hill, Smith, and Mann (1987) showed the importance of efficacy beliefs in the decision to adopt an innovation. They demonstrated the impact of computer self-efficacy on adoption, independent of the beliefs relating to the instrumental value of doing so. It has been argued that self-efficacy is crucial for adaptive behavior and performance. If employees lack confidence regarding new behaviors they are unlikely to try these out (Griffin & Hesketh, 2003). Wanberg and Banas (2000) found that change-related self-efficacy, self esteem, optimism and a sense of control predicted openness to change, while openness predicted outcomes such as job satisfaction, irritation and turnover intentions. Ashford (1988) found that people with high self-esteem were better at coping with stress during organizational change than people low on self-esteem. Campbell (2006) showed that employees with a high learning orientation were more positive and proactive towards change than employees with a low learning orientation. Holt et al. (2007) used change efficacy in their model for individual readiness for change. Change-related efficacy was found to partially mediate the relationship between change-related information and well-being. Furthermore, self-efficacy was found to buffer stress during the change process (Jimmieson, Terry, & Callan, 2004).

It has been suggested that promotion focus is associated with more engagement in change-related behaviors than prevention focus (Dewett & Denisi, 2007). Also, Liberman, Idson, Camacho, and Higgins (1999) found that promotion-focused individuals showed more openness to change than individuals with a prevention focus. Avey, Wernsing, and Luthans (2008) found that the predictive value of PsyCap on change attitudes was mediated by positive emotions. Mindfulness had a moderating role and was found to compensate for low PsyCap. Stark, Thomas, and Poppler (2000) found that self-esteem moderated the effects of organizational change on job satisfaction. Employees with high self-esteem reported higher job satisfaction than those with low self-esteem. Personal resources have also been studied as mediators in organizational change settings. For example, Martin, Jones, and Callan (2005) found a relationship between psychological climate and adjustment indicators (well-being, job satisfaction, commitment, absenteeism, and turnover intention). This relationship was mediated by change-efficacy, control, and change-related stress. Frayne and Geringer (2000) found that self-efficacy partially mediated the relationship between self-management training, outcome expectancies, and job performance.

Employee Attitudes to Organizational Change

Attitudes to specific behaviors have been shown to have predictive value for behavior (Petty & Cacioppo, 1981). Many organizational change studies include attitudinal constructs such as resistance or willingness to change (e.g. Metselaar, 1997; Rafferty & Griffin, 2006; Van Dam, Oreg, & Schyns, 2007). One of the earliest influential studies dealing with employees' resistance to change was that of Coch and French (1948), which showed the positive impact of employee participation on reducing employee resistance to change. More recently, studies have also included positive attitudes, such as willingness and readiness for change (Armenakis et al., 1993; Piderit, 2000). Readiness for change is defined as employees' beliefs, attitudes and intentions regarding the necessity and the chance of successful implementation of organizational change. It is seen as the cognitive precursor to resistant or supporting behaviors in relation to the change. Willingness to change refers to a positive behavioral intention towards the implementation of change in the structure, culture, or work processes of an organization, resulting in efforts to support or enhance the change process (Metselaar, 1997). Other constructs that focus on positive attitudes and beliefs include commitment to change (Herscovitch & Meyer, 2002) and openness to change (e.g., Miller, Johnson, & Grau, 1994). In our approach we include the relationship and interaction between change attitudes and personal resources. Furthermore, we include attitudes not as outcomes but as driving forces predicting actual behaviors towards the change.

Dealing with Organizational Change: Strategies

What do employees actually do in terms of interacting with the change, managing themselves and their working environment? Organizational change impacts the work environment which, in turn, demands a response from the employee. Employees make an effort to maintain the fit between their abilities and the external demands of the environment. These strategies range from those aimed at regulating the external environment to those regulating intrapersonal processes. Reactive responses have been described as those efforts where employees try to change themselves in order to manage changing demands. Active or proactive responses are those strategies that entail employees initiating behaviors that positively impact their working environment and restore the fit (Griffin & Hesketh, 2003).

Strategies to cope

Coping can be defined as the conscious cognitive and behavioral efforts to manage the internal and external demands of situations that are appraised as stressful (Folkman & Lazarus, 1980; Lazarus & Folkman, 1984). Coping strategies can be problem-focused; aimed at eliminating the stressor, or emotion-focused; aimed at managing emotional responses. Aspinwall and Taylor (1992) showed that the impact of psychological control and self-esteem on adjustment and performance was mediated by specific forms of active, problem-focused coping. In organizational change research, support has been found for the mediating role of coping strategies in the relationship between personal resources and positive employee outcomes (Callan, 1993; Judge et al., 1999). Main effects of coping strategies on well-being have also been found, irrespective of the level of stress (Callan et al., 1994). Recently, researchers have suggested a move away from the broad distinction of problem-focused vs. emotion-focused coping (Connor-Smith & Flachsbart, 2007; Skinner, Edge, Altman, & Sherwood, 2003). A focus is needed on more specific coping strategies and personality facets. In line with the person-situation perspective, it is important to view coping as an ongoing, *interactive* process between employees and their working environment (Briner, Harris, & Daniels, 2004). Our approach provides scope to do this and it may provide insights concerning the specific relationships between different personal resources and specific strategies they predict. Strategies represent the measurable behaviors employees engage in. We differentiate strategies to manage the external change environment (job crafting and active coping) versus strategies to manage oneself (self-regulation and self-leadership).

Job crafting and self-leadership

Self-regulation is a broad term that illustrates the evolving focus on employees as "purposeful, goal-striving individuals" (Vancouver & Day, 2005, p.156). The idea of behavioral self-regulation refers to a mechanism that monitors progress towards desired states or goals. When a discrepancy is detected, an effort is made to change behavior in order to reduce the discrepancy and move towards desired end states (Carver & Scheier, 1981, 1998). There is no consensus on a uniform definition of self-regulation. It has been broadly defined as "the processes involved in attaining and maintaining internally represented desired states" (goals) (Vancouver & Day, 2005, p.158). Goal establishment, planning, striving and revision have been identified as key components of self-regulation processes. Where coping is a reactive process to a demanding, stressful situation, self-regulation processes view employees as goal-oriented, active agents. Individuals who are resourceful in terms of being confident and hopeful were found to persist when faced with obstacles in attaining their goals, as opposed to disengaging or searching for alternative goals (Carver & Scheier, 1998). Employees are not mere products of their environment, but actively sculpt their environments (Bell & Staw, 1989). This notion is part of both job-crafting theory and self-leadership theory.

Job Crafting is defined as "the physical and cognitive changes individuals make in the task or relational boundaries of their work" (Wrzesniewski & Dutton, 2001, p. 179). The concept of job crafting recognizes that employees are continuously interacting with their environments, regardless of their hierarchical position within an organization. Different types of crafting have been identified; firstly employees can change the number, scope and type of job tasks. Secondly, employees can craft the quality and the amount of social encounters with other people encountered at work. Thirdly, cognitive task boundaries can be changed, by thinking differently about which tasks are and aren't part of the role, and how these fit together (Wrzesniewski & Dutton, 2001). In a change situation these dynamic processes are likely to be even more salient.

Self-leadership was introduced as an expansion on the concept of self-management, which refers to the degree to which an employee takes responsibility for the managerial aspects of his or her job over and above the content and production-related responsibilities (Manz & Sims, 1980; Markham & Markham, 1995). Self-leadership emphasizes intrinsic work motivation and rewards. It is related to job resources such as autonomy, in that it allows employees to influence how a task is carried out. Self-leadership focuses on *what* to do and *why* (goal selection and setting), and also *how* to attain these goals. Self-leadership is defined as "a process through which individuals control their own behavior, influencing and leading themselves through the use of specific sets of behavioral and cognitive strategies" (Neck & Houghton, 2006, p.270). The main components of self-leadership include behavior-focused strategies (i.e., self-observation, self-goal-setting, self-reward, self-punishment), and self-cueing (i.e., reminding oneself of important goals). Secondly, natural reward strategies that focus on building intrinsically pleasurable or motivating aspects into a task or working environment. These strategies can range from changing lighting or decoration at work to focusing on particular enjoyable aspects of a job. The theory suggests that these strategies will lead to feelings of self-control, purpose and increased performance (Houghton & Neck, 2002). Thirdly, constructive thought patterns pertain to "the creation and maintenance of functional patterns of habitual thinking" (Houghton & Neck, 2002, p. 674). These strategies lean on theories from therapeutic settings such as rational emotive therapy (Ellis, 1977) and are nowadays widely used in interventions outside clinical contexts such as in coaching, which is also focused on facilitating self-regulation behaviors (self-observation, self-management, goal-setting) (e.g., Costa & Garmston, 2002; Wasylyshyn, 2003). A positive relationship was found between personal resources and the use of self-leadership strategies (Norris, 2008). We expect personal resources to positively influence employees' use of self-leadership strategies in order to work productively while having positive work experiences. Since self-leadership is presented as a normative theory, these strategies may be particularly relevant for intervention studies in change research.

Outcomes: Adaptive Performance and Work Engagement during Change

Although many studies focus on attitudes to change as outcomes, there seem to be fewer studies that include both individual characteristics and behavioral outcomes in terms of adaptive performance. In our model we propose that personal resources can boost work engagement and adaptive performance during change processes in organizations. We expect this process to be partially mediated by change attitudes and behavioral strategies. Below, outcome variables included in our model are described.

Work engagement is defined as a positive, fulfilling, work-related state of mind that is characterized by vigor, dedication, and absorption (Schaufeli, Salanova, González-Romá, & Bakker, 2002). Vigor refers to high levels of energy and mental resilience while working, the willingness to invest effort in one's work, and persistence in the face of difficulties. Dedication refers to a sense of significance, enthusiasm, inspiration, pride, and challenge. The third dimension of engagement is absorption, or flow, and is characterized by being fully concentrated and happily engrossed in one's work, so that time passes quickly and one has difficulties with detaching from work. Job and personal resources are found to be the main predictors of engagement; these resources gain their salience in the context of high job demands (Bakker, Demerouti, & Verbeke, 2004). Engaged workers are more creative, more productive, and more willing to go the extra mile. Work engagement has been shown to be contagious and may therefore be of special importance during change, as a counterforce for possible change-cynicism.

Employees typically engage in in-role and extra-role performance. In-role or task performance is defined as those officially required outcomes and behaviors that directly serve the goals of the organization (Motowidlo & Van Scotter, 1994). In-role performance includes meeting organizational objectives and effective functioning (Behrman & Perreault, 1984). Extra-role or contextual performance is defined as employees' discretionary behaviors that are believed to directly promote the effective functioning of an organization, without necessarily directly influencing a person's target productivity (Podsakoff & MacKenzie, 1994). Examples include willingness to help colleagues who have heavy workloads or the avoidance of problems with colleagues (this is also known as a specific form of organizational citizenship behavior; Organ & Paine, 1999). According to Dewett and Denisi (2007), a specific form of extra-role performance is change-related citizenship behavior. This refers to the expression of constructive challenge intended to improve rather than undermine the functioning of an organization undergoing change.

In our model we use *adaptive performance* as an outcome variable that expresses the change content. Since our level of analysis is the employee, the content of organizational change can be anything from cultural change to implementation of new software, as long as it affects the way in which people are required to behave at work. We define adaptive performance as work behaviors related to the new way of working, which is part of the organizational change. Adaptive performance can be understood as in-role performance in a change context. Pulakos, Arad, Donovan, and Plamondon (2000) developed an eight-dimension behavioral taxonomy for adaptive performance, including such aspects as learning new tasks, technologies and procedures, handling work stress, demonstrating interpersonal adaptability and creative problem solving. Our approach to adaptive performance is different from this and other general conceptualizations (e.g., Griffin & Hesketh, 2003) in that we view adaptive performance as a specific measure of change-related behavior. Ideally this should be captured both by self-assessment and other ratings. The measure is specified based on the specific change content. For example, when the change is related to multidisciplinary team-working, a measure is used that specifies team-working behaviors. Examples include discussing project progress with the team, designing methods as a team, and soliciting feedback from the team. Employees are consequently asked how often they engage in these behaviors. This type of measure allows us to capture behavior change and, thus, employee adaptive performance.

Personal Resources Adaptation Model

As argued above, when it comes to understanding adaptation to organizational change, employees' personal resources are relevant factors. Our model (Figure 7.2) departs from the assumption that organizational change will result in changes in the work environment. For example, employees may be confronted with increased

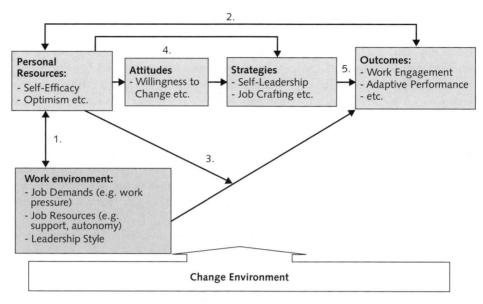

Figure 7.2   Personal Resources Adaptation Model

demands (e.g., more time pressure, higher workload, etc.) and more ambiguous operating environments (Armenakis & Bedeian, 1999; Campbell, 2006). People are expected to show new behaviors, process new information, and/or utilize new equipment during change (Armenakis & Bedeian, 1999). At the same time, the change may positively impact job resources, for example by increasing efficiency, facilitating communication, or possibilities for learning. The example of a Dutch regional college illustrates this. Teachers were confronted with a new policy that required them to change their didactic approach in order to help students to develop their talents. This resulted in having to use new materials and having to coach students, which was far-removed from more traditional methods of transferring knowledge. As a result of this change, teachers were exposed to higher cognitive demands, but they may have also perceived more task variety. Below we discuss the relationships represented in the "Personal resources adaptation model" (Figure 7.2.)

Personal resources and the work environment: Reciprocal influences

The model suggests a reciprocal relationship between employees' personal resources and job demands/resources. In line with the work of Kohn and Schooler (1982), we expect that personal resources will influence job demands/resources. This is also in line with the suggestions of Zapf, Dormann, and Frese (1996) regarding reversed causal effects of well-being on (perceived) working conditions and the drift hypothesis (people in a bad state drift to worse jobs). Employees with more personal resources will create job resources for themselves. For example, Scheier, Weintraub, and Carver (1986) found that people high in optimism were more likely to seek and receive social support. This may be influenced by employees' self-regulation strategies. Personal resources may also influence perceptions of the changed work environment. Resilient employees are more likely to perceive a new requirement as a challenge, while less resilient employees will experience changed requirements as taxing demands (Maddi, 2005).

Secondly, we expect job demands/resources in the working environment to influence the presence of personal resources. Many studies have established that job demands and job resources can impact employee health and well-being (e.g., Bakker & Demerouti, 2008; Hackman & Oldham, 1980; Karasek, 1979; Schaufeli & Salanova, 2007). We expect that job resources (e.g., support) may enhance the presence of personal resources (e.g., self-efficacy). These relationships should be tested in a longitudinal design.

Personal resources as mediators in the relationship between work environment and outcomes

The model suggests that personal resources may act both as mediators and moderators in explaining the relationship between the work environment and outcomes (i.e., work engagement and adaptive performance) while direct effects can also be observed.

A *direct* positive effect of personal resources on work engagement and performance is expected. Aspinwall and Taylor (1992) found that optimism had a direct effect on college adjustment. This direct effect can work for other personal resources as well. For example, self-efficacy makes employees feel competent, confident, and motivated. Self-efficacious employees therefore experience more engagement towards their work and eventually perform better (Xanthopoulou et al., 2009a).

In addition to this, we expect personal resources to *mediate* the influence of changes in the work environment on work engagement and performance. The model proposes that job resources (e.g., support, autonomy) will influence and build personal resources, which in turn will have a direct favorable impact on work engagement and performance. This process was observed in a study by Xanthopoulou et al. (2008), which showed that support enhanced self-efficacy which consequently increased work engagement. This mediated relationship between work environment, personal resources and positive organizational outcomes, has also been shown for organizational-based self-esteem (Pierce & Gardner, 2004) and PsyCap (Luthans et al., 2006).

Reciprocal relations between personal resources and outcomes

We expect that over time there will be a beneficial impact of work-engagement and adaptive performance on personal resources. This is in line with the broaden-and-build theory, that outlines how the presence of positive emotions triggers an upward spiral towards broadminded coping (i.e., taking a broad perspective and finding positive meaning), which in turn leads to more positive affect (Fredrickson & Joiner, 2002). In our model this would mean that positive emotions that accompany work engagement and performance can build enduring personal resources.

Personal resources as moderators

The model also suggests that personal resources will moderate the influence of job resources on performance and engagement. Personal resources can form a buffer against the adverse impact of job demands. This has been shown in a study where self-efficacy moderated the relationship between job demands and psychological health outcomes (Van Yperen & Snijders, 2000). This effect has also been shown for job resources, which buffered the negative impact of job demands on work engagement (Bakker et al., 2007). In addition, we expect that personal resources will enhance the positive impact of job resources on well-being and performance. We expect more resourceful employees to be more motivated and better able to spot resources in the changing environment and use them to their advantage, resulting in improved performance and engagement.

Role of Change Attitudes and Strategies

Most studies in this area have focused on the impact of change context variables (e.g., communication, participation, and trust) on attitudes to change (e.g., Kotter & Schlesinger, 1979). We focus on the presence of personal resources and how this influences attitudes to change. We expect the presence of more resources to lead to a more positive change attitude. In turn, change attitudes will influence employees' choice of strategies for interacting with the change.

The model suggests that personal resources are translated into (cognitive) behavioral strategies. For example, self-efficacy beliefs are linked to a strategy of remembering previous mastery experiences and using these in evaluating one's current capacities to deal with a situation (Bandura, 1997). Maddi (2005) studied responses to radical organizational change and found that resilient employees used more adaptive behavioral and cognitive strategies than less resilient employees. They were more proactive in initiating support and were able to change their thinking on the situation, which allowed them to develop more understanding and more effective plans. Similar dynamic processes are described in Aldwin et al.'s (1996) Deviation Amplification Model, which suggests that high base-levels of general personal resources lead to more adaptive coping strategies, which lead to high situational and personal resources and ultimately this builds up general levels of personal resources. This idea of a positive gain spiral has also been applied to the workplace (e.g., Llorens, Schaufeli, Bakker, & Salanova, 2007; Xanthopoulou et al., 2009a). In spite of the fact that it may be the practical ways of using and creating resources that will promote well-being and engagement in times of change, strategies haven't been studied widely in this process as of yet.

In our view it is useful to include personal resources separately, as opposed to combining them into a higher-order construct (such as PsyCap). Being able to distinguish between the impact of different personal resources will inform the design of targeted interventions.

We expect strategies used to deal with a changing environment will predict work engagement and adaptive performance. Problem-focused strategies were shown to predict higher levels of job satisfaction during a merger (Amiot, Terry, Jimmieson, & Callan, 2006). Also, self-leadership strategies were shown to be related to innovative behaviours at work (Carmeli, Meitar, & Weisberg, 2006).

Conclusion

The aim of this chapter was to outline why it is relevant to include the role of the person in studies on organizational change. Change has become a constant and may form a risk factor for employee health and well-being (Saksvik et al., 2007). Healthy organizational change requires both the creation of positive working conditions and the development of employee personal resources and strategies such as self-efficacy, optimism and self-leadership, which in turn may positively influence organizational change-ability. Our model proposes that employees are active agents who shape their environment using behavioral strategies, influenced by personal resources and change attitudes. These employee-level processes influence positive employee outcomes, i.e., work engagement and adaptive performance. This type of research will inform the design of employee-level change interventions. Behavior change at this level is often the missing link in large-scale change interventions. Research in this area will help organizations to balance top-down with bottom-up initiatives to facilitate positive change.

Practical implications

This chapter emphasizes the need for organizations and managers to be aware of individual differences in employee personal resourcefulness. Besides the widely known steps involving communication, participation and skills training, it is important to be aware that employees are resourceful, active agents who do not generally think of themselves as resisting. Managers should focus on bringing self-managing behaviors to the fore, helping employees to see the positive sides of the change, giving support to less self-efficacious employees, etc. Employees should be encouraged to find meaning in the change. This could be achieved by discussing how the changes will affect personal and work-related goals, and how to best manage this impact. Being open to negative change attitudes and actively leveraging positive attitudes is important in monitoring progress. Negative attitudes may hold important information, and it has been suggested that resistance can be a sign of commitment. Soliciting feedback on the change content and process is important. Methods such as appreciative enquiry may be used to involve all employees in a positive change effort

(Cooperrider & Sekerka, 2003). Employers might consider training their managers to develop coaching leadership styles that support and encourage employees' self-leadership strategies. Employees and managers could jointly map the working environment in terms of job demands/resources, including both the physical and psychosocial working environment (support, task variety, etc.). Finally, it is important for managers to be aware of their own personal resources, attitudes and strategies, and how these may impact their leadership behaviors.

Future research

In order to develop practical interventions, research should focus on further investigating the development process of personal resources over time, and the role of traits, self-awareness, and other relevant variables. Also, research might focus on which behavioral strategies are most conducive to adaptive performance (taking into account moderation effects, i.e., which strategies are most suitable for which employees). Another topic relevant during organizational transitions is the positive gain spiral or learning cycle in which general levels of personal resources are built, based on successful strategies, mastery experiences, and performance. Also, the interaction between leaders' and followers' personal resources, attitudes and strategies, and the impact of this interplay on successful adaptation would be interesting for future organizational change research. This could result in practical guidelines to facilitate the adoption of new work practices. Multiple measurement methods, like quantitative diary studies, can make these micro-processes more transparent by examining how they unfold on a daily or weekly level.

Final note

Managing change will always be a challenging, dynamic process where different perspectives at different levels need to be taken into account. We have argued here that an individual-level focus ought to be a crucial element in any change process, since transitions to new ways of working are nearly always accompanied by ambiguity and uncertainty. Besides the obvious aspects of knowledge and skills training, employees' personal resources, attitudes, and strategies can and should be actively managed to facilitate adaptive performance and work engagement. Organizational change cannot be successful without individual change, and individual change requires personal resourcefulness.

Acknowledgement

This work was supported by a HIPO (High Potential) grant from Utrecht University.

References

Abramis, D. J. (1994). Work role ambiguity, job satisfaction, and job performance: Meta-analysis and review. *Psychological Reports*, 75, 1411–1433.

Aldwin, C. M., Sutton, K. J., & Lachman, M. (1996). The development of coping resources in adulthood. *Journal of Personality*, 64, 837–871.

Amabile, T. A., & Conti, R. (1999). Changes in the work environment for creativity during downsizing. *Academy of Management Journal, 42,* 630–640.

Amiot, C. E., Terry, D. J., Jimmieson, N. L. & Callan, V. J. (2006). A longitudinal investigation of coping processes during a merger: implications for job satisfaction and organizational identification. *Journal of Management, 32,* 552–574.

Antonovsky, A . (1979). *Health, stress and coping.* San Francisco: Jossey-Bass.

Armenakis, A. A., & Bedeian, A. G. (1999). Organizational change: A review of theory and research in the 1990s. *Journal of Management, 25,* 293–315.

Armenakis, A. A., Harris, S. G., & Mossholder, K. W. (1993). Creating readiness for organizational change. *Human Relations, 46,* 681–703.

Ashford, S. J., (1986). Feedback-seeking in individual adaptation: A resource perspective, *The Academy of Management Journal, 29,* 465–487.

Ashford, S. J. (1988). Individual strategies for coping with stress during organizational transitions. *The Journal of Applied Behavioral Science, 24,* 19–36.

Aspinwall L. G., & Taylor, S. E. (1992). Modeling cognitive adaptation: A longitudinal investigation of the impact of individual differences and coping on college adjustment and performance. *Journal of Personality and Social Psychology, 63,* 989–1003.

Aspinwall, L. G., & Taylor, S. E. (1997). A stitch in time: Self-regulation and proactive coping. *Psychological Bulletin, 121,* 417–436.

Avey, J. B. Wernsing, T. S., & Luthans, F. (2008). Can positive employees help positive organizational change? Impact of psychological capital and emotions on relevant attitudes and behaviors, *Journal of Applied Behavioral Science, 44,* 48–70.

Bakker, A. B., & Demerouti, E. (2007). The job demands-resources model: state of the art, *Journal of Managerial Psychology, 22,* 309–328.

Bakker, A. B., & Demerouti, E. (2008). Towards a model of work engagement. *Career Development International, 13,* 209–223.

Bakker, A. B., Demerouti, E., & Verbeke, W. (2004). Using the Job Demands – Resources model to predict burnout and performance. *Human Resource Management, 43,* 83–104.

Bakker, A. B., Hakanen, J. J., Demerouti, E., & Xanthopoulou, D. (2007). Job resources boost work engagement particularly when job demands are high. *Journal of Educational Psychology, 99,* 274–284.

Bakker, A. B., & Schaufeli, W. B. (2008). Positive organizational behaviour: Engaged employees in flourishing organizations. *Journal of Organizational Behavior 29,* 147–154.

Bakker, A. B., Schaufeli, W. B., Leiter, M. P. & Taris, T. (2008). Work engagement: An emerging concept in occupational health psychology. *Work & Stress, 22,* 187–200.

Bandura, A. (1989). Human agency in social cognitive theory. *American Psychologist, 44,* 1175–1184.

Bandura, A. (1997). *Self-efficacy: The exercise of control.* New York: Freeman.

Baumeister, R. F., & Vohs, K. D. (2002). The pursuit of meaningfulness in life. In C. R. Snyder and S. J. Lopez (Eds.), *Handbook of positive psychology* (pp. 608–618). New York: Oxford University Press.

Behrman, D. N., & Perreault, W. D. J. (1984). A role stress model of the performance and satisfaction of industrial salespersons. *Journal of Marketing, 48,* 9–21.

Bell, N. E., & Staw, B. M. (1989). People as sculptors versus sculpture. In M. B. Arthur, D. T. Hall, & B. S. Lawrence (Eds.), *Handbook of career theory* (232–251). New York: Cambridge University Press.

Block, J., & Kremen, A. M. (1996) IQ and ego-resiliency: conceptual and empirical connections and separateness. *Journal of Personality and Social Psychology, 70,* 349–61.

Bovey, W. H., & Hede, A. (2001) Resistance to organisational change: the role of defence mechanisms. *Journal of Managerial Psychology*, 16, 534–548.

Briner, R. B., Harris, C., & Daniels, K. (2004). How do work stress and coping work? Toward a fundamental theoretical reappraisal. *British Journal of Guidance & Counselling*, 32, 223–234.

Brockner J., & Higgins, E. T. (2001). Regulatory focus theory: Implications for the study of emotions at work. *Organizational Behavior and Human Decision Processes*, 86, 35–66.

Callan, V. J. (1993). Individual and organizational strategies for coping with organizational change. *Work and Stress*, 7, 63–75.

Callan, V. J., Terry, D. J., & Schweitzer, R. (1994). Coping resources, coping strategies and adjustment to organizational change: Direct or buffering effects? *Work and Stress, 8*, 372–383.

Campbell, D. J. (2006). Embracing change: Examination of a "capabilities and benevolence beliefs model" in a sample of military cadets. *Military Psychology, 18*, 131–148.

Carmeli, A., Meitar, R., & Weisberg, J. (2006). Self-leadership skills and innovative behaviors at work. *International Journal of Manpower, 27*, 75–90.

Cartwright, S., & Holmes N. (2006). The meaning of work: The challenge of regaining employee engagement and reducing cynicism. *Human Resource Management Review, 16*, 199–208.

Carver, C. S., & Scheier, M. F. (1981). *Attention and self-regulation: A control theory approach to human behavior*. New York: Springer-Verlag.

Carver, C. S., & Scheier, M. F. (1998). *On the self-regulation of behavior*. New York: Cambridge University Press.

Chalofsky, N. (2003). An emerging construct for meaningful work. *Human Resource Development International, 6*, 69–83.

Coch, L., & French, J. (1948). Overcoming resistance to change. *Human Relations, 1*, 512–532.

Connor-Smith, J. K., & Flachsbart, C. (2007). Relations between personality and coping. *Journal of Personality and Social Psychology*, 93, 1080–1107.

Cooperrider, D. L., & Sekerka, L. E. (2003). Toward a theory of positive organizational change. In K. S. Cameron, J. E. Dutton, & R. E. Quinn (Eds.), *Positive organizational scholarship: Foundations of a new discipline* (pp. 225–240). San Francisco: Berrett-Koehler.

Costa, A. L., & Garmston, R. J. (2002). *Cognitive coaching: A foundation for renaissance schools*, 2nd edition. Norwood, MA: Christopher-Gordon Publishers.

Demerouti E., Bakker, A. B., Nachreiner, F., & Schaufeli, W. B. (2001). The Job Demands–Resources model of burnout. *Journal of Applied Psychology 86*, 499–512.

Dewett, T., & Denisi, A. S. (2007). What motivates organizational citizenship behaviours? Exploring the role of regulatory focus theory. *European Journal of Work and Organizational Psychology, 16*, 241–260.

EarvolinoRamirez, M. (2007). Resilience: A concept analysis. *Nursing Forum, 42*, 73–82.

Ellis, A. (1977). *The basic clinical theory of rational-emotive therapy*, New York: Springer-Verlag.

Fernandez, S., & Rainey, H. G. (2006). Managing successful organizational change in the public sector. *Public Administration Review, 66*, 168–176.

Folkman S., & Lazarus R. S. (1980). An analysis of coping in a middle-aged community sample. *Journal of Health and Social Behavior, 21*, 219–39.

Frankl, V. (1963). *Man's search for meaning*. London: Hodder & Stoughton.

Frayne, C. A., & Geringer, J. M. (2000). Self-management training for improving job performance: A field experiment involving salespeople. *Journal of Applied Psychology, 85*, 361–372.

Fredrickson, B. L., & Joiner, T. (2002). Positive emotions trigger upward spirals toward emotional well-being. *Psychological Science, 13*, 172–75.

Gist, M. E., & Mitchell, T. R. (1992). Self-efficacy: A theoretical analysis of its determinants and malleability. *Academy of Management Review, 17*, 183–211.

Griffin, B., & Hesketh, B. (2003). Adaptable behaviours for successful work and career adjustment. *Australian Journal of Psychology, 55*, 65–73.

Hackman, J. R., & Oldham, G. R. (1980). *Work redesign.* Reading, MA: Addison Wesley.

Hakanen, J. J., Bakker, A. B., & Demerouti, E. (2005). How dentists cope with their job demands and stay engaged: The moderating role of job resources. *European Journal of Oral Sciences, 113*, 479–487.

Head, J., Kivimaki, M., Martikainen, P., Vahtera, J., Ferrie, J. E. & Marmot, M.G. (2006). Influence of change in psychosocial work characteristics on sickness absence: The Whitehall II study. *Journal of Epidemiology Community & Health, 60*, 55–61.

Helgeson, V. S. (1999). Cognitive adaptation as a predictor of new coronary events after percutaneous transluminal coronary angioplasty. *Psychosomatic medicine, 61*, 488–495.

Helgeson, V. S. (2003). Cognitive adaptation, psychological adjustment, and disease progression among angioplasty patients: 4 years later. *Health Psychology, 22*, 30–8.

Herold, D. M., Fedor, D. B., & Caldwell, S. D. (2007). Beyond change management: A multi-level investigation of contexual and personal influences on employees' commitment to change. *Journal of Applied Psychology, 92*, 942–951.

Herscovitch, L., & Meyer, J. P. (2002). Commitment to organizational change: Extension of a three-component model. *Journal of Applied Psychology, 87*, 474–487.

Hill, T., Smith, N. D., & Mann, M. F. (1987). Role of efficacy expectations in predicting the decision to use advanced technologies. *Journal of Applied Psychology, 72*, 307–314.

Hobfoll, S. E. (1986). *Stress, social support, and women.* London: Taylor & Francis.

Hobfoll, S. E. (2002). Social and psychological resources and adaptation. *Review of General Psychology, 6*, 307–324.

Hobfoll, S. E., Johnson, R. J., Ennis, N., & Jackson, A. P. (2003). Resource loss, resource gain, and emotional outcomes among inner city women. *Journal of Personality and Social Psychology, 84*, 632–643.

Hodgkinson, G. P., & Healey, M. P. (2007). Cognition in organizations. *Annual Review of Psychology, 59*, 387–417.

Holt, D. T., Armenakis, A. A., Feild, H. S., & Harris, S. (2007). Readiness for organizational change: The systematic development of a scale. *Journal of Applied Behavioral Science. 43*, 232–255.

Houghton, J. D., & Neck, C. P. (2002). The revised self-leadership questionnaire: testing a hierarchical factor structure for self-leadership, *Journal of Managerial Psychology, 17*, 672–91.

Jahoda, M. (1958). *Current concepts of positive mental health.* New York: Basic Books.

Jerusalem, M. (1993). Personal resources, environmental constraints, and adaptational processes: The predictive power of a theoretical stress model. *Personality and Individual Differences, 14*, 15–24.

Jimmieson, N. L., Terry, D. J., & Callan, V. J. (2004). A longitudinal study of employee adaptation to organizational change: The role of change-related information and change-related self-efficacy. *Journal of Occupational Health Psychology, 9*, 11–27.

Judge, T. A., Thoresen, C. J., Pucik, V., & Welbourne, T. M. (1999). Managerial coping with organizational change: A dispositional perspective. *Journal of Applied Psychology, 84*, 107–122.

Karasek, R. (1979). Job demands, job decision latitude and mental strain: Implications for job design. *Administrative Science Quarterly, 24*, 285–306.

Kark, R., & Van Dijk, D. (2007). Motivation to lead, motivation to follow: The role of the self regulatory focus in leadership processes. *Academy of Management Review, 32*, 500–528.

Kohn, M. L., & Schooler, C. (1982). Job conditions and personality: a longitudinal assessment of their reciprocal effects. *American Journal of Sociology, 87*, 1257–1289.

Korunka, C., Weiss, A., & Karetta, B. (1993). Effects of new technologies with special regard for the implementation process per se. *Journal of Organizational Behavior, 14*, 331–348.

Kotter, J. P. (1996). *Leading change*. Boston, MA: Harvard Business School Press.

Kotter, J. P (2005). *Our iceberg is melting: Changing and succeeding under any conditions*. New York: St. Martin's Press.

Kotter, J. P., & Schlesinger, L. A. (1979). Choosing strategies for change. *Harvard Business Review, 106*, 14.

Lam, T., Cho, V., & Qu, H. (2007). A study of hotel employee behavioral intentions towards adoption of information technology. *Hospitality Management, 26*, 49–65.

Lazarus, R. S., & Folkman, S. (1984). Stress, appraisal, and coping. New York: Springer Verlag.

Liberman, N., Idson, L. C., Camacho, C. J., & Higgins, E. T. (1999). Promotion and prevention choices between stability and change. *Journal of Personality and Social Psychology, 77*, 1135–1145.

Little, L. M., Gooty, J., & Nelson, D. (2007). Positive psychological capital: Has positivity clouded measurement rigor? In D. L. Nelson and C. L. Cooper (Eds.), *Positive organizational behaviour* (pp. 191–210). London: Sage.

Llorens, S., Schaufeli, W. B., Bakker, A. B., & Salanova, M. (2007). Does a positive gain spiral of resources, efficacy beliefs and engagement exists? *Computers in Human Behavior, 23*, 825–841.

Luthans, F. (2002). Positive organizational behavior: Developing and managing psychological strengths. *Academy of Management Executive, 16*, 57–72.

Luthans, F., Avey, J. B., Avolio, B. J., Norman, S. M., & Combs, G. J. (2006). Psychological capital development: towards a micro-intervention. *Journal of Organizational Behavior, 27*, 387–93.

Luthans, F., Avolio, B. J., Avey, J. B., & Norman, S. M. (2007). Positive psychological capital: Measurement and relationship with performance and satisfaction. *Personnel Psychology, 60*, 541–572.

Luthans F., Avolio, B., Walumbwa, F., & Li, W. (2005). The psychological capital of Chinese workers: Exploring the relationship with performance. *Management and Organization Review, 1*, 247–269.

Luthans, F., Norman, S. M., Avolio, B. J., & Avey, J. B. (2008). The mediating role of psychological capital in the supportive organizational climate–employee performance relationship. *Journal of Organizational Behavior, 29*, 219–238.

Luthans, F., & Youssef, C. M. (2004). Human, social, and now positive psychological capital management: Investing in people for competitive advantage. *Organizational Dynamics, 33*, 143–160.

Luthans, F., Youssef, C. M., & Avolio, B. J. (2007). Psychological capital: Investing and developing positive organizational behaviour. In D. L. Nelson & C. L. Cooper (Eds.), *Positive organizational behaviour* (pp. 9–24). London: Sage.

Luthar, S., Cicchetti, D., & Becker, B. (2000). The construct of resilience: A critical evaluation and guidelines for future work. *Child Development, 71*, 543–562.

Lyubomirsky, S., Sousa, L., & Dickerhoof, R. (2006). The costs and benefits of writing, talking, and thinking about life's triumphs and defeats. *Journal of Personality and Social Psychology, 90*, 692–708.

Maddi, S. R. (2005). *Resilience at work: How to succeed no matter what life throws at you*. New York: Amacom.

Manz, C. C., & Sims, H. P., Jr. (1980). Self-management as a substitute for leadership: A social learning perspective. *Academy of Management Review, 5*, 361–367.

Markham, S. E., & Markham, I. S. (1995). Self-management and self-leadership reexamined: a levels of analysis perspective. *Leadership Quarterly, 6*, 343–359.

Martin, A. J., Jones, E. S., & Callan, V. J. (2005). The role of psychological climate in facilitating employee adjustment during organizational change. *European Journal of Work and Organizational Psychology, 14*, 263–289.

Maslow, A. H., (1968). *Toward a psychology of being*, Princeton, NJ: Van Nostrand.

Masten, A. S. (2001). Ordinary magic: Resilience process in development. *American Psychologist, 56*, 227–239.

May, D. R., Gilson, R. L., & Harter, L. M. (2004). The psychological conditions of meaningfulness, safety and availability and the engagement of the human spirit at work. *Journal of Occupational and Organizational Psychology, 77*, 11–37.

Meijman, T. F., & Mulder, G. (1998). Psychological aspects of workload. In P.J. Drenth, H. Thierry & C. J. de Wolff (Eds.) *Handbook of work and organizational psychology* (pp. 5–33). Hove, U.K.: Erlbaum.

Metselaar, E. E. (1997). *Assessing the willingness to change; construction and validation of the DINAMO*. Amsterdam: VU.

Microsoft (2005) *Digital work style: The new world of work*. Microsoft white paper. Retrieved from www.microsoft.com

Miller, V. D., Johnson, J. R., & Grau, J. (1994). Antecedents to willingness to participate in a planned organizational change. *Journal of Applied Communication Research, 11*, 365–386.

Mischel, W. (2004). Toward an integrative science of the person (prefatory chapter). *Annual Review of Psychology, 55*, 1–22.

Motowidlo, S. J., & Van Scotter, J. R. (1994). Evidence that task performance should be distinguished from contextual performance. *Journal of Applied Psychology, 79*, 475–480.

Neck, C. P., & Houghton, J. D. (2006). Two decades of self-leadership theory and research: Past developments, present trends, and future possibilities. *Journal of Managerial Psychology, 21*, 270–295.

Nolen-Hoeksema, S. (2000). The role of rumination in depressive disorders and mixed anxiety/depressive symptoms. *Journal of Abnormal Psychology. 109*, 504–11.

Norris, S. E. (2008). An examination of self-leadership. *Emerging Leadership Journeys, 1*, 43–61.

Organ D. W., & Paine, J. B. (1999). A new kind of performance for industrial and organizational psychology: Recent contributions to the study of organizational citizenship behavior. In C. L. Cooper & I. T. Robertson (Eds.), *International Review of Industrial and Organizational Psychology* (Vol. 14; pp. 337–368). Chichester, U.K.: John Wiley & Sons.

Pearlin L., & Schooler C. (1978). The structure of coping. *Journal of Health and Social Behavior, 19*, 2–21.

Peterson, C. (2000). The future of optimism. *American Psychologist, 55*, 44–55.

Peterson, C., & Barrett, L. C. (1987). Explanatory style and academic performance among university freshmen. *Journal of Personality and Social Psychology, 53*, 603–607.

Peterson, S., & Luthans, F. (2003). The positive impact of development of hopeful leaders. *Leadership and Organization Development Journal, 24*, 26–31.

Peterson, C., & Seligman, M. (2004). *Character strengths and virtues: A handbook and classification*. New York: Oxford University Press.

Petty, R. E., & Cacioppo, J. T. (1981). *Attitudes and persuasion: Classic and contemporary approaches*. Boulder, CO: Westview Press Inc.

Piderit, S. (2000). Rethinking resistance and recognizing ambivalence: A multidimensional view of attitudes toward an organizational change. *The Academy of Management Review, 25*, 783–794.

Pierce, J. L., & Gardner, D. G. (2004). Self-esteem within the work and organizational context: A review of the organizational-based self-esteem literature. *Journal of Management, 30*, 591–622.

Podsakoff, P. M., & MacKenzie, S. B. (1994). Organizational citizenship behaviors and sales unit effectiveness. *Journal of Marketing Research, 31*, 351–363.

Pulakos, E. D., Arad, S., Donovan, M. A., & Plamondon, K. E. (2000). Adaptability in the workplace: Development of a taxonomy of adaptive performance. *Journal of Applied Psychology, 85*, 612–624.

Rabkin, J. G., & Streuning, E. L. (1976). Life events, stress, and illness. *Science, 194*, 1013–1020.

Rafferty, A., & Griffin, M. (2006). Perceptions of organizational change: A stress and coping perspective. *Journal of Applied Psychology, 91*, 1154–1162.

Rogers, C. R. (1961). The process equation of psychotherapy. *American journal of psychotherapy, 15*, 27–45.

Rutter, M. (1985). Resilience in the face of adversity: protective factors and resistance to psychiatric disorder. *British Journal of Psychiatry, 147*, 598–611.

Ryff, C. D., & Singer, B. (1996). Psychological well-being: Meaning, measurement, and implications for psychotherapy research, *Psychotherapy and Psychosomatics, 65*, 14–23.

Saksvik, P. Ø., Tvedt, S. D., Nytrø, K., Andersen, G. R., Andersen, T. K., Buvik, M. P., et al. (2007). Developing criteria for healthy organizational change. *Work & Stress, 21*, 243–263.

Schaufeli, W. B., & Salanova, M. (2007). Work engagement: an emerging psychological concept and its implications for organizations. In S. W. Gilliland, D. D. Steiner & D. P. Skarlicki (Eds.), *Research in social issues in management: Managing social and ethical issues in organizations, Vol. 5*, Greenwich, CT: Information Age Publishers.

Schaufeli, W. B., Salanova, M., González-Romá, V., & Bakker, A. B. (2002). The measurement of engagement and burnout: A two sample confirmatory factor analytic approach. *Journal of Happiness Studies, 3*, 71–92.

Scheier, M. F., Weintraub, J. K., & Carver, C. S. (1986). Coping with stress: Divergent strategies of optimists and pessimists. *Journal of Personality and Social Psychology, 51*, 1257–1264.

Scheier, M. F., & Carver, C. S. (1985). Optimism, coping and health: Assessment and implications of generalized outcome expectancies. *Health Psychology, 4*, 219–247.

Seligman, M. E. P. (1991) *Learned optimism*, New York: Knopf.

Seligman, M. E. P., & Schulman, P. (1986). Explanatory style as a predictor of productivity and quitting among life insurance sales agents. *Journal of Personality and Social Psychology, 50*, 832–838.

Skinner, E. A., Edge, K., Altman, J., & Sherwood, H. (2003). Searching for the structure of coping: A review and critique of category systems for classifying ways of coping. *Psychological Bulletin, 129*, 216–269.

Snyder, C. R. (2000). *Handbook of hope.* San Diego: Academic Press.

Sorge, A., & Van Witteloostuijn, A. (2004). The (non)sense of organizational change: An essay about universal management hypes, sick consultancy metaphors and healthy organization theories. *Organization Studies, 25,* 1205–31.

Stajkovic A. D., & Luthans F. (1998). Self-efficacy and work-related performance: A meta-analysis. *Psychological Bulletin, 124,* 240–261.

Stark, E., Thomas, L. T., & Poppler, P. (2000). Psychological disposition and job satisfaction under varying conditions of organizational change: Relevance and meaning from survivors and walking wounded. Paper presented at the annual meeting of the Western Academy of Management, Kona, Hawaii.

Stewart-Black, J., & Gregersen, H. B. (2008). *It starts with one, changing individuals changes organizations.* Upper Saddle River, NJ: Wharton School Publishing.

Taylor, S. E., Kemeny, M. E., Reed, G. M., Bower, J. E., & Gruenewald, T. L. (2000). Psychological resources, positive illusions, and health. *American Psychologist, 55,* 99–109.

Taylor, S. (1983). Adjustment to threatening events: a theory of cognitive adaptation. *American psychologist, 38,* 1161–1173.

Vahtera, J., Kivimaki, M., Pentti, J., & Theorell, T. (2000). Effect of change in the psychosocial work environment on sickness absence: a seven year follow-up of initially healthy employees. *Journal of Epidemiology and Community Health, 54,* 484–93.

Vancouver, J. B., & Day. D. V. (2005). Industrial and organisation research on self-regulation: from constructs to applications. *Applied Psychology: An International Review, 54,* 155–185.

Van Dam, K., Oreg, S., & Schyns, B. (2007). Daily work contexts and resistance to organizational change: The role of leader-member exchange, perceived development climate and change process quality. *Applied Psychology: An International Review. 57,* 313–334.

Van den Heuvel, M., Demerouti, E., Schreurs, B. H. J., Bakker, A. B., & Schaufeli, W. B. (2009). Does meaning-making help during organizational change? Development and validation of a new scale. *Career Development International, 14,* 508–533.

Van Yperen, N. W., & Snijders, T. A. (2000). A multilevel analysis of the demands–control model: Is stress at work determined by factors at the group level or the individual level? *Journal of Occupational Health Psychology, 5,* 182–90.

Wanberg, C. R., & Banas, J. T. (2000). Predictors and outcomes of openness to changes in a reorganizing workplace. *Journal of Applied Psychology, 85,* 132–42.

Wasylyshyn, K. M. (2003). Executive coaching: An outcome study. *Consulting Psychology Journal: Practice & Research, 55,* 94–106.

Wheaton, B. (1983). Stress, personal coping resources, and psychiatric symptoms: An investigation of interactive models. *Journal of Health & Social Behavior 24,* 208–229.

Woodman, R. W., & Dewett, T. (2004). Organizationally relevant journeys in individual change. In M. S. Pool & A. H. Van de Ven (Eds.), *Handbook of organizational change and innovation* (pp. 32–49). Oxford: Oxford University Press.

Wrzesniewski, A., & Dutton, J. E. (2001). Crafting a job: revisioning employees as active crafters of their work. *Academy of Management Review, 26,* 179–201.

Wrzesniewski, A., Dutton, J., & Debebe, G. (2003). Interpersonal sensemaking and the meaning of work. *Research in Organizational Behaviour, 25,* 93–135.

Xanthopoulou, D., Bakker, A. B., Demerouti, E., & Schaufeli, W. B. (2007). The role of personal resources in the job demands-resources model. *International Journal of Stress Management, 14,* 121–41.

Xanthopoulou, D., Bakker, A. B., Demerouti, E., & Schaufeli, W. B. (2009a). Reciprocal relationships between job resources, personal resources, and work engagement. *Journal of Vocational Behavior, 74,* 235–244.

Xanthopoulou, D., Bakker, A. B., Demerouti, E., & Schaufeli, W. B. (2009b). Work engagement and financial returns: A diary study on the role of job and personal resources. *Journal of Occupational & Organizational Psychology, 82,* 183–200.

Xanthopoulou, D., Bakker, A. B., Heuven, E., Demerouti, E. & Schaufeli, W. B. (2008). Working in the sky: A diary study among flight attendants. *Journal of Occupational Health Psychology, 13,* 345–356.

Zapf, D., Dormann, C., & Frese, M. (1996). Longitudinal studies in organizational stress research: A review of the literature with reference to methodological issues. *Journal of Occupational Health Psychology, 1,* 145–169.

8

Work and Health
Curvilinearity Matters

Maria Karanika-Murray
Nottingham Trent University, U.K.

Interest in work-related health and well-being has developed into a rich area of enquiry over the last few decades (Barling & Griffiths, 2003; Cooper, 1998; Cooper, Dewe, & O'Driscoll, 2001; Quick & Tetrick, 2003; Schabracq, Winnubst, & Cooper, 2002). The plethora of theoretical models that aim to describe the relationships between characteristics of work and health outcomes is complemented by a large volume of empirical work that has exploded in this short period of time. Simultaneously, a small body of empirical work has emerged that indicates that relationships between work and health may be more complex than initially presumed, and that they do not always or necessarily follow a stable linear pattern. A number of models from psychology's rich theoretical repository allude to possible curvilinear effects of work characteristics on health and well-being. Evidence that such effects may be curvilinear prompts a need to re-examine available theory. This chapter is about the curvilinearity hypothesis in the relationships between work characteristics and health and well-being outcomes.

Any proposition of an optimal level of the effects of work characteristics on an individual's health and performance entails an assumption of curvilinear relationships. It suggests that this relationship is not linear and stable over time, but rather that an individual's health and well-being can change according to the way that they experience particular work characteristics (Karanika-Murray, Antoniou, Michaelides, & Cox, 2009). It has often been proposed that optimal levels lie away from extremes of work characteristics (e.g., Cox, 1978; French, Caplan, & Harrison, 1982; Selye, 1975; Warr, 1987, 1990). Specifically, inverted-U models of stress and performance imply that some level of stress is necessary for optimal performance and therefore functional. Increasing stress can lead to improved performance; after a certain point, however, increasing levels of stress can become dysfunctional (McGrath, 1976; Selye, 1975; Warr, 1987, 2007). The inflation or upward slope of the curve is consistent with the positive linear theory of stress, which views stress as motivating and therefore a challenge; the deflation or downward part is consistent with the negative linear theory, which holds that stress at any level is harmful and reduces performance (Jamal, 1985; Muse, Harris, & Feild, 2003). Of course, curvilinearity exists in many different forms and is not a new concept in psychology (see Carver & Scheier, 1998). For example, discontinuous effects, such as ceiling effects or thresholds (i.e., increase of a predictor has no effect on an outcome until a critical level is reached), disproportionate effects (i.e., an outcome changes as a response to a predictor, but at different or varying rates), and interaction and moderation effects have all been investigated in psychological research.

The curvature of the effects of a specific work characteristic on a particular health outcome can indicate how stable this effect is and when it is positive or negative, at which point(s) where it can have its optimal effect, at which point(s) it changes, and what this change means for the way that the outcome is experienced by an individual. It can also inform practitioners how best to design interventions to improve health and well-being, and which groups of individuals to target. Thus, the important question is not how costly work-related stress is; this has been well-established (e.g., Cooper et al., 2001, p. 1). Rather, if we accept that relationships between work and health are not necessarily linear and stable but effects can change, and that there can be too much of a beneficial work characteristic or too little of a harmful one, then the important question from a practical point of view becomes what are the optimal levels of this work characteristic for health and well-being. Such a focus can reformulate our understanding of how work impacts on health and well-being.

Available empirical evidence provides support for curvilinear relationships between a range of work characteristics and job satisfaction. These include skill discretion (Fletcher & Jones, 1993), social support (de Jonge & Schaufeli, 1998), job tension (Zivnuska, Kiewitz, Hochwarter, Perrewé, & Zellars, 2002), and decision latitude (Rydstedt et al., 2006). Job scope and complexity (Xie & Johns, 1995), job autonomy, and social support (Borg, Kristensen, & Burr, 2000) have also been found to impact on emotional exhaustion in a curvilinear way. Furthermore, the effects of psychological demands and social support on self-reported health have been found to be curvilinear (Borg et al., 2000), as has the effect of supportive management on job tension (Harris & Kacmar, 2006). Although a review of this literature is beyond the aims of this chapter, there is evidence to support the assertion that the effects of a range of work characteristics on health and well-being outcomes can be positive (or negative), but only up to a certain threshold, after which extreme levels of these work characteristics can have different effects to those expected.

Although there is some consensus for the existence of curvilinear effects of work characteristics on health and well-being, empirical support has not always been consistent (for a discussion see Karanika, 2006; McGrath, 1976; Muse et al., 2003). This has led some scholars to contest the possibility of curvilinearity and to label it as an urban myth in occupational health psychology (Taris, 2006). However, the existence of contradictory findings is not evidence for the absence of curvilinear effects. Strong evidence comes from studies that have explicitly and simultaneously examined both linear and curvilinear models, indicating that the latter provide better fit than linear-only models. Effects can be small (e.g., Fletcher & Jones, 1993; Jeurissen & Nyklíček, 2001; Rydstedt et al., 2006; Xie & Johns, 1995) or substantial (e.g. de Jonge & Schaufeli, 1998; Karanika-Murray et al., 2009; Warr, 1990), but are nevertheless present.

This chapter looks at curvilinearity in the effects of work characteristics on health and well-being. It starts by discussing the linearity assumption, outlines a number of theoretical models that suggest curvilinear effects, whose tenets have often been overlooked in this line of research, and closes by discussing some underlying themes and opportunities for moving away from the linearity assumption. It is hoped that this chapter will draw attention to, and refresh interest in, the nature of the effects of work on health.

The Linearity Assumption

True linear relationships, where an outcome changes as a response to a stimulus in a stable and proportionate manner, are rare in nature and among psychosocial phenomena. They can only be observed at a restricted range around the middle of the standard normal distribution (Guion, 1998) and at a particular point in time. Possible reasons for the scarcity of investigations and lack of attention to possible curvilinear relationships pertain to both methodological and conceptual issues. Methodological limitations can also shape the types of questions that researchers ask or answer with the available tools (Frese & Zapf, 1988; Zapf, Dormann, & Frese, 1996). Thus there may exist a general underlying tendency in occupational health psychology to view relationships as stable and linear, the so-called linearity assumption (e.g., Abbott, 1988; Ferris et al., 2006; Guion, 1998; Muse et al., 2003; Schrader-Frechette, 1998), and consequently to use linear data-analysis methods. Although methodological limitations are difficult to overcome, the tendency to ask the wrong questions cannot be justified given the rich theoretical repository available in occupational health psychology.

Scholars in psychology and the social sciences have voiced a growing discontent with the preoccupation with linearity, in both theory and research. In his seminal paper *Transcending General Linear Reality*, sociologist Andrew Abbott (1988) argued that implicit assumptions about how social events occur can thwart the examination and appropriate analysis of many important problems. Other disciplines have witnessed a similar upheaval. Mendenhall, Macomber, Gregersen, and Cutright (1998), for example, have expressed concerns with the conventional linear approach as used in human resource management, noting that the static nature of linear models creates a view of reality that is incongruent with its dynamic nature. In health psychology, Karanika-Murray and Michaelides (2008) also argued that the underlying dynamics of health necessitate the use of nonlinear approaches. Guion (1998) used the term 'Procrustean approach' to describe this widespread phenomenon of working on problems to fit established methods rather than developing methods that are most appropriate to the questions being asked. This general linear reality (Abbott,

1988; Ferris et al., 2006) may provide an incomplete representation of the whole spectrum of possible effects of the work environment on employee health.

In occupational health psychology, Ferris and his colleagues (2006) argued that "the field is building a science of stress that is disproportionately linear" and "this inherent bias has had a considerable influence on shaping the knowledge base in this area of enquiry" (p. 204). Furthermore, Frese and Zapf (1988) highlighted the complex nature of work-related health and provided some methodological recommendations for improving research in the area including, among others, more attempts at curve fitting (i.e. examining curvilinear relationships) and exploring change over time. Zapf et al. (1996) also observed that "linear data analysis methods would usually underestimate the true strength of the relationships", adding that "we are not aware of articles taking such considerations into account" (p. 147; see also Sullivan & Bhagat, 1992).

Most of the statistical analyses used in social sciences research are founded on the general linear model[1] (Trochim, 2000). An examination of the standard statistics textbooks in psychology shows that they tend to cover linear data analysis methods; also most research published in mainstream academic journals tends to rely on correlational approaches and their derivatives. It is, of course, acceptable to use linear approaches to model curvilinear relationships, as in the case of the polynomial regression technique. Our understanding has been hindered not by the use of linear methods, but by the use of such methods in place of more appropriate alternatives. Reliance on linear methods can limit research to the examination of stable and linear relationships, routinely attributing anomalies to external error or chance. Most importantly, it can constrain the ways in which researchers routinely conceptualize the relationships between work and health. Although robust, linear methods "in too many cases rule out the possibility for discovering … more complex aspects of [the] mind" (Toomela, 2007, p. 18).

Although linear analytical approaches are powerful methods that have generated theory and influenced understanding, the general linear model overlooks many principles of the reality of psychosocial phenomena and cause-effect relationships (Mendenhall et al., 1998). These concern, for example, direction of causality, aggregativity among system elements (such that there are no emergent phenomena or interactions), and independence of variables (Abbott, 1988). The fact that variable y can change as variable χ changes does not necessarily mean that this change happens at the same constant rate. Since they involve observations that are related to many facets of their context (Everitt, 1978), data in occupational health psychology are almost invariably complex and multivariate, permitting a wide range of possible relationships and effects between χ and y. For example, if the rate at which χ increases in relation to increases in y slows, the y value will eventually stop increasing (asymptotic relationship). If change of χ is faster than the change of y but then becomes slower, then it is possible to have a sigmoidal relationship. Finally, the relationship where χ increases as y also increases, but only up to a certain point after which it starts to decrease, describes a quadratic function (inverted-U shaped) (some examples are given in the next section)—the possibilities are endless.

Although empirical evidence exists, it tends to be scarce. A major review of the literature on the relationships between work stressors and their effects (Rick, Thomson, Briner, O'Regan, & Daniels, 2002) indicated that there is evidence for nonlinear relationships, but also noted that only two out of the 45 studies included in the review explicitly looked at such relationships. Karanika (2006) also found only 18 published studies from 1986 to 2006 that looked at quadratic relationships between work and health. Of course, the scarcity of evidence is not indicative of the quality of these studies but, rather, may show a lack of attention on possible curvilinear relationships.

In addition, the current state of psychosocial research has been criticized for the lack of fair designs that enable investigators to assess curvilinearity (Muse et al., 2003). This may explain why the majority of effect sizes reported are small or average (see next section for a discussion), which are to be expected given the loss of correlational power accrued (Frese & Zapf, 1988). A review by Karanika (2006) revealed explained variance between 7% and 81% for the nonlinear models (and between 5% and 39% for the linear models). Although the additional variance explained by a curvilinear model may not necessarily be substantially larger than that explained by its linear equivalent, the resulting model will be truer to the nature of the data, and this can have important implications for practice. Failure to account for possible curvilinear effects can lead to inconsistent or insignificant results when data are examined in linear terms (Zapf et al., 1996; Karanika et al., 2009). Karasek (1979) referred to this as the "paradox of disappearance", the phenomenon of curvilinear or interactive findings vanishing in small populations when relationships are summarized linearly.

Curvilinear Effects in Theory

A rich repository of theoretical models is available to researchers in occupational health psychology to explain curvilinear effects of work characteristics on health and well-being. It is worth exploring some of the most prominent of the models that suggest such effects. They are outlined below in chronological order with some empirical evidence where available. It should be noted that although some models refer to stress, strain, and stressors, rather than work characteristics and health and well-being, the principles discussed earlier apply.

Yerkes–Dodson law

In 1908, Yerkes and Dodson described an inverted-U relationship between aversive reinforcement and discrimination learning under varied task difficulty, observed in a sample of mice. Although Yerkes and Dodson did not intend to apply their observations to human psychology, these were later construed as the Yerkes–Dodson law of a general relationship between arousal (or motivation, drive, or tension) and performance, reflecting popular concepts of learning and motivation in modern psychology (Hancock & Ganey, 2003; Teigen, 1994). The Yerkes–Dodson law has been construed as a hypothesis that predicts a negative quadratic relationship between stress and health (such that $y = \alpha + \beta\chi^2$) (the inverted-U hypothesis). Although the validity of the Yerkes–Dodson law has been questioned on the grounds of its poor experimental design and a failure to replicate the original studies (Hancock & Ganey, 2003; Neiss, 1988; Teigen, 1994), the inverted-U hypothesis has served as an important catalyst for research and theory. The concept is broad enough to be used in different contexts (for instance in motivation, emotion, and stress) and has a strong intuitive appeal. Propositions known to be true based on observation are merely data and not theory (Kukla, 2001). As Teigen (1994) astutely notes, "a more benevolent interpretation would be to assume that the Yerkes–Dodson curves reflect a basic relationship to be observed between a variety of psychological variables" (p. 542).

Catastrophe model of anxiety and performance

An extension of the inverted-U hypothesis is the catastrophe model of anxiety and performance (Fazey & Hardy, 1988; Hardy & Parfitt, 1991; Hardy, Parfitt, & Pates, 1994). This model distinguishes between cognitive anxiety, the mental component of state anxiety, and somatic anxiety, or physiological arousal, to explain dramatic decrements in performance for different levels of cognitive anxiety and physiological arousal. Based on catastrophe theory, and specifically the cusp catastrophe model (see Carver & Scheier, 1998; Guastello, 2002; Stewart & Peregoy, 1983; Woodcock & Davis, 1978), the model describes when sudden changes in performance can happen. At low levels of cognitive anxiety, the relationship between physiological arousal and performance resembles a linear shape. At high levels of cognitive anxiety, the shape of this relationship becomes sigmoidal or discontinuous and can lead to dramatic decrements in performance (the hysteresis hypothesis). When cognitive anxiety is high, smaller increases in physiological arousal can result in catastrophic changes in performance, and it takes more effort to restore peak performance. Developed and applied in sport psychology, the model demonstrates a successful application of psychological theory to practice. It is worth noting that catastrophe theory has aided the understanding of an array of aspects of human behavior, including relationship formation, persuasion (Carver & Scheier, 1998), leadership, group behavior (Guastello, 2002), learned helplessness, political involvement, and schizophrenia (Woodcock & Davis, 1978).

General adaptation syndrome

According to Selye (1975), "stress is the non-specific response of the body to any demand made upon it" (p. 27). Selye's general adaptation syndrome (GAS) is a description of the stages that an individual goes through in response to stimuli and includes an alarm reaction, a stage of resistance, and a stage of exhaustion. It describes the stereotypy and generality of the response to a wide range of physical, environmental, psychological, and biological stimuli. The principal contributions of the GAS are: (1) the specification of eustress (the positive and motivating aspect of stress) and distress ("damaging or unpleasant stress", Selye, 1975, p. 31) as two distinctive states, and (2) the implication that effects are nonmonotonic (i.e., curvilinear). Although Selye did not prescribe the existence of an optimal level of stress in a continuum from eustress to distress, these can be viewed as representing the two axes of the quadratic relationship.

Holistic model of stress

As an extension of the GAS, the holistic model of stress (Nelson & Simmons, 2003) incorporates the notions of eustress and distress into a process model that describes the impact of stressors on strain and outcomes. It takes into account possible positive and negative effects, acknowledges the role of individual differences, and presents "savoring eustress" as the opposite of "coping with distress". It also posits that a particular stressor can elicit both positive and negative responses at the same time, depending on the level of the stressor experienced (again, implying a quadratic or curvilinear effect).

Activation theory

Activation theory (Gardner & Cummings, 1988; Scott, 1966) postulates that (1) each individual has a characteristic level of activation, (2) experienced stimulation, performance and affect depend on the individual's characteristic level of activation, and (3) an activation level that results in optimal performance is associated with different environmental, physiological, or cognitive stimuli. As an individual's experienced activation level deviates from their optimal activation level for the task, their performance declines and motivation to maintain the preferred activation level increases. Such a deviation can be either positive or negative, indicating an inverted-U effect. Research based on activation theory has indicated curvilinear effects of work demands and tension on task performance (explaining 15% variance in the outcomes, twice as much as the linear model: Gardner, 1986), job satisfaction (explaining between 19% and 28% variance: Jansen, 2001), turnover intention, and value attainment (explaining between 12% and 23% of variance: Zivnuska et al., 2002) (see also Gardner & Cummings, 1988; Xie & Johns, 1995).

Cognitive activation theory

In the same vein, the cognitive activation theory of stress (Eriksen, Olff, Murison, & Ursin, 1999) suggests that stress reactions are triggered by a perceived discrepancy between what an individual expects and their actual experience of an event, which provides motivation for goal-directed behavior. External states are evaluated against internal expectations through feedback and feedforward mechanisms, such that too much or too little of an experienced event can trigger behavior to restore the ideal homeostatic state.

Person–environment fit theory

The basic premise of the person–environment fit (PE fit) theory (Caplan & Harrison, 1993; Cooper et al., 2001; Edwards, Caplan, & Harrison, 1998) is that a misfit between the individual's characteristics (abilities and values) and aspects of their environment (demands and resources) can lead to unmet needs, which in turn can lead to experienced strain. A situation where the environmental provisions for fulfilling an individual's needs are inadequate, or where their abilities to meet external demands are insufficient, may lead to strain. When demands exceed abilities or when needs exceed supplies, the theory specifies that the relationship is linear and monotonic or stable. However, when supplies exceed needs or when abilities exceed demands, three possible relationships between PE fit and strain are hypothesized, depending on the degree of needs: an asymptotic relationship, a monotonic relationship (linear) and a quadratic relationship (inverted-U). The possibility for curvilinear effects derives from the fact that although supplies can decrease strain, after a certain point "excess supplies may increase strain when they inhibit the fulfillment of needs on other dimensions" (Edwards et al., 1998, p. 34). Similarly, "excess abilities may increase strain by creating insufficient supplies for motives" (ibid., p. 36). PE fit theory is the only theory known that explicitly prescribes the conditions for expected curvilinear effects. Xie and Johns (1995) found J-shaped relationships between job scope (skill variety, task identity, task significance, autonomy, and feedback) and emotional exhaustion (explaining between 8% and 11% of the variance in emotional exhaustion). Similarly, PE fit has been successfully applied to understanding the effects of workload, job complexity, and role ambiguity in a range of occupations (French et al., 1982). However, the theory has been criticized for overlooking the role of the social context (Cooper et al., 2001), and reinforcing a tendency to assume that environments are either positive or negative and that individuals will always function either above or below optimum (Lazarus, 1991).

Equity theory

One of the most influential social exchange theories, equity theory (Adams, 1965; Walster, Berscheid, & Walster, 1973), states that individuals evaluate exchange relationships with others and with their organization in terms of the ratio between efforts (investment or input spent, such as time, effort, skill) and rewards (returns or outcomes received, for example, esteem, status, money, appreciation). A situation will be viewed as equitable when this ratio equals that of a comparison other. Thus, feeling either advantaged or deprived can lead to distress (Adams, 1965; Walster et al., 1973). Furthermore, there is a bias towards positive outcomes, such that reactions to perceived under-reward are stronger than reactions to perceived over-reward (Mowday, 1991), implying a curvilinear relationship between perceived inequity and distress. Van Dierendonck, Schaufeli, and Buunk (2001) examined the impact of perceived inequity in professional–recipient relationships on emotional exhaustion and revealed curvilinear effects of inequity at Time 1 on emotional exhaustion at

Time 2. An advantaged relationship had a stronger negative affect on emotional exhaustion than a deprived relationship.

Effort–reward imbalance model

The more recent effort–reward imbalance (ERI) model (Siegrist, 1996; Siegrist et al., 2004) emphasizes the central role of cognition and the balance between efforts and rewards as instrumental for the development of dissatisfaction and ill-health. "The focus of the [ERI] model is on reciprocity of exchange in occupational life where high-cost/low-gain conditions are considered particularly stressful" (Siegrist, 1996, p. 27). Asymmetric exchange can lead to strain (Siegrist et al., 2004; van Vegchel, de Jonge, Bosma, & Schaufeli, 2005). The ERI model is an extension of equity theory in the context of occupational stress; the discrepancy between what is offered and what is received can be harmful, both too much or too little can be unwanted and have negative effects, and homeostasis is necessary for optimal functioning.

Job strain model; demand–control–support model

Karasek's (1979) job strain model posits that the interaction between job demands and job decision latitude is the primary source of work-related stress, and that the risk of strain will be higher in situations where demands are high and decision latitude is low (the interaction hypothesis). The model suggests that there is an optimal balance between demands (including workload, work scheduling) and control (such as skill discretion, decision authority). Its extended version, the demand–control–support (DCS) model (Karasek & Theorell, 1990), also includes social support as a crucial component in this relationship. The DCS model is currently the most influential and widely cited model of the relationship between work characteristics and health outcomes (Barling & Griffiths, 2003), as numerous reviews and empirical work attest. Despite its appeal, it has also received equivocal support (e.g., Landsbergis, 1988; van der Doef & Maes, 1999) due to the problematic nature of the variables used, the nature of the measures used, the diversity of the groups studied, and a lack of support for the interaction hypothesis (e.g., de Jonge, Reuvers, Houtman, & Kompier, 2000; de Lange, Taris, Kompier, Houtman, & Bongers, 2003; Fletcher & Jones, 1993; Parkes, 1991; van Veldhoven, Taris, de Jonge, & Broersen, 2005). Perhaps recognizing the fact that interactions can represent curvilinear relationships, Karasek (1979) explicitly acknowledged the possible existence of curvilinear effects of work characteristics on outcomes and recommended that research should examine such effects, although he did not incorporate this explicitly in the model.

Vitamin model

Along with PE fit theory, Peter Warr's (1987, 2007) vitamin model offers an explicit conceptualization of the shape of the effects of work characteristics on well-being. Warr used the vitamin analogy to argue that job features can affect employee well-being (anxiety, depression, and happiness) in the same way as vitamins do. Some job features are desirable only up to certain levels, after which an additional decrement in their effects occurs, analogous to an inverted-U relationship. Too much or too little of these may contribute to reduced well-being (for example, opportunity for personal control, opportunity for skill use, variety, and opportunity for interpersonal contact). In contrast, some job features can have a constant effect on well-being (such as availability of money, valued social position, and physical security), which is analogous to a ceiling effect; a positive linear relationship that reaches a plateau after a certain point. He groups these job features into 12 broad categories that are comprised of more specific job features (Warr, 2007). The vitamin model has inspired a large body of research on a variety of job features and health outcomes, in a range of homogeneous and heterogeneous occupational groups. For example, De Jonge and Schaufeli (1998) found curvilinear effects of job demands, job autonomy, and workplace social support on three indicators of well-being (job satisfaction, emotional exhaustion, and anxiety), but linear effects of job autonomy on emotional exhaustion. Warr (1990) found evidence for curvilinear effects of job demands on job satisfaction (explaining 45% of its variance). Finally, de Jonge et al. (2000) indicated that the effects of work characteristics on job satisfaction, psychosomatic health complaints, and sickness absence were best explained by linear additive models, whereas the effects of work characteristics on emotional exhaustion and depression were curvilinear, concluding that "it seems sensible to pay more attention to curvilinear relationships in future research" (p. 266).

Some Challenges and Opportunities

Despite strong conceptual bases for possible curvilinear effects of work characteristics on health and well-being, there seems to be a gap between the tendency to look at linear effects in research and available theory. Properties of these models that pertain to curvilinear effects have often been neglected in research, with some notable exceptions. It is hoped that advances in research methods and approaches will lead to resolution of contradictory findings and a deeper understanding of curvilinear effects. It will also help to delineate the boundary conditions within which specified work characteristics exert their optimal effects on various health outcomes in a range of occupations and contexts. This section highlights some issues concerning research and theorizing in this area, and provides some recommendations for developing approaches that properly attend to the possibility of curvilinear effects.

Although some of these models are useful for summarizing observations, they fail to address the important questions of how, why, and when; "many are post hoc and few are predictive" (Cox & Mackay, 1981, p. 91), and few discuss the boundary conditions for the impact of work characteristics on health outcomes. Mohr (1982) has usefully distinguished between factor, or variance, and process models: variance models aim to explain the variance in the outcomes and provide sufficient conditions for the outcome, whereas process models (e.g., GAS) describe how and when things happen and the necessary conditions for an outcome. Variance models have dominated research traditions in the social sciences, to the extent that true process theories are rare (Gilbert, 1995). Process theories are of great value for developing theory because they acknowledge the importance of context and time.

Along these lines, scholars have stressed the importance of developing process and transactional accounts of the interplay among work and health over time, observing that "much job stress research can in fact be depicted as reflecting an interactional model of stress, where the various components (stressors, strain, and coping) are treated as static constructs and as having unidimensional effects" and that "research methods need to explore the ongoing interplay among these components over time and to examine the possibility of multidimensional (mutual) causality" (Cooper et al., 2001, p. 213). For example, expressing the need for conceptualizing relationships as they unfold over time in a complex transaction between the individual and their environment, Lazarus and Folkman's (1989) model of coping places appraisal as central for determining coping reactions. Similarly, the cybernetic theory of stress, coping and well-being (Edwards, 1998) defines stress as a perceived goal discrepancy and coping as efforts to reduce that discrepancy. By describing this process as a negative feedback loop, it combines the way that an individual experienced strain and well-being with individual and situational factors to explain coping behaviors.

This available theoretical repository provides good grounds for developing research and theory on possible curvilinear relationships between work and health. For example, PE fit theory and the vitamin model espouse a more complex view of work and health by describing the needed conditions when the effect of a work characteristic on well-being will be optimal, as well as the boundaries for such an effect. Similarly, activation theory and the effort–reward imbalance model highlight the importance of continuous appraisal, which can reveal discrepancies between perceived and ideal states leading to motivation to re-establish homeostasis. The interactive perspective is also not uncommon in some models (e.g., Cooper et al., 2001; Quick & Tetrick, 2003), which present individuals as active agents rather than passive actors and recipients (Cox & Mackay, 1981). Developments in theory can transform research and build strong bridges with practice.

Furthermore, since curvilinearity can take many distinct forms, research into curvilinear effects of work characteristics on health outcomes should be sensitive to the conditions for detecting such effects. These include a multitude of issues to be taken into consideration, such as the population being studied, range of occupations, work characteristic of interest, specific health or well-being outcome examined, and range of scores (e.g., Fletcher & Jones, 1993; Jeurissen & Nyklíček, 2001; Warr, 1990). The latter is extremely important, as a narrow range of scores may only represent part of the curve or a distorted curve, and thus not reflect the full array of effects. The fact that not all studies have found support for expected curvilinearity may be due to such contingencies, which also make it difficult to integrate findings. For example,

Jeurissen and Nyklíček (2001) acknowledged that range restriction in their sample did not provide the wide distribution of scores necessary to detect curvilinear relationships (see also Warr, 1990). In addition, the whole spectrum of the phenomenon should be sampled, both extreme and normal conditions, and both the upward and downward parts of the curve (Muse et al., 2003). It has also been suggested that large heterogeneous samples of employees and jobs would enable the detection of curvilinear effects (Jeurissen & Nyklíček, 2001; Warr, 1990; Xie & Johns, 1995). Of importance is also the expected life-cycle of the effect of a particular work characteristic on a particular outcome. Longitudinal studies have indicated lagged effects of the former on the latter, and effects weakening over time (specifically, weaker effects after 3 to 12 months, depending on the particular work characteristic or stressor, and the outcome examined; Garst, Frese, & Molenaar, 2000; Sonnentag & Frese, 2003). Important impact can go undetected unless researchers pay attention to the appropriate time-lag in the impact of work characteristics on well-being outcomes. Such methodological considerations should be taken into account when choosing measures and analytical methods, and when evaluating existing research. Beyond Mendenhall et al.'s (1998) suggestion that we should re-evaluate the appropriateness of examining curvilinear phenomena using research methods based on the linearity assumption, it would be appropriate to recommend an eclectic approach to research. Such an approach should be based on the underlying assumptions of data analysis methods, the requirements and nature of the data, and the anticipated nature of the phenomena being studied.

In terms of practical implications, an advantage of explicitly modeling curvilinear effects is the estimation of the points where the effects of a work characteristic change or where their impact on health and job satisfaction is optimal. Critical points indicate when the effect of, for example, job demands on job satisfaction levels off, slows down, or changes direction, and are thus invaluable for practice. Applied to managing work-related health, they can help to identify the points when a beneficial work characteristic can become a hazard and a risk to health. For example, Karanika-Murray et al. (2009) developed a technique for multivariate curvilinear risk estimation, which is based on the premise that in the presence of curvilinear relationships, risk can change depending on an individual's experience with a particular job characteristic. This technique estimates the range of values where risk is positive or negative, and the point of optimal functioning where risk is zero. Identifying these optimal levels has significant predictive and practical utility; it provides a way for identifying priority groups and prioritizing interventions to manage work-related health, thus helping to improve the relevance of policies and interventions (Guastello, 1992).

The curvilinearity hypothesis is sustained by both theory and a small body of available research on the relationships between work and health. Despite considerable progress in the last few decades, there are some methodological challenges still to overcome (for excellent discussions of methodological problems in the area see Frese & Zapf, 1988; Hochwarter, 2004; Jex, Beehr, & Roberts, 1992; Kahn & Byosiere, 1992; Kasl, 1987; Muse et al., 2003; Sullivan & Bhagat, 1992; Zapf et al., 1996). One of these challenges is related to underlying assumptions about the nature of psycho-social phenomena and the type of effects of work on health and well-being. Recourse to the curvilinearity hypothesis can help to reformulate our understanding of the boundary conditions for the effects of work characteristics on health and well-being. To strengthen the interface between theory and data, it is important that researchers (1) are aware of the underlying assumptions of available data analysis methods, (2) are attentive to the nature of the data and phenomena under investigation, and (3) build on current theories on the relationships between work and health.

Conclusions

This chapter has highlighted the limitations of the linearity assumption in examinations of the relationships between work characteristics and health and well-being. It argues that researchers in the field have become accustomed to thinking in linear terms and have neglected the rich theory that supports curvilinear effects. The chapter provides a focused overview of the available theoretical models that explicitly or implicitly incorporate the possibility of curvilinear effects, and discusses some challenges and opportunities for the development of research in this area. Conflicting findings in this small body of empirical research are indicative of the need for further examinations with appropriate designs and analytical tools. By articulating the underlying assumptions of our research methods and tools and by updating our practices, while at the same time building on the theoretical models and insights accrued over the last decades, we can realize the benefits of the curvilinearity hypothesis for advancing our understanding and opening new avenues for action and intervention. It is hoped that this discussion will draw attention to the transformative leverage that overcoming underlying assumptions of linearity can bring in order to explore the complexity of relationships between work and health.

Note

1. The general linear model specifies the relationship between predictor and outcome such that $y = \alpha + \beta\chi + e$, where α is a constant, β is the effect coefficient, and e is the error term. By assuming that χ and y are linearly related and that the distribution of y is of the normal Gaussian form, this represents a line, so that as χ increases y also increases at a stable and proportionate rate. Variance not explained by the linear term is subsumed within the error term.

References

Abbott, A. (1988). Transcending general linear reality. *Sociological Theory, 6*, 169–186.
Adams, J. S. (1965). Inequity in social exchange. *Advances in Experimental Social Psychology, 2*, 267–299.

Barling, J., & Griffiths, A. (2003). A history of occupational health psychology. In J. C. Quick & L. E. Tetrick (Eds.), *Handbook of occupational health psychology* (pp. 19–33). Washington, DC: American Psychological Association.

Borg, V., Kristensen, T. S., & Burr, H. (2000). Work environment and changes in self-rated health: A five year follow-up study. *Stress Medicine, 16,* 37–47.

Carver, C. S., & Scheier, M. F. (1998). *On the self-regulation of behavior.* Cambridge: Cambridge University Press.

Caplan, R. D., & Harrison, R. V. (1993). Person-environment fit theory: Some history, recent developments, and future directions. *Journal of Social Issues, 49,* 253–275.

Cooper, C. L. (1998). *Theories of organizational stress.* New York: Oxford University Press.

Cooper, C. L., Dewe, P. J., & O'Driscoll, M. P. (2001). *Organizational stress: A review and critique of theory, research and applications.* Thousand Oaks, CA: Sage Publications.

Cox, T. (1978). *Stress.* London: Macmillan Press.

Cox, T., & Mackay, C. (1981). A transactional approach to occupational stress. In E. N. Cortlett & J. Richardson (Eds.), *Stress, work design, and productivity.* Chichester: John Wiley & Sons.

De Jonge, J., & Schaufeli, W. B. (1998). Job characteristics and employee well-being: A test of Warr's Vitamin Model in health care workers using structural equation modelling. *Journal of Organizational Behavior, 19,* 387–407.

De Jonge, J., Reuvers, M. M. E. N., Houtman, I. L. D., & Kompier, M. A. J. (2000). Linear and non-linear relations between psychosocial job characteristics, subjective outcomes, and sickness absence: Baseline results from SMASH. *Journal of Occupational Health Psychology, 5,* 256–268.

De Lange, A. H., Taris, T. W., Kompier, M. A. J., Houtman, I. L. D., & Bongers, P. M. (2003). "The very best of the millennium": Longitudinal research and the Demand-Control-(Support) model. *Journal of Occupational Health Psychology, 8,* 282–305.

Edwards, J. R. (1998). Cybernetic theory of stress, coping and well-being: Review and extension to work and family. In C. L. Cooper (Ed.), *Theories of organizational stress.* New York: Oxford University Press.

Edwards, J. R., Caplan, R. D., & Harrison, R. V. (1998). Person–environment fit theory: Conceptual foundations, empirical evidence, and directions for future research. In C. L. Cooper (Ed.), *Theories of organizational stress* (pp. 28–67). New York: Oxford University Press.

Eriksen, H. R., Olff, M., Murison, R., & Ursin, H. (1999). The time dimension in stress responses: Relevance for survival and death. *Psychiatry Research, 85,* 39–50.

Everitt, B. S. (1978). *Graphical techniques for multivariate data.* New York: North-Holland.

Fazey, J., & Hardy, L. (1988). *The inverted-U hypothesis: A catastrophe for sport psychology?* British Association of Sports Sciences Monograph No. 1. Leeds: The National Coaching Foundation.

Ferris, G. R., Bowen, M. G., Treadway, D. C., Hochwarter, W. A., Hall, A. T., & Perrewé, P. L. (2006). The assumed linearity of organizational phenomena: Implications for occupational stress and well-being. In P. L. Perrewé & D. C. Ganster (Eds.), *Research in occupational stress and well-being, Vol. 5* (pp. 203–232). Oxford: Elsevier Science.

Fletcher, B. C., & Jones, F. (1993). A refutation of Karasek's demand–discretion model of occupational stress with a range of dependent measures. *Journal of Organizational Behavior, 14,* 319–330.

French, J. R. P., Caplan, R. D., & Harrison, R. V. (1982). *The mechanisms of job stress and strain.* New York: John Wiley & Sons.

Frese, M., & Zapf, D. (1988). Methodological issues in the study of work stress: Objective vs. subjective measurement of work stress and the question of longitudinal studies. In C. L. Cooper & R. Payne (Eds.), *Causes, coping and consequences of stress at work* (pp. 375–411). Chichester: John Wiley & Sons.

Gardner, D. G. (1986). Activation theory and task design: An empirical test of several new predictions. *Journal of Applied Psychology, 71*, 411–418.

Gardner, D. G., & Cummings, L. L. (1988). Activation theory and job design: Review and reconceptualization. In B. M. Staw & L. L. Cummings (Eds.), *Research in organizational behavior, Vol. 10* (pp. 81–122). Greenwich, CT: JAI Press.

Garst, H., Frese, M., & Molenaar, P. C. M. (2000). The temporal factor of change in stressor-strain relationships: A growth curve model on a longitudinal study in East Germany. *Journal of Applied Psychology, 85*, 417–438.

Gilbert, G. N. (1995). Emergence in social simulation. In G. N. Gilbert & R. Conte (Eds.), *Artificial societies: The computer simulation of social life* (pp. 144–156). London: UCL Press.

Guastello, S. J. (1992). Accidents and stress-related health disorders: Forecasting with catastrophe theory. In J. C. Quick, L. M. Murphy, & J. J. Hurrell (Eds.), *Stress and well-being at work: Assessments and interventions for occupational mental health* (pp. 252–269). Washington, DC: American Psychological Association.

Guastello, S. J. (2002). *Managing emergent phenomena: Non-linear dynamics in work organizations.* Mahwah, NJ: Laurence Erlbaum.

Guion, R. M. (1998). Some virtues of dissatisfaction in the science and practice of personnel selection. *Human Resource Management Review, 8*, 351–365.

Hancock, P. A., & Ganey, H. C. N. (2003). From the inverted-U to the extended-U: The evolution of a law in psychology. *Journal of Human Performance in Extreme Environments, 7*, 5–14.

Hardy, L., & Parfitt, G. (1991). A catastrophe model of anxiety and performance. *British Journal of Psychology, 82*, 163–178.

Hardy, L., Parfitt, G., & Pates, J. (1994). Performance catastrophes in sport: A test of the hysteresis hypothesis. *Journal of Sports Science, 12*, 327–334.

Harris, K. J., & Kacmar, K. M. (2006). Too much of a good thing? The curvilinear effect of leader–member exchange on stress. *Journal of Social Psychology, 146*, 65–84.

Hochwarter, W. A. (2004). Social influence and job stress: Direct, intervening and non-linear effects. In P. L. Perrewé & D. C. Ganster (Eds.), *Research in occupational stress and well-being, Vol. 3* (pp. 167–206). Oxford: Elsevier Science.

Jamal, M. (1985). Relationship of job stress to job performance: A study of managers and blue-collar workers. *Human Relations, 38*, 409–424.

Janssen, O. (2001). Fairness perceptions as a moderator in the curvilinear relationship between job demands, and job performance and job satisfaction. *Academy of Management Journal, 44*, 1039–1050.

Jeurissen, T., & Nyklíček, I. (2001). Testing the Vitamin Model of job stress in Dutch health care workers. *Work & Stress, 15*, 254–264.

Jex, S. M., Beehr, T. A., & Roberts, C. (1992). The meaning of occupational stress items to survey workers. *Journal of Applied Psychology, 77*, 623–628.

Kahn, R. L., & Byosiere, P. (1992). Stress in organizations. In M. D. Dunnette & L. M. Hough (Eds.), *Handbook of work and organizational psychology, Vol. 3* (pp. 571–650). Palo Alto, CA: Consulting Psychologists Press.

Karanika, M. (2006). *An appeal to reality: Modeling non-linear work–health relationships in the context of risk management* (Unpublished doctoral dissertation). University of Nottingham, Nottingham, UK.

Karanika-Murray, M., Antoniou, A. S., Michaelides, G., & Cox, T. (2009). Expanding the risk assessment methodology for work-related health: A technique for incorporating multivariate curvilinear effects. *Work & Stress, 23*, 99–119.

Karanika-Murray, M., & Michaelides, G. (2008). Conceptualizing nonlinear dynamic systems for health psychology research. *Health Psychology Update, 7*, 28–36.

Karasek, R. A. (1979). Job demands, job decision latitude and mental strain: Implications for job redesign. *Administrative Science Quarterly, 24*, 285–308.

Karasek, R. A., & Theorell, T. (1990). *Healthy work: Stress, productivity and the reconstruction of working life*. New York: Basic Books.

Kasl, S. V. (1987). Methodologies in stress and health: Past difficulties, present dilemmas, future directions. In S. V. Kasl & C. L. Cooper (Eds.), *Stress and health: Issues in research methodology* (pp. 307–318). New York: John Wiley & Sons.

Kukla, A. (2001). *Methods of theoretical psychology*. Cambridge, MA: The MIT Press.

Landsbergis, P. A. (1988). Occupational stress among health care workers: A test for the job demands-control model. *Journal of Organizational Behavior, 9*, 217–239.

Lazarus, R. S. (1991). Psychological stress in the workplace. *Journal of Social Behavior & Personality, 6*, 1–13.

Lazarus, R. S., & Folkman, S. (1989). *Stress, appraisal and coping*. New York: Springer.

McGrath, J. E. (1976). Stress and behavior in organizations. In M. D. Dunnette (Ed.), *Handbook of industrial and organizational psychology* (pp. 1351–1395). Chicago: Rand McNally College Publishing.

Mendenhall, M. E., Macomber, J. H., Gregersen, H., & Cutright, M. (1998). Non-linear dynamics: A new perspective on IHRM research and practice in the 21st century. *Human Resource Management Review, 8*, 5–22.

Mohr, M. (1982). *Explaining organizational behavior*. San Francisco: Jossey-Bass.

Mowday, R. T. (1991). Equity theory predictions of behavior in organizations. In R. M. Steers & L. W. Porter (Eds.), *Motivation and work behavior* (pp. 111–151). New York: McGraw-Hill.

Muse, L. A., Harris, S. G., & Feild, H. S. (2003). Has the inverted-U theory of stress and job performance had a fair test? *Human Performance, 16*, 349–364.

Neiss, R. (1988). Reconceptualizing arousal: Psychobiological states in motor performance. *Psychological Bulletin, 34*, 977–1001.

Nelson, D. L., & Simmons, B. L. (2003). Health psychology and work stress: A more positive approach. In J. C. Quick & L. E. Tetrick (Eds.), *Handbook of occupational health psychology* (pp. 97–117). Washington, DC: American Psychological Association.

Parkes, K. R. (1991). Locus of control as a moderator: An explanation for additive versus interactive findings in the demand-discretion model of work stress? *British Journal of Psychology, 82*, 291–312.

Quick, J. C., & Tetrick, L. E. (2003). *Handbook of occupational health psychology*. Washington, DC: American Psychological Association.

Rick, J., Thomson, L., Briner, R., O'Regan, S., & Daniels, K. (2002). *Review of existing supporting scientific knowledge to underpin standards of good practice for key work-related stressors—Phase 1* (Research Report RR024). Sudbury, UK: HSE Books.

Rydstedt, L. W, Ferrie, J., & Head, J. (2006). Is there support for curvilinear relationships between psychosocial work characteristics and mental well-being? Cross-sectional and long term data from the Whitehall II study. *Work & Stress, 20*, 6–20.

Schabracq, M. J., Winnubst, J. A. M., & Cooper, C. L. (2002). *Handbook of work and health psychology*. Chichester: John Wiley & Sons.

Schrader-Frechette, K. S. (1998). *Risk and rationality: Philosophical foundations for populist reforms*. Berkeley, CA: University of California Press.

Scott, W. E. (1966). Activation theory and task design. *Organizational Behavior & Human Performance, 1*, 3–30.

Selye, H. (1975). *Stress without distress*. London: Hodder & Stoughton.

Siegrist, J. (1996). Adverse health effects of high-effort/low-reward conditions. *Journal of Occupational Health Psychology, 1*, 27–41.

Siegrist, J., Starke, D., Chandola, T., Godin, I., Marmot, M., Niedhammerd, I., & Petere, R. (2004). The measurement of effort–reward imbalance at work: European comparisons. *Social Science & Medicine, 58*, 1483–1499.

Sonnentag, S., & Frese, M., (2003). Stress in organizations. In W. C. Borman, D. R. Ilgen, & R. J. Klimoski (Eds.), *Comprehensive handbook of psychology, Vol. 12: Industrial and organizational psychology* (pp. 453–491). Hoboken: Wiley.

Stewart, I. N., & Peregoy, R. (1983). Catastrophe theory modeling in psychology. *Psychological Bulletin, 94*, 336–362.

Sullivan, S. E., & Bhagat, R. S. (1992). Organizational stress, job satisfaction and job perform-ance: Where do we go from here? *Journal of Management, 18*, 353–374.

Taris, T. W. (2006). Bricks without clay: On urban myths in occupational health psychology. *Work & Stress, 20*, 99–104.

Teigen, K. H. (1994). Yerkes-Dodson: A law for all seasons. *Theory & Psychology, 4*, 525–547.

Toomela, A. (2007). Culture of science: Strange history of the methodological thinking in psychology. *Integrative Psychological & Behavioral Science, 41*, 6–20.

Trochim, W. M. K. (2000). *The research methods knowledge base* (2nd ed.). Cincinnati, OH: Atomic Dog Publishing. Retrieved from http://trochim.human.cornell.edu/kb/index. htm

Van der Doef, M., & Maes, S. (1999). The job demand-control(-support) model and psycho-logical well-being: A review of 20 years of empirical research. *Work & Stress, 13*(2), 87–114.

Van Dierendonck, D., Schaufeli, W. B., & Buunk, B. P. (2001). Burnout and inequity in the human service professionals: A longitudinal study. *Journal of Occupational Health Psychology, 6*, 43–52.

Van Vegchel, N., de Jonge, J., Bosma, H., & Schaufeli, W. (2005). Reviewing the effort–reward imbalance model: Drawing up the balance of 45 empirical studies. *Social Science & Medicine, 60*, 1117–1131.

Van Veldhoven, M., Taris, T., de Jonge, J., & Broersen, S. (2005). The relationship between work characteristics and employee health and well-being: How much complexity do we really need? *International Journal of Stress Management, 12*, 3–28.

Walster, E., Berscheid, E., & Walster, G. W. (1973). New directions in equity research. *Journal of Personality & Social Psychology, 25*, 151–176.

Warr, P. B. (1987). *Work, unemployment and mental health*. Oxford: Clarendon Press.

Warr, P. B. (1990). Decision latitude, job demands, and employee well-being. *Work & Stress,* *4*, 285–294.

Warr, P. B. (2007). *Work, happiness and unhappiness.* Mahwah, NJ: Lawrence Erlbaum.

Woodcock, A., & Davis, M. (1978). *Catastrophe theory.* New York: E.P. Dutton.

Xie, J. L., & Johns, G. (1995). Job scope and stress: Can job scope be too high? *Academy of Management Journal, 38*, 1288–1309.

Zapf, D., Dormann, C., & Frese, M. (1996). Longitudinal studies in organizational stress research: A review of the literature with reference to methodological issues. *Journal of Occupational Health Psychology, 1*, 145–169.

Zivnuska, S., Kiewitz, C., Hochwarter, W. A., Perrewé, P. L., & Zellars, K. L. (2002). What is too much or too little? The curvilinear effects of job tension on turnover intent, value attainment, and job satisfaction. *Journal of Applied Social Psychology, 32*, 1344–1360.

9

Peer Assistance Programs in the Workplace

Social Support Theory and the Provision of Effective Assistance to Employees in Need

Maya Golan
Technion, Israel Institute of Technology

Yael Bacharach
Cornell University

Peter Bamberger
Technion, Israel Institute of Technology

Peer assistance programs (PAPs), also known as member assistance programs (MAPs), are voluntary, peer-based frameworks that motivate employees experiencing personal problems to seek help, facilitate the process of help-seeking, and, in some cases, directly provide support and assistance to those employees (Bacharach, Bamberger, & Sonnenstuhl, 1996). While their roots stretch back over a century, contemporary PAPs emerged in American workplaces as a union-based response to employee assistance programs (EAPs)—management-based frameworks for helping employees in need (Bacharach, Bamberger, & Sonnenstuhl, 2001; French, Dunlap, Roman, & Steele, 1997; Hartwell et al., 1996; Hayghe, 1991; Trice & Beyer, 1978). Recently, such programs have begun to attract the attention of managers and unions outside of the USA (Berridge, Cooper, & Highley-Marchington, 1997; Buon, 2006; Buon & Taylor, 2008; Kirk, 2005).

In this chapter, we seek to provide an overview of the historical development of PAPs and their core technology, and examine how such programs have been adapted for implementation in organizations outside of the USA. After reviewing the history of PAPs and the theoretical frameworks upon which they are based, we will draw from an Israeli experience in applying this technology in two organizations to: (a) identify the program parameters likely to require cultural fitting, (b) review practical methods for training and guiding the peer counselors who operate such programs, and (c) highlight significant program outcomes and key factors likely to determine program success.

Historical Development of PAPs

The workplace has long been recognized as a convenient and potentially highly effective forum for detecting and helping employees deal with personal problems, especially those stemming from substance abuse (Blocker, 1989; Sonnenstuhl, 1996). Indeed, for over a century, both labor and management have recognized the power of work and workplace relations as a basis for motivating those in need of assistance to seek help, and for providing help to those seeking it.

The first assistance programs appeared in the U.S. during the nineteenth century, when industrial organizations began to flourish. These programs embodied Americans' historical reliance on voluntary association and mutual aid (De Toqueville, 1976; Clawson, 1989). In these early programs, labor unions rather than management took responsibility for helping employees in need (Commons & Gilmore, 1910). Indeed, as noted by others (e.g., Clawson, 1989; Bacharach et al., 2001), many of the early craft unions (particularly those representing railroad crafts) organized around the theme of mutual aid and assistance. Such assistance was typically provided informally, with coworkers taking up "collections" for their colleagues in need, or serving as a "sounding board" for those in need of someone to talk to (Bacharach et al., 2001).

Although labor unions continued to offer helping services to their members, in the second half of the twentieth century the nature of these services underwent an important transformation, with informal, peer-based assistance being replaced by more formal and structured *peer assistance programs* (PAPs) (Trice & Schonbrunn, 1981; Ferguson & Fersing, 1965). Indeed, the peer counseling program of the American Federation of Labor and Congress of Industrial Organizations (AFL-CIO), which was established in 1955, is considered the oldest work-based assistance program in the United States (Perlis, 1980; Perlow, 1979). Union interest in peer-based assistance programs intensified in the 1980s, with unions representing employees in such firms as United Airlines, US Airways, CSX Transportation, Amtrak, General Motors and Ford Motors developing their own PAPs. This renewed union interest in peer assistance was in part stimulated by the recognition of union members and leaders that such programs provide a basis for building and maintaining member solidarity.

During the nineteenth century, assistance to employees in need was also provided by the management of some of the larger industrial organizations as part of the industrial betterment movement (Sonnenstuhl, 1996). However, it was only in the second half of the twentieth century that such management-based assistance services became widespread in the United States as the provision of such services became embedded in mainstream collective bargaining agreements. According to Steele (1995) the "push" for management to provide such services stemmed from the Taft-Hartley Act—a federal law legislated in 1947, which greatly restricted the activities and power of labor unions. However, Bacharach et al. (2001) suggest that unions saw advantages in having such services included as part of the employee benefits package and increasingly negotiated for the incorporation of such services as a management-provided benefit to their members. Consequently, by the 1970s labor had effectively dropped mutual aid and informal peer-to-peer assistance as a basis for union organizing and solidarity, and transferred the responsibility for such services to management. Moreover, during the 1970s and 1980s, following a National Institute on Alcohol Abuse and Alcoholism campaign for promoting their EAP model, there was an immense increase in the number of management-sponsored assistance programs in the USA. Although EAPs originated in programs providing help to alcoholics, these programs also dealt with other personal problems (Hartwell et al., 1996), such as mental health problems, family violence, marital and parenting conflicts, occupational stress, legal services, elder care, maternity care, and critical incident stress (Hopkins, 1997, Spell & Blum, 2005).

By the late 1980s employee assistance (EA) services were offered by the vast majority of the Fortune 1000 firms, most often with credentialed/professional counselors offering on-site assistance. Scholars (e.g., Maiden, 1998) emphasize that management was motivated to provide EA services because it expected that such services would enhance workers' performance and productivity and reduce employee turnover. However, with employers becoming increasingly concerned with the rising costs of employee health-related benefits, by the 1990s many firms opted to contract such services out to external mental health agencies and insurance companies; a move that further formalized the work-based assistance process and limited coworkers from assisting one another (Bacharach et al., 1996, 2001; Sonnenstuhl & Trice, 1987; Steele, 1995; Steele & Trice, 1995).

Nonetheless, labor unions did not give up on their historical responsibility for assisting employees in need. From the late 1980s to date, a growing number of labor unions have regained an interest in helping employees manage their personal problems. Bacharach et al. (1996) claim that the trigger for labor unions' renewed interest in peer-based assistance was the widespread adoption of drug testing and managed care by management. Indeed, by the early 1990s, most employers had adopted some form of drug testing (Blum, Fields, Milne, & Spell, 1992; Denenberg & Denenberg, 1991; Seeber & Lehman, 1989; Spell & Blum, 2005), a move perceived by labor unions as coercive and limiting employees' access to other helping services (Jacobs & Zimmer, 1991; AFL-CIO, 1993). Furthermore, Bacharach et al. (2001) argue that by the late 1980s, unions recognized that the servicing approach to union–member relations adopted after World War II was no longer an effective means by which to retain members and increase union density, and that such an approach had to be replaced by more of an organizing logic. Mutual aid, particularly in the form of peer assistance, became recognized as an important element of such logic.

Accordingly, labor unions activists such as McCabe (1992) and McKay (1993) argued that despite the exposure of a growing number of employees to EA services, reforms such as managed care, patient matching, and drug testing have made helping more bureaucratic, expensive, and remote from employees' needs (Bacharach et al., 2001). These activists claimed that PAPs, rather than EAPs, constitute an important alternative for helping employees, not just in unionized workplaces but in other community-based institutions such as schools and churches. Indeed, during the nineties, schools began using the mechanism of peer helping to improve students' well-being. For example, Black, Tobler, and Sciacca (1998) describe the advantage of a peer intervention program over programs led by teachers and researchers in preventing drug abuse among school students. A second example is provided by Tanaka and Reid's (1997) positive evaluation of a student peer helping program. This program is based on the same underlying logic of a PAP. In other words, students help each other by listening, providing information and referring to professional help when required.

American labor unions' criticism of management sponsored programs was translated into action in 1991, when union representatives decided to withdraw from the professional association for employee assistance professionals (EAPA), and established a new independent association called Labor Assistance Professionals (LAP) which continues to promote the PAP model in the USA.

PAP Core Technology

As noted earlier, PAPs are defined as typically voluntary, peer-based programs designed to motivate employees suffering from substance abuse and other personal problems to seek help and to provide support and assistance to those seeking help (Bacharach et al., 1996). PAPs rely on one or more groups of employees volunteering to serve as *peer counselors* and, in that role, assisting employees in need to manage their personal problems by referring them to external self-help and professional helping services in the community, and in the case of substance abuse problems, by educating them to maintain long-term abstinence and sobriety (Bamberger & Sonnenstuhl, 1995).

PAPs are considered one of the various frameworks for EAP services provision (Cagney, 1999). However, in contrast to traditional EAPs, which are staffed with credentialed professionals (for an overview on EAPs see Sonnenstuhl & Trice, 1990), PAPs rely on networks of workers who volunteer their time to assist employees in need (Bacharach, Bamberger, & McKiney, 2000). Based on their study of a flight attendants' assistance program, Bamberger and Sonnenstuhl (1995: pp. 295–296) offer a brief description of what is entailed in the role of peer counsellor:

> In their passive role, the peer counselors provide troubled co-worker with solicited information. They wait for troubled flight attendants to ask them for help, assess their problems and refer them to community agencies for assistance. In their active role, peer counselors seek out their troubled colleagues and provide them with unsolicited advice about their behavior, confront them with evidence of their problems and encourage them to accept help before they get "out of hand". In either case the objective of the peer counselor is the same—to motivate the flight attendants to change their troubling behavior.

While all PAPs are grounded on the notion of volunteerism and peer delivery of service, PAPs vary along several dimensions (Bacharach et al., 1996). For example, the program may be funded by labor, management, or both. The services provided may include substance abuse education, assessment, referral to community treatment providers, follow-up and aftercare or in-house counseling. Programs may, in addition to a network of employee volunteers in the field, be staffed by in-house contracted professionals and/or union members or officers compensated for their time. Also, programs may focus on different types of problems such as substance abuse, stress, general mental health, trauma or critical incidents. Finally, some PAPs operate in worksites in which employees lack access to EA services, while others are implemented in firms with an operating EAP (Bacharach et al., 1996). In the case of the latter, the PAP may operate as an alternative to the EAP or as a "funnel" leading employees in need to the EA professional.

Scholars have identified a number of advantages offered by PAPs (Bacharach et. al., 1994; 1996). First, PAPs are often cheaper to run because they are structured around a network of peer volunteers rather than relying upon paid professionals. Second, employees may be more willing to seek help from a peer than from a professional employed by the management. For example, even if confidentiality is assured, employees may be reluctant to seek help for a drug problem from a management-employed professional out of concern that management will ultimately be made aware of the matter. Additionally, employees may prefer to seek assistance from someone with an experience similar to their own as opposed to a professional who, while perhaps highly skilled, may be viewed as lacking first-hand experience with the kind of problem faced by the worker. Third, peers having constant access to the employee need may be better positioned to provide critical long-term follow-up. Finally, because PAPs can be structured around occupations rather than organizations, they may be offered to employees working in firms that are too small to operate EAP.

The precise prevalence of PAPs in the USA is unknown since almost all the prevalence data on assistance programs focuses on EAPs. PAP prevalence was reported as 10% of all assistance programs in America in 1990 (Hayghe, 1991) and six years later reached 17% of all assistance programs (Hartwell et al., 1996). According to a national study conducted in 2008 by the EAPA, 65% of all American organizations provide EA services (EAPA, 2008). Assuming that the current prevalence of PAPs is similar to Hartwell et al's estimation, then PAPs represent some 11% of employee assistance service frameworks in existence among American enterprises. Regardless of their exact prevalence, recent evidence suggests that the distribution of all types of assistance programs including PAPs has been increasing both in the USA, as well as in Europe (Buon & Taylor, 2008).

The Diffusion of Work-Based Assistance Programs Outside of the USA

Globalization has stimulated the diffusion of work-based assistance programs beyond North America with many American-based firms interested in ensuring a common set of human resource services in all of their international facilities

(Buon, 2006). Additionally, over the past decade, European firms have also begun to offer employee assistance services to their employees (Reddy, 2005), with EAPs being particularly prevalent in the U.K. (Buon & Taylor, 2008). One result of this trend was the establishment of the Employee Assistance European Forum (EAEF) in 2002, an organization mandated to develop standards of practice for European workplace assistance programs. Nowadays, EAEF represents members from 23 European countries and has three European "chapters" (i.e., professional branches) in the U.K., Ireland and Greece (EAEF, 2008). A market survey founded by the EAEF for the purpose of expanding EA services in Europe (Buon & Taylor, 2008) reported that 10% of British employees, 25% of Danish employees and employees in more than 500 German companies have access to EA services.

Unlike EAPs, PAPs remain a phenomenon that is unique to North American enterprises. Several factors may account for the failure of PAPs to diffuse beyond the boundaries of North America. First, there is no European professional association such as the American LAP that is capable of supporting the promotion and development of PAPs outside of the USA. Second, given the lack of such an association, local PAP initiatives or other similar peer-based assistance programs may be operating outside of the USA without being publicly announced and recognized. Finally, it may be that while formal, professional assistance efforts, such as those represented by employee assistance programs, may be tailored to meet the demands of local norms and laws, such tailoring may be more difficult to achieve when the basis of assistance is less formal as in the case of peer assistance.

Indeed, while the research on cross-cultural workplace assistance is limited, (e.g., Grossmark, 1999; Buon & Taylor, 2008) and focuses only on management-based EAPs, a number of studies suggest that tailoring assistance across national boundaries tends to focus on more technical matters such as adopting referral practices so as to take into account differences in health coverage, and adopting program foci to reflect local employee needs. For example, Roman (1983) compared American and Australian EAPs, and explained the differences between them as stemming from the nature and structure of local health benefits, an explanation more recently endorsed by Kirk (2005). Cross-cultural differences have also been found with regard to the trigger for program adoption. For example, British programs were usually established in order to support employees in dealing with high stress levels and create a caring impression by the company management (Berridge et al., 1997), while Australian programs usually started as a response to a rare or dramatic incident that posed a challenge to existing organizational resources (Kirk, 2005).

The relative absence of PAPs outside of North America does not mean this framework cannot be adapted to meet the needs of labor and management in other countries. Indeed, our current research, focusing on how the North American PAP model was implemented in two Israeli enterprises, demonstrates that this approach to work-based assistance may offer significant global potential and important advantages to both labor unions and managements in a variety of enterprises outside of North America.

PAPs in Israel

During the years 2004 to 2008, we were given the opportunity to follow and evaluate the implementation and operation of the first two PAPs established in Israel—a country whose enterprises for the most part did not offer any type of assistance programs (Bamberger & Biron, 2006). In this section, we describe the two programs (referred to as Alpha and Beta), with respect to their establishment, peer counselor training, utilization rate, and typical case handling. We will also describe the nature of the relations between the program's peer counselors (on the one hand) and management and labor (on the other), and discuss some of the noncounseling activities in which peer counselors engaged in the effort to promote their program and build a culture of caring.

Program establishment

Alpha, the first PAP established in Israel, was launched in December 2004 and has been operating since then. It was established in a manufacturing factory, an Israeli branch of a global European food corporation, employing 350 unskilled operators and packers. We collected data on the program between the years 2004 and 2008 by observing program-related activities and by interviewing the peer counselors and the employees who approached them.

Alpha was established as a joint union–management project, based on the proto-typical American PAP. In order to start the program, a steering committee that included union and management representatives consulted with a team of experts who were involved in establishing some of the largest PAPs in the USA, as to how the program should be structured and operated. The opening words of Alpha's mission, written by the steering committee, express the underlying logic of self-help the program is built upon:

> Alpha management and labor recognize that factory workers may suffer from a variety of personal problems that can take a toll on their well being, their family lives, and their job performance. Examples of personal problems are alcohol and other drug problems, family and marital difficulties, and emotional and stress-related disorders. In order to assist workers manage their personal problems and improve their job performance, labor and management are implementing a comprehensive assistance program designed to assist workers in finding help for their personal problems from professional and self-help services in the community. The program is staffed by peer counselors knowledgeable about the Israeli community services available to workers and the procedures for getting help from these valuable resources.

In order to start operating the program, the steering committee appealed to the enterprise's employees to volunteer as peer counselors. Twenty-five employees responded. Ten of them, representing the various informal social networks in the factory, were selected by the steering committee and participated in a three-day training workshop that provided basic skills in peer counseling and referral. In addition to the workshop, the steering committee hired a subcontracted social worker, who owned a company offering EA services in Israel, to provide the peer counselors with periodic post-training professional guidance as they interacted with employees in need.

The peer counselors advertised the new program in the factory newspaper, on company message boards, by distributing flyers and "business cards", and by holding informative meetings with groups of workers. The message communicated to the employees focused on the program guidelines and on practical information explaining how the peer counselors could be reached. Furthermore, employees were encouraged to approach the peer counselors if required, and they were promised that total confidentiality would be kept.

Beta, the second Israeli program, was established in a community hospital employing approximately 1,000 workers in October 2006. The initiative for establishing Beta came from the in-house social service manager who heard about Alpha and was interested in offering similar PAP services to the hospital employees as a supplement to the hospital social services that had a low utilization rate. We studied the adoption and administration of the program at Beta between the years 2006 and 2008 by conducting interviews with the peer counselors and by observing on-going program activities.

The stages involved in establishing Beta were similar to those undertaken to establish Alpha—with two substantial differences. First, being the second program established in Israel enabled Beta operators to both consult with the team of experts that supported Alpha's establishment and profit from the experience and knowledge accumulated by Alpha's steering committee and peer counselors. Second, unlike Alpha, Beta's steering committee did not hire a subcontracted social worker to professionally guide the peer counselors, but rather nominated one of the social workers already working in the hospital for this task. This decision was a double-edged sword. On one hand, the social worker's familiarity with the organization's bureaucracy and with the peer counselors was helpful in quickly and efficiently launching the program. On the other hand, shortly after the program began operating, it was perceived by the hospital workers as competing with the hospital social service department in receiving employees' help requests. Consequently, the peer counselor's professional guide had a clear conflict of interest, which may account for Beta's low utilization rate as discussed below.

Training and guiding the Israeli peer counselors

At both Alpha and Beta, peer counselors participated in a three-day preliminary hands-on, skills-based training program aimed at providing them with the necessary skills, techniques and information required for facilitating the PAP help-seeking and referral processes. The training was prepared and conducted by several experienced consultants who had been involved in the establishment of some of the largest PAPs in the USA. The training content was identical for the Alpha and Beta programs and included four modules: introduction to PAP mechanism, counseling skills and techniques, clarification and discussion of the type of problems that were likely to arise and available community helping resources, and the promotion of the PAP in the organization.

In the first module, the purpose of the PAP and its mechanism were presented by familiarizing the peer counselors with existing models of PAPs in the USA, the program mission, and specific organizational procedures and policies that were written and approved in order to operate the program (e.g., policies regarding substance abuse among workers, procedures for record keeping of program activities and supervisory referral processes). In this module, the peer counselors' role was presented as a support system, designed to assist employees to manage personal problems by referring employees in need to external self-help and professional helping services in the community. Particular attention was paid to the notion that peer counselors were not expected to become professional therapists or experts in solving personal problems. In the case of substance abuse problems, the peer counselors' role was extended to include education regarding the effects of substance abuse on users and those around them, as well as activities required for the post-treatment after-care, monitoring, and follow up.

The purpose of the second module was to teach the peer counselors basic counseling skills and raise their awareness of the importance of gaining the employees' trust and attentively listening to them. This part of the training included opportunities to learn and practice counseling techniques. However, since counseling skills require long-term practice, the peer counselors continued to practice in the follow-up professional guiding meetings and training that took place after Alpha and Beta programs were launched.

The skill-based module focused on teaching the peer counselors four skills labeled by the consultant who conducted the training as "being present", "being empathic", "listening with empathy" and "confronting constructively". *Being present* reflects a psychological approach (DeYoung, 2003) emphasizing the need to let go of past or future thoughts and to be "here and now," giving full attention to the person with whom one interacts. Accordingly, the peer counselors practiced experiential exercises during which they were shown how to "be present," a skill that consequently helps peer counselors refrain from judgments, criticism, or expectations.

The second skill, *being empathic*, was drawn from therapy literature. Empathy comes from the German word *Einfühlung* meaning: "to project yourself into what you observe" and is used in therapy "to feel in to the other" (Johnson, 2004). The humanistic approach stresses the importance of empathy in therapy (Bohart & Greenberg, 1997; Rogers, 1975) to help the client feel safe, develop trust in the therapist and to allow self disclosure and vulnerability. Accordingly, the connection between the peer counselors' empathy and the employees' trust, sense of safety, and acceptance of help were repeatedly emphasized. The peer counselors practiced this skill by brainstorming what seeking help feels like and then simulating help-seeking; a process that enabled them to experience employees' thoughts and feelings while they engage in help seeking.

The third skill, *listening with empathy*, involved three steps. The first, titled "listen with curiosity", encouraged peer counselors to be genuinely curious while they listen to employees and to convey interest in the latter's experiences, feelings, thoughts, and beliefs without judgment. Peer counselors were encouraged to use their tone of voice and other nonverbal cues such as posture, gestures, facial expression, and eye contact in order to convey their curiosity to employees. The second step titled "take in what you hear" literally means that the peer counselors were instructed to absorb what employees say by hearing their words, reading their gestures, and taking in their thoughts, ideas, and emotions. It was emphasized that in order to do this, the peer counselors may need to slow down the pace of the conversation by politely interrupting the employees and employing a third step called "reflect with accuracy". This technique consists of repeating the employees' words to show that their perspective is understood, and also giving employees an opportunity to clarify any misunderstanding and summarize their main ideas (Thompson, 2003).

Empathic listening was taught by performing experiential exercises involving a simulated interaction between a peer counselor and an employee need. During the exercises, peer counselors were encouraged to share authentic personal experiences with each other, so that they could actually experience the value of empathic listening. While practicing their listening, the peer counselors experienced the struggle between the need to give advice, "be an expert," and present their own experience, and the necessity of being a good listener. The role-playing exercises demonstrated several advantages of empathic listening versus a common dialogue. First, empathic listening increases the employees' 'trust in the peer counselor and the counselor's commitment to the helping process. Consequently, the likelihood that they will return to the peer counselor for additional help or follow-up referral recommendations increases. Second, empathic listening results in positive feelings such as comfort, being understood and feeling safe. Finally, it promotes further exploration of the employees' understanding of their difficulties and allows them to find solutions on their own.

The fourth skill, *confronting constructively*, which is relevant mainly for dealing with substance abuse or violence problems, is widely discussed in the EAP (e.g. Sonnenstuhl & Trice, 1987) and the counseling literatures (e.g., Thompson, 2003). Since such problems might involve high denial levels (Bacharach et al. 2001), the peer counselors practiced how to convince employees to accept help and how to provide them with a rehabilitation treatment program as soon as possible using role-play exercises. It was emphasized that peer counselors must have some reliable evidence regarding the employees' problematic behavior prior to conducting the confrontation. Without proper evidence, the peer counselors were warned not to confront employees but rather limit themselves to expressing concern and trying to find out more details about the employees' condition. While confronting employees, the peer counselors were instructed to be caring, yet compelling, about the influence of the problematic behaviour, its consequences on employees and others. Also, the peer counselors were taught to voice their concern about the possibility that employees might lose their job, particularly if there was evidence of inappropriate behaviors such as absenteeism and lateness that could be used to support this concern.

The aim of the third module was to familiarize peer counselors with different types of problems that employees may have and with the community-based helping services available to them. This module was conducted by several specialists operating local helping services providing help in case of substance and alcohol abuse, family violence, and teenage problems. The specialists advised the peer counselors to establish a working relationship with their respective services in order to refer potential help seekers to them. Also, representatives from local municipal social services agencies participated in this part of the training and presented the social services available for Alpha and Beta organizations.

Finally, the fourth training module consisted of preparing a work plan for different actions aimed at promoting the PAP in the organizations. Peer counselors were requested to brainstorm future scripts related to the intra-organization PAP marketing, and prepared a work plan to carry out the relevant actions.

Post-training interviews with the programs' peer counselors revealed several differences between the Alpha and Beta training sessions. In Alpha, all peer counselors attended the training and the atmosphere was formal and festive. For example, the training period began with a short ceremony in the presence of several officials from local municipalities. In addition, the Alpha steering committee hired subcontractors to film the training session for further study and as a souvenir for the participants. Finally, Alpha participants were awarded with a graduation diploma. Alpha interviewees consistently remarked that this small token served as a powerful and important empowering and motivational device. In Beta, attendance in the training sessions was less than full, and several peer counselors (including the physician participants) missed most of the training due to work obligations. Also, the Beta training sessions were perceived as an optional, routine activity, rather than as a significant prerequisite for volunteering in the PAP.

After the preliminary training, the Alpha and Beta peer counselors participated in monthly team meetings. The meetings were conducted by a professional PAP expert in Alpha and by an in-house social service worker in Beta. Both professional guides were constantly available to the peer counselors, offering answers to questions raised by peer counselors. During the meetings the peer counselors focused on ways to advertise the PAP, increase utilization rates and further develop the counselors' help-giving skills using similar exercises to those used in the initial training sessions. Also, the peer counselors shared their experiences in case handling and discussed different intervention possibilities offered by other peers and the professional guide. Because of the low utilization rate in Beta, there were fewer discussions on case handling and more attention was paid to PAP promotion compared with the team meetings conducted in Alpha. However, in both programs the team meetings were an important practical continuation of the preliminary training session which improved the peer counselors' ability to help employees in need.

Program utilization and case handling

During the four years we documented Alpha activity, its peer counselors handled 86 requests for help. Thirty-four (40%) of these cases related to financial distress and 15 (17%) to substance abuse. Other type of problems included coworker or supervisor relations, health, family disputes, spousal unemployment, workplace violence, bereavement, child adoption, family violence, sexual harassment, and legal aid. Beta's utilization rate was substantially lower than Alpha's, particularly when one takes into account that Beta's peer counselors were servicing an employee base about three times that of Alpha's. By the time we completed data collection, two years after program establishment, Beta's peer counselors had handled only 9 cases involving the following problems: financial distress, coworker or supervisor relations, family disputes, and health crises. Table 1 shows the number of cases by problem type, for both programs.

The Israeli peer counselors were trained and expected to help employees by empathically listening to them. referring them if necessary, to professional help services, and following up on their condition. While providing help, peer counselors were encouraged to consult with the social worker guiding them and with other peer counselors, without revealing confidential details. In most cases, in both programs, peer counselors followed the modus operandi described above, with one significant difference: in only19% of the cases in Alpha and none of the cases in Beta, did peer counselors refer employees to professional services. In all other cases, peer counselors tried to help employees by themselves. In some cases, help was provided

Table 9.1   Number of Cases by Problem Type

Problem description	Number of cases in Alpha	Number of cases in Beta
Financial difficulties	34	3
Substance abuse	15	
Employment relation	8	2
Family disputes	6	2
Health	7	1
Unknown	5	
Unemployment	3	
Workplace violence	2	
Bereavement	2	1
Child adoption	1	
Family violence	1	
Sexual harassment	1	
Legal aid	1	
Total	86	9

regardless of ethical or even legal concerns that emerged. For example, a Beta peer counselor helped an employee who was prosecuted to prepare documents for the court discussion and accompanied the employee to court. One Alpha peer counselor took food supplies from the factory kitchen and prepared a package for an employee with financial difficulties. Another Beta peer counselor, who was suffering from financial difficulties himself, agreed to give cash money from his own savings to an employee in need. An extreme example of questionable help was a case in which an Alpha peer counselor prepared a home remedy for an employee suffering from hemorrhoids; a remedy which he admitted might increase blood pressure.

Managerial support

Alpha enjoyed substantial and consistent management support, which was publicly expressed during several meetings with employees and senior management and manifested in approval for most of the peer counselors' budget and resource requests. Furthermore, the management encouraged and funded the participation of program representatives in an Israeli competition for innovative human resource projects, in which Alpha won third place. Also, on several occasions, peer counselors were allowed by their managers to participate in program activities during working shifts, without being requested to make up the time. Interestingly, despite management's extensive backing and support, we saw no evidence of employees viewing management as the program's main sponsor. Moreover, Alpha's managers took every possible effort to ensure that peer counselors were given the autonomy to run the program as they wished.

The situation at Beta was different. Although the hospital management formally announced its support of the program, and despite its presence in steering committee meetings, support was never translated into action. Peer counselors had difficulty securing funding and resources, and simple requests such as securing a room for program activities or getting a budget for publishing information about the program were postponed and ultimately denied. Also, several peer counselors complained that they were forbidden by their managers to attend program meetings during working hours. One peer counselor even claimed that she was encouraged to retire earlier than planned because her manager complained that participating in the program had a negative influence on her work performance. The approach adopted by Beta's management had an obvious, negative influence on the peer counselors' motivation. Indeed, in the interviews we conducted, several peer counselors expressed the opinion that the lack of management support was largely to blame for the program's low utilization rate.

Union support

Alpha's labor union was highly involved and supportive of the program in its first months. However, triggered by a series of cases in which Alpha peer counselors helped employees with problems that the union deemed traditional union matters (e.g., scheduling shifts and conflicts with supervisors), the union's attitude toward the program changed and became antagonistic. Union representatives argued that the peer counselors' activity undermined their position and presented the union as weak and incompetent. It should be noted that in order to avoid such conflicts, clear guidelines prohibiting involvement of peer counselors in union matters were formulated before the program began operating. However, some of the peer counselors chose to ignore these guidelines because they did not believe in the union's ability to help employees and were concerned about disappointing those who requested help. Hostility between Alpha's peer counselors and the union was manifested both in the peer counselors' critical comments against the union, as well as in union representatives' attempts to interfere with several of Alpha's activities.

Beta's labor union was also involved in and supportive of the program at first, and took an active role in the steering committee. In fact, Beta's union was so enthusiastic about the program that one of its leaders volunteered to join the group of peer counselors. Despite the initial concerns of some peer counselors regarding potential conflicts of interest, no such conflicts emerged. However, after a few months, the union's involvement in, and advocacy of, the program declined for no apparent reason. Moreover, the peer counselor who was also a union representative withdrew from the program. Beta peer counselors speculated that the union's disengagement stemmed from the program's low utilization rate and the recognition that the program was not having the kind of impact that they had initially hoped for.

Additional activities

In addition to helping employees, peer counselors in both programs engaged in other activities aimed at improving employees' well-being and the general atmosphere in the organizations. These activities were also designed to improve employees' perception of the program and their positive reputation as a means by which to ultimately increase the program utilization rate. It is noteworthy that the employees in both organizations were free to choose among the peer counselors and consequently some peer counselors were never approached by any employees. For them, the additional activities were the sole opportunity to fulfill their desire to help their co-workers.

Given the high prevalence of help requests due to financial difficulties, Alpha's main additional activity was the collection of secondhand clothes, furniture, and baby equipment for needy employees. In order to help employees overcome their embarrassment when receiving them, such donations were stored in an isolated warehouse. Those in need of such resources were thus able to access them in a confidential manner. This project was an enormous success; it became the program's symbol in the factory, and was perceived by the employees as its main activity. Subsequently, the project was implemented in several other Israeli subsidiaries of the corporation. Several employees who left the factory and started working in other organizations also initiated similar donation projects in their new workplaces. Beta peer counselors tried to implement similar projects, but encountered difficulties in getting management approval for a room to be devoted to the storage of donations. Their solution was to transfer donations directly to employees with financial difficulties without giving recipients the option to choose what they needed in private. Alpha's peer counselors also collected donations of dry food packages for needy employees. Since the factory was producing food, the peer counselors had access to food products that were suitable for eating but not for sale (e.g., due to damaged packaging), and were also able to get similar products from some of the factory's subcontractors.

A further activity carried out by Alpha's peer counselors involved visiting employees absent from work for long periods due to chronicle illness or maternity. Each month, a human resource representative gave one of the peer counselors a list of relevant employees, and the peer counselors arranged shifts of home visits to these employees. The same activity was deemed unsuitable for Beta's peer counselors as it was feared that it would generate absenteeism among the hospital's workers. Instead, Beta's peer counselors visited mourning employees during the Jewish ritual *shiv'a'* (the seven days of mourning after the death of a family member).

Finally, peer counselors did not limit themselves to the direct provision of services or resources. In both enterprises, peer counselors organized events designed to increase awareness of the program's existence. Alpha's peer counselors arranged a series of in-plant workshops on topics such as family financial planning, adolescent substance abuse, and the early diagnosis of breast cancer. Employees were not charged for participating in these workshops. Moreover, they provided peer counselors with additional opportunities to encourage help-seeking and the utilization of their services. Similarly, Beta's peer counselors arranged for free tutoring services in math and English to be provided by employees for the children of fellow employees.

Discussion

Our aim in this chapter was to review the history of PAPs in the workplace, to examine their core technology and to provide a detailed description of how such programs were established and operated in a non-North American cultural context. Several conclusions can be drawn from the Israeli experience in applying the PAP technology. First, given the lack of literature on PAPs outside of the USA and the strong reliance of these programs on American voluntarism and mutual aid norms (DeToqueville, 1976), the Israeli experience provides unique empirical evidence on the feasibility of applying PAP overseas. Despite the several shortcomings of the Israeli PAPs highlighted in our description, their achievements illustrate that PAP technology is flexible and adaptable in accordance with local norms. This being the case, it is very likely that the prevalence of PAPs around the globe will continue to grow and local forms of PAP will emerge in other countries in the near future.

However, our observations with regard to Beta's low utilization rate and the Israeli peer counselors' self-help provisions, suggest that such programs are likely to be culture-bounded, and call for further understanding of the complexities involved in transferring this technology across cultures. The Israeli experience, in other words, suggests that while it is possible to implement the American PAP model in other countries, cross-cultural factors might limit its direct transferability, particularly with regard to peer counselors' perception of their role and responsibilities. In order to increase the likelihood of the program's institutionalization and survival and to extend its utilization and effectiveness, local practitioners should attempt to identify salient cultural differences prior to implementation, and ensure that they are reflected in the guidelines framing the program's establishment, the training and on-going guidance provided to peer counselors, and the material used to promote the program to the broader workforce.

Second, whereas American labor unions played a dominant role not only in establishing the programs, but also in operating them, the Israeli unions were either indifferent or antagonistic. Consequently, while the Israeli trade union movement may eventually recognize the potential offered by peer assistance as a basis for organizing and enhancing union–member relations, the programs that ultimately emerged in the two enterprises explored here may reflect a form of peer assistance that is not necessarily based on intense, union involvement. The ability of such peer-based programs to develop and grow despite the lack of union support suggests that employers may be able to initiate and support the development of peer-based assistance frameworks even in the absence of a trade union.

Third, on-going and intense management support appears to have been the critical factor explaining the difference between Alpha and Beta utilization rates. Indeed, our findings show that management support increased the motivation of peer counselors, and enabled them to engage in additional activities that ultimately strengthened the reputation of the program and improved its utilization rate.

However, management support should be provided with caution to avoid management being identified as the program's main sponsor. Such identification may jeopardize the program's success and sustainability since it undermines the basic concept of self-help among peers, raises suspicion regarding program confidentiality, and heightens employee concerns that the program serves simply as a mechanism of normative control.

Finally, by providing detailed descriptions of the measures taken to establish the programs, training session content, and the different program activities, we hope to begin bridging the gap between theories of social support and practical organizational interventions. While the literature is saturated with practical recommendations for the establishment and operation of management-based and professionally staffed EAPs, to the best of our knowledge, there is only a very limited literature regarding peer assistance in the workplace and the practical aspects of PAP establishment and operation (e.g., Bacharach et al. 2000). We are hopeful that this chapter will contribute to an understanding of such programs, encourage additional research, and help both occupational health scholars and practitioners diffuse this important work-based helping technology to enterprises and their employees around the globe.

Acknowledgements

We are grateful to Rachel Bar Hamburger, Ada Divon and Mickey Horowitz for their valuable contribution to this study. We also appreciate and respect the late Michal B. for being an exemplary peer-counselor. We acknowledge the support of the Smithers Institute for Alcohol-Related Workplace Studies and the Israel Anti-Drug Authority.

References

AFL-CIO. (1993). *Helping to overcome addiction: A union representative's guide for dealing with substance abuse.* Washington, DC: AFL-CIO.

Bacharach, S. B., Bamberger, P. A., & Sonnenstuhl, W. J. (1994). *Member assistance programs in the workplace.* Ithaca, NY: ILR Press.

Bacharach, S. B., Bamberger, P. A., & Sonnenstuhl, W. J. (1996). Member assistance programs: An emergent phenomenon in industrial relations. *Industrial Relations, 35,* 261–275.

Bacharach, S. B., Bamberger, P. A., & Mckiney, V. (2000). Boundary management tactics and logics of action: The case of peer support providers. *Administrative Science Quarterly, 45,* 704–736.

Bacharach, S. B., Bamberger, P. A., & Sonnenstuhl, W. J. (2001). *Mutual aid and union renewal: Cycles of logic of action.* Ithaca and London: Cornell University Press.

Bamberger, P. A. & Biron, M. (2006). The prevalence and distribution of employee substance-related problems and programs in the Israeli workplace. *Journal of Drug Issues, 36,* 755–786.

Bamberger, P. A. & Sonnenstuhl, W. J. (1995). Peer referral networks and utilization of a union-based EAP. *The journal of Drug Issues, 25,* 291–312.

Berridge, J., Cooper, C. L., & Highley-Marchington, C. (1997). *Employee assistance programs and workplace counseling.* Chichester: John Wiley & Sons.

Black, D. R., Tobler, N. S. & Sciacca, J. P. (1998) Peer helping/involvement: An efficacious way to meet the challenge of reducing alcohol, tobacco and other drug use among youth? *Journal of School Health, 68,* 87–93.

Blocker, J. (1989) *American temperance movements: Cycles of reform.* Boston: Twayne.

Blum, T., Fields, D., Milne, H., & Spell, C. (1992). Workplace drug testing programs: A review of research and a survey of worksites. *Journal of Employee Assistance Research, 1*(2), 315–349.

Bohart, A. C., & Greenberg, L. S. (1997) *Empathy reconsidered: New directions in psychotherapy.* Washington, DC: APA Press.

Buon, T. (2006). Non-English speaking countries, adjusting to cultural differences. *Journal of Employee Assistance, 36,* 27–28.

Buon, T., & Taylor, J. (2008). A review of the EAP market in the United Kingdom and Europe. *Journal of Workplace Behavioral Health, 23,* 425–444.

Cagney, T. (1999). Models of service delivery. In J. M. Oher, (Ed.), *The employee assistance handbook* (pp. 59–70). New York: John Wiley and Sons?.

Clawson, M. A. (1989) *Constructing brotherhood: class, gender, and fraternalism.* Princeton, NJ: Princeton University Press.

Commons, J., & Gilmore (1910). *A documentary history of American industrial society.* Cleveland: A.H. Clark Company.

Denenberg, T. S., & Denenberg, R. V. (1991). *Alcohol and other drugs: issues in arbitration.* Washington, DC: Bureau of National Affairs.

DeToqueville, A. (1976) *Democracy in America.* New York: Anchor-Doubleday.

DeYoung, P. A (2003). *Relational psychotherapy: A primer.* New York and Hove: Brunner-Routledge Press.

EAEF (2008). Employee Assistance European Forum. Retrieved from http://www.eaef.org/index.php?site=abouteaef

EAPA (2008). Employee Assistance Professionals Association. Retrieved May 2, 2009, from http://www.eapassn.org/public/pages/index.cfm?pageid=825

Ferguson, C., & Fersing, J. (1965). *The legacy of neglect.* Fort Worth, TX: Industrial Mental Health Associates.

French, M. T., Dunlap, L. J., Roman, P. M., & Steele, P. D. (1997). Factors that influence the use and perceptions of employee assistance programs at six worksites. *Journal of Occupational Health Psychology, 2,* 312–324.

Grossmark, R. (1999). Cultural diversity and employee assistance programs. In J. M. Oher, (Ed.), *The employee assistance handbook* (pp. 71–90). New York: John Wiley and Sons.?

Hartwell, T. D., Steele, P., French, M. T., Potter, F. J., Rodman, F. N., & Zarkin, G. A. (1996). Aiding troubled employees: The prevalence, cost, and characteristics of employee assistance program in the United States. *American Journal of Public Health, 86,* 804–808.

Hayghe, H. V. (1991). Anti-drug programs in the workplace: Are they here to stay? *Monthly Labor Review, 114,* 26–28.

Hopkins, K. M. (1997). Supervisor intervention with troubled workers: A social identity perspective. *Human Relations, 50,* 1215–1238.

Jacobs, J., & Zimmer, L. (1991). Drug treatment and workplace drug testing: politics, symbolism, and organizational politics. *Behavioral Sciences and the Law, 9,* 345–360.

Johnson, S. M. (2004). *The practice of emotionally focused couple therapy.* New York and Hove: Brunner-Routledge Press.

Kirk, A. K. (2005). Employee assistance program adoption in Australia: Strategic human resource management or "knee-jerk" solutions? *Journal of Workplace Behavioral Health, 21*(1), 79–95.

McCabe, J. (1992). Getting the word out. *EAPA Exchange,* January, 12.

McKay, J. (1993). Boston LAP program promotes expansion. *EAPA Exchange,* July, 10.

Maiden, R. P. (1998). EAP evaluation in a federal government agency. *Employee Assistance Quarterly, 3*(3& 4), 191–203.

Perlis, L. (1980). Labor and employee assistance programs. In R. Egdahl and D. C. Walsh (Eds.), *Mental wellness programs for employees* (pp. 78–84). New York: Springer-Verlag.

Perlow, A. (1979). *What have you done for me lately?* New York: Routledge.

Reddy, M. (2005). The once and future EAP. In D. Masi, (Ed.), *The international employee assistance compendium* (3rd ed.). London: Masi Research Consultants, Inc.

Roman, P. M. (1983). Employee assistance programs in Australia and the United States: comparisons of origin, structure and the role of behavioral science research. *The Journal of Applied Behavioral Science, 19,* 367–379.

Rogers, C. (1975). Empathy: An unappreciated way of being. *The Counseling Psychologist, 5,* 2–10.

Seeber, R., & Lehman, M. (1989). The union response to employer-initiated drug-testing programs. *Employee Responsibilities and Rights Journal, 2*(1), 39–48.

Sonnenstuhl, W. (1996) *Working sober: The transformation of an occupational drinking culture.* Ithaca, NY: ILR Press.

Sonnenstuhl, W. J., & Trice, H. M. (1987). The social construction of alcohol problems in a union's peer counseling program. *Journal of Drug Issues, 17*, 223–254.

Sonnenstuhl, W. J., & Trice, H. M. (1990). *Strategies for employee assistance programs: The crucial balance* (2nd ed.). Ithaca, NY: ILR Press.

Spell, C. S., & Blum, T. C. (2005). Adoption of workplace substance abuse programs: strategic choice and institutional perspectives. *Academy of Management Journal, 48*, 1125–1142.

Steele, P. D. (1995). Worker assistance programs and labor process: Emergence and development of the employee assistance model. *Journal of Drug Issues, 25*, 423–450.

Steele, P. D., & Trice, H. (1995). History of job-based alcoholism programs: 1972–1980. *Journal of Drug Issues, 25*, 397–422.

Tanaka, G., & Reid, K. (1997). Peer helpers: Encouraging kids to confide. *Educational leadership, 55*(2), 29.

Thompson, R. A. (2003). *Counseling techniques: Improving relationships with others, ourselves, our families, and our environment* (2nd ed.). New York & Hove: Brunner-Routledge.

Trice H. M., & Beyer, J. M. (1978). *Implementing change. Alcoholism policies in work organizations.* New York: The Free Press.

Trice, H. M. & Schonbrunn. M. (1984). A history of job-based alcoholism programs: 1900–1955. *Journal of Drug Issues, 11*, 171–198.

10

Individual Adaptation to the Changing Workplace
A Model of Causes, Consequences, and Outcomes

Jane D. Parent
Merrimack College, USA

Change is disturbing when it is done to us; exhilarating when it is done by us.
Rosabeth Moss Kanter

Many organizations are continuously implementing major changes to the way they do business in response to growing international competition, a changing workforce, increasingly complex and changing work environments, the global economic downturn, and other external pressures (Lawler, 1986; Manz, 1992; Ployhart & Bleise, 2006). As organizations strive to maintain their competitive edge, they are reorganizing, downsizing, outsourcing, shifting from manufacturing to knowledge-based work, and facing more competition than ever. With this, new and additional job demands are placed on individuals within these organizations. Large-scale change is a feature of today's work environment (Robinson & Griffiths, 2005). Also inevitable is the fact that employees must adapt to these constantly changing environments in order to survive and prosper. Development of a body of knowledge about managing change is an important priority for both academics and general managers (Beer, 1987; Saksvik et al., 2007). The need for adaptive workers has become increasingly important due to the fact that today's organizations are characterized by changing, dynamic environments (Ilgen & Pulakos, 1999; Pulakos, Arad, Donovan, & Plamondon, 2000).

This chapter analyzes the causes, consequences and outcomes of individual adaptation to a changing work environment. A theoretical model is introduced to broaden and refine our understanding of the process of adaptation to organizational change. This chapter also analyzes both individual differences and organizational factors affecting individual responses to change. The concept of an array of adaptive responses (dive, survive, revive, and thrive) is introduced to the theoretical research on organizational changes as well as the idea that better adaptors will experience better work outcomes.

Introduction

The question at the heart of much of the research on individual responses to change in organizations is why there is so much variance in individuals' response to change. Why do some individuals thrive on change and adapt to function at a higher level after an organization change? Why are there individuals at the other extreme of the spectrum that fail to adapt at all and, in fact, function at a much lower level (or exit an organization) after a change occurs? The purpose of this chapter is to explore the theory that there is an array of adaptive responses individuals experience when change occurs within their organizations, with a view toward making recommendations as to how managers and practitioners can facilitate organizational change. Many empirical studies have been conducted into responses to changes in organizations with regard to coping with change, being open to change, handling stress associated with change, the effects of positive and negative communication during change, perceptions of change, and adaptive and maladaptive responses to change (e.g., Ashford, 1988; Bellou, 2006; Bond, Flaxman, & Bunce, 2008; Bordia, Jones, Gallios, Callan, & Difonzo, 2006; Chan & Schmidt, 2000; Chang, 2006; Kirton, 1989; Kohler, Munz, & Grawitch, 2006; Moyle & Parkes, 1999; Wanberg & Banas, 2000; Watson & Chadwick, 2003). And while there have been numerous studies that review various aspects of change and the individual's response within the organization there are still conceptual and empirical gaps in the research on individual adaptation at work (Chan, 2000; Ployhart & Bleise, 2006).

This chapter broadens and refines our understanding of the individual's process of adaptation to organization change. Specifically, both internal (i.e., psychological) differences and external (i.e., environmental or organizational) factors that affect individual responses and that have an effect on a person's ability to change and thrive in organizations are investigated. Additionally, the idea that "better" adapters will be "better" performers in the workplace is examined. Further, the model developed seeks to apply the concept of thriving (change that leads to growth) to an organizational setting. The notion that changes in organizations can lead to individual growth and thriving is a concept that has not been explored in depth in the field of occupational health psychology.

Gaining insight into the causes, consequences and outcomes of individuals' adaptation to workplace changes is theoretically important to the occupational health psychology field for many reasons. This chapter combines literatures from both organization studies and psychology to gain better insight into the concepts of adaptability and thriving. The marriage of the theoretical literature about response to trauma (Janoff-Bulman, 1992; O'Leary & Ickovics, 1995; Scheier & Carver, 1992) provides a different framework from which to analyze how individuals adapt to organizational change.

This chapter suggests the expansion of previous empirical research conducted on adaptation to organizational change. Previous studies on individual adaptation to change have taken place surrounding newcomer adaptation (Chan & Schmitt, 2000), adjustment to a college setting (Aspinwall & Taylor, 1992; Brissette, Scheier, & Carver, 2002), and openness to change in a reorganizing workplace (Wanberg & Banas, 2000). This chapter seeks to expand on previous theory and research by providing examples of both individual attributes and context-specific organizational factors affecting the ability of a person to adapt to organizational changes. Most studies of individual adaptation have not included both individual and organizational factors. Context specific variables are potentially more malleable or responsive to organizational intervention efforts than dispositional variables. Managers and practitioners can gain valuable insight into the factors that affect one's ability to adapt to change making organizational change interventions more successful.

Adapting to Change

Organizational change can occur in varying ways. Change can come about in the form of a merger, an acquisition, or a reorganization. While most changes are designed and implemented to generate long-term benefits to both the individual and the organization, change is often perceived as stressful while it is taking place. Both good (process improvement, acquisitions, etc.) and bad (layoffs, reorganizations, etc.) changes necessitate adaptation for individuals. Change for individuals in organizations can mean a loss of power, as responsibility and accountability are shifted. It can also mean that critical relationships are lost as new patterns of interaction are demanded. More responsibility might be placed upon individuals at lower levels of the organization. Additionally, there are potential losses in rewards, particularly status and monetary rewards as power shifts, and losses in identity as the meaning people make of their work lives is threatened by changes in the organization (Beer, 1987; Saksvik, et al, 2007). Theory and past research suggest that change (whether positive or negative) is traumatic for individuals within an organization (Ashford, 1988; Burke, 1988; Callan, Terry, & Schweitzer, 1994, Kanter, 1983). Trauma is defined as an event or situation that causes great distress or disruption. The degree of trauma an individual experiences will depend on the nature of the change. In the psychological literature, there has been much discussion surrounding how traumatic events shatter our fundamental schemas (Janoff-Bulman, 1992). Schemas are characterizations of our primary assumptions about ourselves and about the world (Fiske & Taylor, 1991). These schemas will effect our interpretations of traumatic events. When trauma occurs, inconsistencies develop in our schemas. These inconsistencies force an individual to develop new "mini-theories" about the world. Change and adaptation occurs through reconstruction of our individual schemas (Janoff-Bulman, 1992). A person's ability to change and adapt will depend on how strong his or her beliefs (schemas) were prior to the change. In addition, how this cognitive process occurs in individuals will dictate how well they adapt to change (Janoff-Bulman, 1992).

In looking at change as trauma, we can associate individuals' responses to organization change in a similar fashion. Carver (1998) and Scheier and Carver (1992) advance a model of adaptive responses to trauma that can be incorporated within an organizational context. While researchers in the field of trauma attend to both physical and mental aspects of the individual faced with trauma, most agree that the key to thriving after a trauma occurs at the mental level and is not dependent on physical recovery (see Carver, 1998; Janoff-Bulman, 1982, 1992; Morgan & Janoff-Bulman, 1994; O'Leary & Ickovics, 1995).

Array of Adaptive Responses

Both Carver (1998) and O'Leary and Icovics (1995) assert that there are four potential responses to change/trauma. These four responses are to succumb, to survive, to be resilient, and to thrive (see Figure 10.1.). Most studies of individual coping or adaptation to organizational change have not included the concept of thriving. Most refer to the idea of coping as a return to the previous state or work level. In this chapter, the notion that there exists an array of adaptive responses, including not only the idea of coping with change, but the idea of thriving on change is advanced. Each state of change is described. Figure 10.2. depicts the potential change to an individual's performance over time after a change event.

Dive/succumb

At the lowest level of functioning, an individual will succumb to a change. The individual continues a downward slide in which the initial detrimental effect is

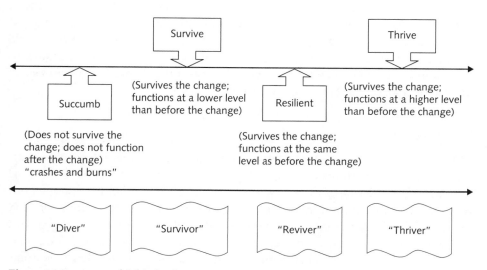

Figure 10.1   Array of Adaptive Responses

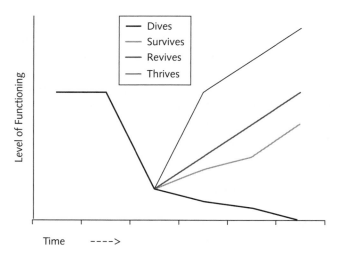

Figure 10.2   Responses to Organization Change

compounded and the individual eventually surrenders (Carver, 1998). Using an example of a person who experiences a heart attack, succumbing will result in death. The individual might suffer additional heart attacks or related health problems. In the organizational sense, the result is that the individual "crashes and burns" because they do not or cannot function after a change occurs. Ultimately, this individual will not be able to perform his or her duties at work and will exit the organization.

Survive/impairment

A somewhat better outcome of a traumatic event is survival, but with impairment. O'Leary (1992) describes survival as continuing to function, but in an impaired fashion. Using our heart attack scenario, an individual will survive the heart attack, but may not be able to complete tasks that he or she could before the attack. In an organization, this means that the individual survives the change but functions at a lower level than s/he did prior to the change.

Revive/resilience

At the next level, considered resilient, an individual survives the change with a decrement associated with the initial challenge then continues to function at the same level as before the change (O'Leary, 1992). After rehabilitation, for example, our heart attack victim will continue to play their weekly tennis match, go for walks, and generally have the same outlook on life at they did before the heart attack. Similarly, after a period of adjustment, our employee picks up where he or she left off, performing at the same level as before the change. No long-term harm has been done; no real gain has occurred either.

Thrive/grow

Finally, there are people who emerge from disruptive events and even traumatic events with newly developed skills that enable them to thrive (Carver, 1998). These individuals go beyond the original level of psychological functioning to grow vigorously and to flourish (O'Leary, 1992). To get through the experience successfully, they were forced to learn something they did not know how to do before. The individual does not merely return to a previous state, but rather goes beyond it, and in that process adds value to life (O'Leary, 1992). Thriving is a dynamic process of adaptation, influenced by numerous individual and social factors (O'Leary & Ickovics, 1995). Heart attack victims who alter their diet by making healthy choices now feel better than before the attack. They are able to exercise more as a result of learning about different food options. Within an organization, an individual embraces the change and learns some new skill (i.e., how to operate a new computer program) that allows him or her to be more efficient than before the change. This person is thriving within the organization and is ultimately what a manager seeks in an employee.

A portion of the literature on psychological thriving refers to reactions to traumatic physical events; that is, a person suffers a debilitating injury or illness. Of course, change in an organization is not physically debilitating, so making comparisons might seem a stretch. However, it is interesting to note that Carver (1998) and O'Leary and Ickovics (1995) both purport that psychological thriving is not dependent on physical thriving. In other words, thriving is a cognitive state which will fit a response to any type of trauma. Researchers agree also that successful adaptation to life changes is the most desirable outcome and will, in the long term, empower individuals to thrive (Morgan & Janoff-Bulman, 1994).

Influences on the Adaptive Response

It is desirable to have people in an organization who are resilient and who adapt to change in a positive manner. It therefore becomes important to understand the reasons why some individuals adapt to change better than others. Research on this matter is diverse and broad. Significant attention has been given to individual adaptability as a composite KSAO (Knowledge, Skill, Ability and Other characteristics) that takes on many forms in both proactive and reactive changes to an environment (Ployhart & Bleise, 2006). Adaptive responses to change by individuals are the result of both individual differences and the effects of certain situational events on the individual. Judge, Thorensen, Pucik, & Welbourne (1999) point out that most studies of change focus on the macro, structure-oriented, organizational level of the change. Interestingly, Judge et al. go on to say that the possibility that successful coping with change (i.e., adaptation) lies within the psychological predispositions of individuals experiencing the change has been largely neglected. A combination of variables will explain much of the variance in individual adaptive responses to

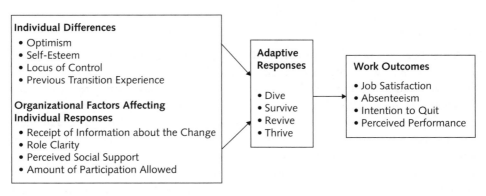

Figure 10.3   A Model of Adaptation to Organization Change

organization change. In a review of the research in this area, Chan (2000) marks this exact point by stating: "Researchers should consider individual differences and training or situational variables when conceptualizing and measuring individual adaptation" (p. 149). Indeed, much of the work on individual adaptation in the workplace has focused on certain individual differences; few studies have encapsulated the necessary variables that enable us to draw conclusions with regard to job performance. In their meta-analysis of planned organizational changes, Robertson, Roberts, and Porras (1993) call for a focus on a common set of individual behaviors to measure the effect of change. This chapter takes this into consideration and develops a model that gives comprehensive insight into individual behaviors with regard to adaptation. Based on a thorough review of the literature on change and adaptability, this model summarizes the key variables that affect an individual's adaptive response to change in an organization (see Figure 10.3). The remainder of this chapter focuses on describing the model in Figure 10.3.

Individual Difference Considerations

Optimism

Optimism is considered the generalized expectancy for positive outcomes to threatening events (Scheier & Carver, 1985, 1987). Optimism can yield benefits on what people do and what people are able to achieve in times of adversity (Scheier & Carver, 1992). It has been found that dispositional optimists display superior adaptation to medical stressors (such as coronary artery bypass surgery, childbirth, failed in-vitro fertilization, and HIV-positive status). Their hopeful view of the future stems from a positive interpretation of the present (Affleck & Tennen, 1996). Greater optimism has been found to be associated with less mood disturbance in response to a variety of stressors (Brissette, Scheier, & Carver, 2002). Optimism is also related to lesser amounts of distress during times of difficulty. There is substantial evidence that optimists use different strategies to cope than do pessimists and that these coping differences contribute to the positive association between optimism and better adjustment (Scheier, Carver, & Bridges, 2001).

Aspinwall and Taylor (1990) examined adjustments made by a group of undergraduate students in their first semester of college. Higher levels of optimism upon entering college were associated with lower levels of psychological distress three months later (cf. Brissette et al., 2002). Aspinwall and Taylor (1992) also found that optimism had a direct positive effect on subsequent adjustment to college. Scheier and Carver (1991) conducted a similar study on adaptation to college life. They, too, found that optimism was a significant predictor of changes in perceived stress, depression, loneliness, and social support over time. Across their first semester of college, optimists became less depressed, less lonely, less stressed and more socially supported then their pessimistic counterparts (Scheier & Carver, 1992).

Most researchers in the field agree that optimism is strongly linked to an individual's ability to adapt to change. Optimism bestows benefits on what people do and what people are able to achieve in times of difficulty or adversity. Brown and Marshall (2001) conducted a number of studies into the relationship between expectancies and performance. They found that individuals with high or medium expectancies of success (a construct similar to optimism) performed better than individuals with low expectancies in solving difficult problems. This allows for the proposition that *individuals with higher levels of optimism will demonstrate better adaptive responses to organizational changes.*

Self-esteem

Self-esteem can be defined as the evaluation that the individual makes and customarily maintains with regard to him/herself expressing an attitude of approval or disapproval (Coopersmith, 1967). It is also the extent to which an individual believes him/herself to be capable, significant, successful and worthy (Coopersmith, 1967). Self-esteem can also be described as the general approval of the self (Pierce, Gardner, Cummings, & Dunham, 1989; cf. Judge, et al., 1999). People with high levels of self-esteem are more resilient in the face of stressful events, because they are less vulnerable to the threatening self-relevant aspects of stressful events (Aspinwall & Taylor, 1992).

Several studies have focused on the relationship between self-esteem and organizational change. Folkman, Lazarus, Gruen, & DeLongis (1986) found a direct effect of self-esteem on adaptation to change on the part of employees. Their study addressed five different stressful situations individuals might encounter in their daily lives. In all situations, Folkman, et al. found that those individuals with higher self-esteem showed a greater ability to adapt to stressful situations. Additionally, Callan, Terry, & Schweitzer (1994) found significant, negative associations between self-esteem and levels of stress, anxiety, and depression among a sample of attorneys who perceived a high degree of change within their respective firms. Finally Aspinwall & Taylor (1992) found that individuals with higher levels of self-esteem demonstrated better long term college adjustment. Individuals with high self-esteem will experience lower levels of stress, anxiety and depression when faced with a high degree of change. This allows for the proposition that *individuals with higher levels of self-esteem will demonstrate better adaptive responses to organizational changes.*

Locus of control

Locus of control is the perception by an individual that he or she has the ability to exercise control over his or her environment. An individual who has an external locus of control tends to attribute work-related successes (and failures) to external causes such as luck or chance. An individual who has an internal locus of control will attribute successes (and failures) to his or her individual efforts. Rotter (1966) completed some early research into internal versus external locus of control for individuals in a series of lab experiments (with mostly college students as participants) designed to gain insight into the relationship between locus of control and resulting behaviors such as performance, achievement motivation, and resistance to subtle suggestion. Rotter summarizes the results of these experiments as follows:

> This research provided strong support for the notion that the individual who has a strong belief that s/he can control his own destiny (internal locus of control) is likely to (a) be more alert to those aspect of the environment which provide useful information for his future behavior; (b) take steps to improve his environmental condition; (c) place greater value on skill or achievement reinforcements and be generally more concerned with his ability, particularly his failures; and (d) be resistive to subtle attempts to influence him. (p. 25)

There have been many empirical studies on the relationship between individual locus of control and change indicating that it is a key factor associated with how an individual will adapt to a traumatic change. Research on locus of control has shown that individuals with internal control beliefs adapt better to stress than individuals with an external locus of control (Callan and Dickson, 1992). In a study of 100 lawyers experiencing organization changes, both self-esteem and locus of control were found to be directly related to their perception of well-being (in terms of lower anxiety and lower depression) after changes occurred (Callan, Terry, & Schweitzer, 1994). In a study involving 124 students, Johnson & Sarason (1978) found that participants who were external in their locus of control orientation experienced significantly greater anxiety and depression surrounding life changes. Further, Ashford (1988) found that feelings of personal control reduced transition-related stress among individuals in the marketing department of a regional Bell Telephone operating company. This allows for the proposition that *individuals with a higher internal locus of control will demonstrate better adaptive responses to organizational changes.*

Previous transition experience

Much of the theory surrounding previous transition experience and adaptability is within the context of newcomer adaptability and individuals entering unfamiliar organizations or situations (Jones, 1983; Louis, 1980; Nicholson, 1984). Nicholson's theory on work role transitions applies to many organizational change situations. For example, when an organization downsizes its staff, many of the people who remain in the organization must transition into new and different roles. New roles, through job redesign or promotion, almost always result when change occurs. Nicholson claims that the influence of prior socialization (having done it before) is an important force in shaping a person's adjustment strategy to a new work role.

Louis (1980) theorized about what newcomers experience on entering unfamiliar organizational settings. In discussing how individuals cope with surprise, she describes a sense-making process which includes the newcomers using past experiences of similar situations to help cope with their current situations.

There is some theoretical evidence that prior stressors may inoculate an individual against extreme trauma following negative life events. Janoff-Bulman (1992) suggests that the individual coping task is to reconstruct fundamental schemas (the shattered assumptive world) in the face of psychological breakdown and that individuals experiencing prior trauma will be able to reconstruct their schemas more effectively.

Although there is little empirical evidence supporting the idea that previous transition experience will positively influence adaptability, there is a strong theoretical case for its influence. In one study that involved job and home relocation, Martin (1995) found that employees showed elevated stress levels ten weeks after a job and home move, but the effect was moderated by the number of moves they had previously made. In other words, individuals who had prior experience changing homes and jobs demonstrated lower stress levels. This allows for the proposition that *individuals with previous transition experience in their current organization will demonstrate better adaptive responses to organizational changes.*

Organizational Factors

Receipt of information about the change

It has been shown that an individual's ability to respond positively to change is affected by how much information is available about the specific change. If adequate information about what specific changes will occur or how a given change will affect their job and organization is not provided, individuals may be uncertain how to respond to a change (Milliken, 1987). Organizational changes generate ambiguity about many things. Much of this uncertainty occurs because individuals do not receive adequate information about impending change. It is often this uncertainty about their futures that makes employees reluctant to adapt to change (Schweiger & DeNisi, 1991). Marks (1982) suggests that during major strategic changes, ambiguity is present surrounding potential terminations, transfers, and the need to survive under a potentially new management team. This ambiguity (resulting from a lack of information about the change) causes individual stress which in turn will have a negative impact on individual adaptation (Ashford, 1988).

Further, the type of information received about the change has an impact on one's ability to adapt to organizational changes. Receiving positive information about a change is likely to reduce the stress surrounding it (Bordia, Jones, Gallois, Callan, & Difonzo, 2006). In a study of positive and negative rumors surrounding change at a large public hospital, it was found that employees who reported having heard negative rumors also reported more change-related stress compared to those who reported having heard positive rumors and those who did not report having heard any rumors (ibid.).

In a longitudinal field experiment (Schweiger & DeNisi, 1991), employees in one plant received a planned program of information concerning a merger with another organization, and employees in a second plant received only limited information. They found that employees in the first plant experienced less uncertainty and perceived the company to be more trustworthy, honest, and caring than did employees in the second plant. In another longitudinal field study, Wanberg and Banas (2000) found that increased information for dealing with proposed changes was associated with greater change acceptance.

Additionally, London (1983) identifies several characteristics of changing organizational environments that enhance career resiliency, a construct similar to adaptability. Among these characteristics is openness of organizational communication. London advances the notion that organizations will create more career-resilient (adaptable) individuals through better communication. This allows for the proposition that *individuals who receive more information about a particular change in an organization will demonstrate better adaptive responses to organizational changes.*

Role clarity

Within organizational role theory (Katz & Kahn, 1978), roles within groups are considered to be a set of prescriptions that define the behaviors required of an individual member who occupies a certain position. Role theory is also often thought of as some combination of role conflict and role ambiguity. Role theory states that role ambiguity is the lack of necessary information available to a given organizational position (Kahn, Wolfe, Quinn, Snoek, & Rosenthal, 1964). Role conflict arises when differing expectations and differing demands are placed on a person's work role. It has long been theorized that as role ambiguity increases an individual's anxiety will increase as well (Rizzo, House, & Lirtzman, 1970).

The concept of role clarity arises from role theory as well. Role clarity reflects having sufficient information about the responsibilities and objectives of one's job in the broader organization and having knowledge of behaviors considered appropriate for achieving these goals (Kahn, et al, 1964). Role clarity provides a sense of direction and purpose to an individual's job (Kammeyer-Mueller & Wanberg, 2003). Role clarity reflects certainty about duties, authority, allocation of time, and relationships with others (Rizzo, et al, 1970).

Role clarity has been empirically tested in many ways. It has been considered an outcome of adjustment (Kammeyer-Mueller & Wanberg, 2003), a moderator in the relationship between job demands and psychological strain (Bliese & Castro, 2000), and an intervening variable mediating the effects of various organizational practices and organizational outcomes (Rizzo, et al., 1970). A recent study concerning the impact of specific sources of organizational change on the individual found that individuals who perceived a change in their job roles (and were clear about the change) also demonstrated lower perceived stress as a result of higher challenge appraisal (versus uncertainty appraisal) (Kohler, Munz, & Grawitch, 2006). In all of the above cases, role clarity is a measured perception of an individual. Role clarity will influence a person's ability to adapt to organizational changes. If individuals are clear on what their role is in the organization, they will better adapt to changes.

In one of the first empirical studies that systematically measured role conflict and role ambiguity, Rizzo et al. (1970) found that individuals who demonstrated higher role ambiguity (low role clarity) had more job-induced anxiety. They studied 290 salaried managerial and technical employees in a research and engineering division of large company. In addition, they found that individuals with greater role conflict had more somatic tension.

In a more recent study of 106 managers experiencing a downsizing, it was found that individuals with higher levels of role clarity demonstrated greater levels of organization commitment (Allen, Freeman, Russell, Reizenstein, & Rentz, 2001). An individual's increased commitment to the organization after a change such as a downsizing indicates that employees have adapted to the change.

In another recent study of enlisted male soldiers (n = 1,538) preparing for a training exercise, Bliese and Castro (2000) found that even when job demands were high (a stressful work environment), individuals with high role clarity demonstrated lower levels of job strain than individuals with low role clarity. High role clarity ameliorated the effects of work overload. Situations that involved work overload are similar to situations of change in organizations.

Finally, Kammeyer-Mueller and Wanberg (2003) found that role clarity was significantly positively related to organizational commitment in their 4-wave longitudinal study of 1,532 exempt employees recently hired to seven organizations (newcomers). Again, increased commitment to an organization is indication of higher levels of adaptability. This allows for the proposition that *individuals with higher levels of role clarity will demonstrate better adaptive responses to organizational changes.*

Perceived social support

In addition to individual factors, social resources contribute to how well or how poorly an individual will adapt to change (O'Leary, 1992). Individuals with greater social support are less likely to be affected by stressful events and are more likely to maintain good physical and mental health (ibid., p. 432). Social support is strongly associated with psychological well-being (Janoff-Bulman, 1992) and refers to the availability of another individual to turn to for information, affection, comfort, encouragement, or reassurance (Wanberg & Banas, 2000). There is much empirical evidence that supports the notion that social support is positively related to adaptability.

In a study of freshman students' adjustment to college, Aspinwall & Taylor (1992) found that students who sought social support throughout their first two years of college demonstrated a greater overall adjustment to college. Social support from all sources can be helpful to an individual attempting to cope with an organizational change that has an impact on his or her daily work life (Shaw, Fields, Thacker, & Fisher, 1993). In their study of 110 American Telephone and Telegraph employees undergoing a major organizational restructuring, Shaw and colleagues found that social support had a positive direct effect on job stressor and strain levels.

It has also been shown that although social support will decrease at the outset of an organizational change (Fugate, Kinicki, & Scheck, 2002; Moyle & Parks, 1999), it is an important coping resource for merger survivors throughout the various stages of a merger. In the context of organization change, research has shown that the availability of social support enhances worker's adjustment to a variety of stressors (Terry, Callan, & Sartori, 1996).

In a recent study of factors strongly related to personal adaptability, O'Connell, McNeely, and Hall (2008) found that managerial support was positively related to an individual's ability to adapt to broad industry changes. Their study focused on a small number of major employers in the nuclear production and maintenance industry. The changes noted were the move from government-sponsored to private installations. This allows for the proposition that *individuals who perceive strong social support during a change will demonstrate better adaptive responses to organizational changes.*

Amount of participation allowed

Participation refers to allowing individuals to have input regarding a proposed change. There is a growing body of research to suggest that encouraging participation with organizational changes will enable workers to adapt to these changes more constructively (Abbasi & Hollman, 1993; Raelin, 1984; Wanberg & Banas, 2000). Kotter and Schlesinger (1979, cf. Wanberg & Banas, 2000) stress that, to increase the acceptance of change, managers need to listen to employees' suggestions and heed their advice. Participant involvement from across and within different echelons of the organization breeds commitment and makes it easier to adapt to change (Abbasi & Hollman, 1993). In a theoretical examination of deviant versus adaptive behaviors in professional careers, Raelin (1984) points out that cutting an individual off from participation in groups will transform that person from being adaptive to being deviant. Further, in conjunction with the idea that more participation brings about more adaptation, we also know that participative goal-setting is positively related to higher rates of performance in work settings (Sagie & Koslowsky, 2000).

There is some empirical support of the notion that participation is positively related to adaptation. In their study of predictors and outcomes of openness to change (defined as change acceptance and positive view of changes) in a reorganizing workplace, Wanberg and Banas (2000) found that a higher level of individual participation was associated with a view that the changes to the organization would be beneficial. This allows for the proposition that *individuals who perceive greater amounts participation in an organization change will demonstrate better adaptive responses to organization changes.*

Work-Related Outcomes: Job Satisfaction, Absenteeism, Intention to Quit, and Perceived Performance

In order for the model described here to make a significant contribution to the study of organizational change, individual adaptability must be related to variables that are consequential and essential to both individuals and organizations. Successful adaptation to change will likely be manifested in a number of different work outcomes. The following is a review of both theoretical and empirical evidence that better adaptation to change is related to more favorable organizational outcomes.

Raelin (1984) presented a theoretical model of deviant/adaptive behaviors in the organizational careers of professionals. His model suggests that either deviant or adaptive behaviors arise when there are conflicting expectations between the organization and the individual. Conflicting expectations can arise when organizations undergo change. Adaptive behaviors are more desirable at all levels of inquiry (individual and organizational). He suggests that adaptive individuals are better performers on the job, are more satisfied with their work, demonstrate less absenteeism, and are less likely to quit the organization.

London (1983) described a theory of career motivation, a multidimensional construct composed of individual characteristics and career dimensions and behaviors. London proposed that the individual characteristics related to career motivation include career identity, career insight, and career resilience, a similar construct to adaptability as described in this literature review. He defined career resilience as "a person's resistance to career disruption in a less than optimal environment" (p. 621). London further suggests that more career-resilient individuals will demonstrate better quality work and better job performance. His model was, in fact, operationalized several times with confirming results (London & Bray, 1984; Noe, Noe, & Bachhuber, 1990; Wolf, London, Casey, & Pufahl, 1995).

Smollan (2006) theorizes that when employees believe that change will be beneficial they experience positive cognitions which lead to positive emotions surrounding the change. It is expected that employees will willingly engage in the tasks expected of them and may even attempt to exceed performance expectations. Further, in a recent study of organizational mergers and acquisitions, it was found that employees who felt able to effectively manage organizational changes believed that both organizational obligations and contributions had changed as a result of the merger or acquisition (Bellou, 2006).

In Schweiger and DeNisi's (1991) longitudinal field experiment with two plants involved in a merger, employees in both the experimental plant (receiving a realistic merger preview) and the control plant (receiving no formal communications concerning the merger) were surveyed before, during, and after the merger. Employees in the experimental plant were significantly lower on global stress and perceived uncertainty than employees in the control plant. Employees in the control plant exhibited significantly decreased levels of job satisfaction and self-reported performance. Individuals in the control plant also reported increased absenteeism and increased intention to quit the organization as a result of the changes occurring within their organizations. Employees in the experimental plant (who received information about the change) exhibited less of a decrease in job satisfaction, a significant decrease in absenteeism and intention to quit, and a significant increase in self-reported performance.

Individuals who can successfully adapt to change should experience more positive work outcomes. Wanberg and Banas (2000) found that a general attitude in favour of change, change acceptance and positive views of organizational change were positively related to job satisfaction. In a quasi-experiment analyzing psychological flexibility (a similar construct to individual adaptability) and work redesign, participants in the study who had higher levels of psychological flexibility perceived higher levels of job control and in turn experienced greater improvements in absence rates and general health after the work redesign (Bond, Flaxman, & Bunce, 2008). In another study examining the effects of pressure for change, Rush, Schoel, and Barnard (1995) collected data from 325 senior level employees working for various state government agencies. They found that pressure for change was linked to increased feelings of stress, subsequent job dissatisfaction, and intention to quit the organization.

For the purpose of this model, four work-related outcomes that the change literature indicates are related to an individual's ability to adapt to a change in their organization are included. They are job satisfaction, performance, withdrawal intentions, and absenteeism. Thus, our final proposition is that *individuals who demonstrate better adaptive responses to organization changes will demonstrate the following with regard to career outcomes: (1) higher job satisfaction, (2) lower withdrawal intentions, (3) lower levels of absenteeism, and (4) higher perceived performance.*

Conclusion

Today's work environment is driven primarily by economic and shareholder pressures to continue to improve the bottom line. Large-scale organizational change, whether in the form of mergers, acquisitions, restructuring, or downsizing is a widespread feature of today's unstable work environment (Robinson & Griffiths, 2005). Although change has been shown to adversely affect an individual's well-being and productivity, research at the individual level on how people adapt to change is not as prominent as macro-level research on organization change (Wanberg & Banas, 2000).

The objective of the model presented herein (Figure 10.3) is to explore the causes, consequences and outcomes of individual adaptation to organization change. At some point in our lives, nearly everyone experiences changes in their work situation.

Understanding of the process of individual change is critical to workplace success. The above model suggests that both individual differences and context-specific factors influence an individual's adaptive response. Given the right set of antecedents, individuals can thrive in the face of adversity and look upon change as a growth experience. The model suggests that it is well within the control of the organizations to enable successful change. Organizations can provide the right atmosphere for their employees by encouraging participation in change, providing ample communication about change, and generally promoting an environment of support and a culture of acceptance that change will be a normal occurrence, not an exception. To some extent organizations can also have an effect on some of the individual difference antecedents to adaptability as well. For example, providing clear communication about how employees' jobs will change will enhance both role clarity and a person's feelings of control (locus of control) over their job.

The review of theory and research on how individuals adapt to change leaves little doubt about the need for additional research in this area. The model outlined herein can be tested in organizations that are undergoing changes. Previous studies on individual adaptation to change have centered on newcomer adaptation (Chan & Schmitt, 2000), adjustment to a college setting (Aspinwall & Taylor, 1992; Brissette, Scheier, & Carver, 2002), and openness to change in a reorganizing workplace (Wanberg & Banas, 2000). Most studies on individual adaptation have not included both individual and organizational factors when studying this phenomenon (see for example, Ashford, 1988; Griffin & Hesketh, 2003; Judge, et al., 1999). This model can serve as a starting point for future research that measures both individual attributes and context specific organizational factors affecting the ability of a person to adapt to organizational changes.

Given that change will be ever-present in all forms of organization, it is imperative to continue both theoretical and empirical pursuits in this area. Scholars and practitioners need to gain greater understanding of how the change process in organizations functions at the individual level.

References

Abbasi, S. M., & Hollman, K. W. (1993). Inability to adapt: The hidden flaw of managerial ineptness. *ARMA Records Management Quarterly, 27*, 22–25.

Affleck, G., & Tennen, H. (1996). Construing benefits from adversity: Adaptational significance and dispositional underpinnings. *Journal of Personality, 64*, 899–922.

Allen, T. D., Freeman, D. M., Russell, J. E. A., Reizenstein, R. C., & Rentz, J. O. (2001). Survivor reactions to organizational downsizing: Does time ease the pain? *Journal of Occupational and Organizational Psychology, 74*, 145–164.

Ashford, S. J. (1988). Individual strategies for coping with stress during organizational transitions. *Journal of Applied Behavioral Science, 24*, 19–36.

Aspinwall, L. G., & Taylor, S. E. (1992). Modeling cognitive adaptation: A longitudinal investigation on the impact of individual differences and coping on college adjustment and performance. *Journal of Personality and Social Psychology, 63*, 989–1003.

Beer, M. (1987). Revitalizing organizations: Change process and emergent model. *Academy of Management Executive, 1*, 51–55.

Bellou, V. (2006). Psychological contract assessment after a major organizational change. *Employee Relations, 29*, 68–88.

Bliese, P. D., & Castro, C. A. (2000). Role clarity, work overload and organizational support: Multilevel evidence of the importance of support. *Work & Stress, 14*, 65–73.

Bond, F. W., Flaxman, P. E., & Bunce, D. (2008). The influence of psychological flexibility on work redesign: Mediated moderation of a work reorganization intervention. *Journal of Applied Psychology, 93*, 645–654.

Bordia, P., Jones, E., Gallois, C., Callan, V. J., & Difonzo, N. (2006). Management are aliens! Rumors and stress during organizational change. *Group & Organization Management 31*, 601–621.

Brissette, I., Scheier, M. F., & Carver, C. S. (2002). The role of optimism in social network development, coping, and psychological adjustment during a life transition. *Journal of Personality and Social Psychology, 82*, 102–111.

Brown, J. D., & Marshall, M. A. (2001). Great Expectations: Optimism and pessimism in achievement settings. In E. C. Chang (Ed.), *Optimism and pessimism: Implications for theory, research, and practice* (pp. 239–255). Washington, DC: American Psychological Association.

Burke, R. J. (1988). Sources of managerial and professional stress in large organizations. In Cooper, C. L. and Payne, R. (Eds.), *Causes, coping and consequences of stress at work* (pp. 77–114). Wiley: Chichester.

Callan, V. J. & Dickson, C. (1992). Managerial coping strategies during organizational change. *Asia-Pacific Journal of Human Resources, 30*, 47–59.

Callan, V. J., Terry, D. J., & Schweitzer, R. (1994). Coping resources, coping strategies and adjustment to organizational change: Direct or buffering effects? *Work and Stress, 8*, 372–383.

Carver, C. S. (1998). Resilience and thriving: issues, models, and linkages. *Journal of Social Issues, 54*, 245–263.

Chan, D. (2000). Conceptual and empirical gaps in research on individual adaptation at work. *International Review of Industrial and Organizational Psychology, 15*, 143–164.

Chan, D., & Schmitt, N. (2000). Interindividual differences in intraindividual changes in proactivity during organizational entry: A latent growth modeling approach to understanding newcomer adaptation. *Journal of Applied Psychology, 85*, 190–210.

Chang, E. C. (2006). Conceptualization and measurement of adaptive and maladaptive aspects of performance perfectionism: Relations to personality, psychological functioning, and academic achievement. *Cognitive Theory Research, 30*. 677–697.

Coopersmith, S. (1967). *Antecedents of self-esteem*. San Francisco: Freeman.

Fiske, S. T., & Taylor, S. E. (1991). *Social cognition*. New York: McGraw-Hill.

Folkman, S., Lazarus, R. S., Gruen, R. J., & De Longis, A. (1986). Appraisal, coping, health status, and psychological symptoms. *Journal of Personality and Social Psychology, 50*, 571–579.

Fugate, M., Kinicki, A. J., & Scheck, C. L. (2002). Coping with an organizational merger over four stages. *Personnel Psychology, 55*, 905–928.

Gow, K., & McDonald, P. (2000). Attributes required of graduates for the future workplace. *Journal of Vocational Education & Training, 52*, 373–394.

Griffin, B., & Hesketh, B. (2003). Adaptable behaviours for successful work and career adjustment. *Australian Journal of Psychology, 55*, 65–73.

Ilgen, D. R., & Pulakos, E. D. (1999). Employee performance in today's organizations. In D. R. Ilgen & E. D. Pulakos (Eds.), *The changing nature of work performance: Implications for staffing, motivation, and development* (pp. 1–20). San Francisco: Jossey-Bass.

Janoff-Bulman, R. (1982). Esteem and control bases of blame: "Adaptive" strategies for victims versus observers. *Journal of Personality, 50,* 180–192.

Janoff-Bulman, R. (1992). *Shattered assumptions: Toward a new psychology of trauma.* New York: Free Press.

Johnson, J. H., & Sarason, I. G. (1978). Life stress, depression and anxiety: Internal–external control as a moderator variable. *Journal of Psychosomatic Research, 22,* 205–208.

Jones, G. R. (1983). Psychological orientation and the process of organizational socialization. *Academy of Management Review, 8,* 464–474.

Judge, T. A., Thorensen, C. J., Pucik, V., & Welbourne, T. M. (1999). Managerial Coping with organizational change. *Journal of Applied Psychology, 84,* 107–122.

Kahn, R. L., Wolfe, D. M., Quinn, R. P., Snoek, J.D., & Rosenthal, R. A. (1964). *Organizational stress.* New York: Wiley.

Kammeyer-Mueller, J. D., & Wanberg, C. R. (2003). Unwrapping the organizational entry process: Disentangling multiple antecedents and their pathways to adjustment. *Journal of Applied Psychology, 88,* 779–794.

Kanter, R. M. (1975). *Men and women of the corporation.* New York: Basic Books Inc.

Kanter, R. M. (1983). *The change masters: Innovations for productivity in the American corporation.* New York: Simon and Schuster.

Katz, D., & Kahn, R. L. (1978). *The social psychology of organizations.* New York: Wiley.

Kirton, M. J. (1989). Adaptors and innovators at work. In Kirton, M. J. (Ed.), *Adaptors and innovators: Styles of creativity and problem solving.* London: Routledge.

Kohler, J. M., Munz, D. C., & Grawitch, M. J. (2006). Test of a dynamic stress model for organisational change: Do males and females require different models? *Applied Psychology: An International Review, 55,* 168–191.

Kotter, J. P., & Schlesinger, L. A. (1979). Choosing strategies for change. *Harvard Business Review, 57,* 106–114.

Lawler, E. E. (1986). *High-involvement management.* San Francisco, CA: Jossey-Bass.

London, M. (1983). Toward a theory of career motivation. *Academy of Management Review, 8,* 620–630.

London, M., & Bray, D. W. (1984). Measuring and developing young managers' career motivations. *Journal of Vocational Behavior, 3,* 3–25.

Louis, M. R. (1980). Surprise and sense making: What newcomers experience in entering unfamiliar organizational settings. *Administrative Science Quarterly, 25,* 226–251.

Manz, C. C. (1992). Self-leading work teams: Moving beyond self-management myths. *Human Relations, 45,* 1119–1142.

Marks, M. L. (1982). Merging human resources: a review of current research, *Mergers and Acquisitions, 17,* 50–55.

Martin, R. (1995). The effects of prior moves on job relocation stress. *Journal of Occupational and Organizational Psychology, 68,* 49–56.

Milliken, F. J. (1987). Three types of perceived uncertainty about the environment. *Academy of Management Review, 12,* 133–143.

Morgan, H. J., & Janoff-Bulman, R. (1994). Positive and negative self-complexity: Patterns of adjustment following traumatic versus non-traumatic life experiences. *Journal of Social and Clinical Psychology, 13,* 63–85.

Moyle, P., & Parkes, K. (1999). The effects of transition stress: A relocation study. *Journal of Organizational Behavior, 20*, 625–646.

Nicholson, N. (1984). A theory of work role transition. *Administrative Science Quarterly, 29*, 172–191.

Noe, R. A., Noe, A. W., & Bachhuber, J. A. (1990). An investigation of the correlates of career motivation. *Journal of Vocational Behavior, 37*, 340–356.

O'Connell, D. J., McNeely, E., & Hall, D. T. (2008). Unpacking personal adaptability at work. *Journal of Leadership and Organizational Studies, 14*, 248–259.

O'Leary, V. E. (1992). Strength in the face of adversity: Individual and social thriving. *Journal of Social Issues, 54*, 425–446.

O'Leary, V. E., & Ickovics, I. R. (1995). Resilience and thriving in response to challenge: An opportunity for a paradigm shift in women's health. *Women's Health: Research on Gender, Behavior, and Policy, 1*, 121–142.

Pierce, J. L., Gardner, D. G., Cummings, L. L., & Dunham, R. B. (1989). Organization-based self-esteem: Construct definition, measurement, and validation. *Academy of Management Journal, 32*, 622–648.

Ployhart, R. E., & Bleise, P. D. (2006). Individual adaptability (I-ADAPT theory): Conceptualizing the antecedents, consequences and measurement of individual differences in adaptability. *Advances in Human Performance and Cognitive Engineering Research, 6*, 3–39.

Pulakos, E. D., Arad, S., Donovon, M. A., & Plamondon, K. E. (2000). Adaptability in the workplace: Development of a taxonomy of adaptive performance. *Journal of Applied Psychology, 85*, 612–624.

Raelin, J. A. (1984). An examination of deviant/adaptive behaviors in the organizational careers of professionals. *Academy of Management Review, 9*, 413–427.

Rizzo, J. R., House, R. J., & Lirtzman, S. I. (1970). Role conflict and ambiguity in complex organizations. *Administrative Science Quarterly, 15*, 150–163.

Robertson, P. J., Roberts, D. R., & Porras, J. I. (1993). Dynamics of planned organizational change: Assessing empirical support for a theoretical model. *Academy of Management Journal, 36*, 619–634.

Robinson, O., & Griffiths, A. (2005). Coping with the stress of transformational change in a government department. *Journal of Applied Behavioral Science, 41*, 204–221.

Rotter, J. B. (1966). Generalized expectancies for internal versus external control of reinforcement. *Psychological Monographs: General and Applied, 80*, 1–28.

Rush, M. C., Schoel, W. A., & Barnard, S. M. (1995). Psychological resiliency in the public sector: "Hardiness" and pressure for change. *Journal of Vocational Behavior, 46*, 17–39.

Sagie, A., & Koslowsky, M. (2000). *Participation and empowerment in organizations*. Thousand Oaks, CA: Sage Publications.

Saksvik, P. O., Tvedt, S. D., Nytro, K., Andersen, G. R., Andersen, T. K., Buvik, M. P., & Torvatn, H. (2007). Developing criteria for healthy organizational change. *Work & Stress, 21*, 243–263.

Scheier, M. F., & Carver, C. S. (1985). Optimism, coping and health: Assessment and implications of generalized outcome expectancies. *Health Psychology, 4*, 219–247.

Scheier, M. F., & Carver, C. S. (1987). Dispositional optimism and physical well-being: The influence of generalized outcome expectancies on health. *Journal of Personality, 55*, 169–210.

Scheier, M. F., & Carver, C. S. (1991). [Dispositional optimism and adjustment to college]. Unpublished raw data for Scheier, M. F., & Carver, C. S. (1992). Effects of optimism on psychological and physical well-being: Theoretical overview and empirical update. *Cognitive Therapy and Research, 16*, 201–228.

Scheier, M. F., & Carver, C. S. (1992). Effects of optimism on psychological and physical well-being: Theoretical overview and empirical update. *Cognitive Therapy and Research, 16*, 201–228.

Scheier, M. F., Carver, C. S., & Bridges, M. W. (2001). Optimism, pessimism, and psychological well-being. In E. C. Chang (Ed.), *Optimism and pessimism: Implications for theory, research, and practice* (pp. 186–216). Washington, DC: American Psychological Association.

Schweiger, D. M., & DeNisi, A. S. (1991). Communication with employees following a merger: A longitudinal field experiment. *Academy of Management Journal, 34*, 110–135.

Shaw, J. B., Fields, M. W., Thacker, J. W., & Fisher, C. D. (1993). The availability of personal and external coping resources: Their impact on job stress and employee attitudes during organizational restructuring. *Work & Stress, 7*, 229–246.

Smollan, R. K. (2006). Minds, hearts, and deeds: Cognitive, affective and behavioural responses to change. *Journal of Change Management, 6*, 143–158.

Terry, D., Callan, V. J., & Sartori, G. (1996). Employee adjustment to an organizational merger: Stress coping and intergroup differences. *Stress and Medicine, 12*, 105–122.

Wanberg, C. R., & Banas, J. T. (2000). Predictors and outcomes of openness to changes in a reorganizing workplace. *Journal of Applied Psychology, 85*, 132–142.

Watson, S. L., & Chadwick, C. (2003). Perceptions and misperceptions of major organizational changes in hospitals: Do change efforts fail because of inconsistent organizational perceptions of restructuring and reengineering? *International Journal of Public Administration, 26*, 1581–1605.

Wolf, G., London, M., Casey, J., & Pufahl, J. (1995). Career experience and motivation as predictors of training behaviors and outcomes for displaced engineers. *Journal of Vocational Behavior, 47*, 316–331.

11

Building Psychosocial Safety Climate

Evaluation of a Socially Coordinated PAR Risk Management Stress Prevention Study

Maureen F. Dollard
University of South Australia, Australia.

Robert A. Karasek
University of Massachusetts Lowell, USA,
and Copenhagen University, Denmark

For several decades the climate of organizations has been driven by an economic rationalist calculus, while the costly consequences of compromised worker psychological health have been largely ignored (Dollard, 2007a; Johnson, 2008; Karasek, 2008). In this chapter we introduce a new construct called psychosocial safety climate (PSC), and describe how it can be developed in an organization to reduce psychological distress and injury. PSC refers to workplace "policies, practices, and procedures for the protection of worker psychological health and safety" (Dollard, 2007b). We argue that low PSC is a pre-eminent cause of work-related psychological distress. We discuss how PSC can be built in an organization to reduce workplace psychological distress and improve productivity outcomes. We argue that it could be built via the Healthy Conducive Production Model. Our conceptualization is drawn from Karasek's (2008) "associationist" Demand–Control Stress Disequilibrium theory. This is the idea that the impact of the stress burden results from the lack of control an individual has over the complex physiological coordination required to respond effectively. The solution is to impose higher level controls. We apply this idea at the level of the organization.

We outline a process whereby an organization can organize itself into higher levels of complexity, and in this way develop more effective alternative actions—which could yield benefits at all levels. This chapter illustrates an example of these general principles applied in the organizational behavior context (the original Stress-Disequilibrium theory formulation focuses on multi-level physiological responses). Benefits occur through the development of a social level collective that in turn builds the conditions for a strong PSC and then health productivity (conducive production). First, we delineate the construct of psychosocial safety climate contrasting it with related constructs to draw out what is uniquely important about PSC. We then sketch an outline of the Stress Disequilibrium theory, the "associationist" Demand–Control model, prior to looking at how resources from the external social and economic environment could combine with those available internally within the organization and through a socially coordinated process develop an "integrated solution," creating a higher level of complexity in the organization and—here relating to PSC—supporting new options for the reduction of stress at work for both the organization and the individual. Finally, we provide a case study that illustrates how a social structure can stimulate changes to policies, procedures, and practices in relation to psychological health (a so-called psychosocial safety climate). Interpretation of the empirical data in the results section is consistent with this stress-disequilibrium approach.

Psychosocial Safety Climate

For over 30 years a strong theoretical and empirical base has developed under the rubric of safety culture, or climate research, which describes, explains, and predicts how the (physical) safety climate in the workplace leads to physical injury, accidents, and errors (Zohar, 1980). The safety climate construct has utility in the field as building safety culture/climate helps organizations meet their occupational safety and health legal obligations. By contrast, a climate construct has not been identified specifically in relation to *psychological* health and safety.

Psychosocial risks at work are aspects of "work design and the organization and management of work, and their social and environmental contexts, which have the potential for causing psychological, social or physical harm" (Cox et al., 2000, p. 14). Psychosocial safety relates to *freedom* from psychological and social risk or harm. We see low PSC as the pre-eminent psychosocial risk factor at work capable of causing psychological and social harm through its direct effect on other psychosocial risk factors, or its moderating effect on psychosocial risk factors.

The general term organizational climate refers to "shared perceptions of organizational policies, practices, and procedures" (Reichers & Schneider, 1990, p. 20). Organizational climate research that uses molar approaches has been criticized as it is difficult to predict specific outcomes from broad climate constructs (Carr, Schmidt, Ford, & DeShon, 2003). Therefore, calls have been made to define elements of climate that are specific to the predicted outcome, for example, a climate for service or a climate for safety (Schneider, 2000). In our framework, PSC is a facet-specific subset of organizational climate, a climate for psychological health and safety.

Safety climate, a facet-specific component of organizational climate, refers to a climate for physical health and safety (Zohar & Luria, 2005). Evidence shows that safety climate is important for predicting individual safety behavior (Coyle, Sleeman, & Adams, 1995) and other important safety outcomes, such as perceived risk, industrial accidents, and injury to physical health (e.g., Silva, Lima, & Baptista, 2004). Despite its long and important history in relation to worker physical health, the safety climate construct does not appear to have been used explicitly to assess or promote policies, practices, and procedures in relation to psychosocial health and safety. Neither has it been used to articulate the reasons for the onset of accidents, incidents, or chronic exposures in the workplace that may lead to psychological or social injury.

Instead, Dollard and Bakker (in press) note that two separate research and practice literatures have emerged; safety climate literature, focusing on workplace climate, work systems, the environment and physical health; and work-related stress literature focusing on psychosocial risk factors and psychological health. Therefore PSC, because of its links to both areas, potentially unifies disparate lines of research.

The relationship between PSC and the team psychological safety construct (Edmondson, 1999) has been discussed elsewhere (Dollard & Bakker, in press). Theoretically, we see psychosocial safety climate as *causally prior* to psychosocial working conditions, such as organizational support and worker control, rather than as an outcome of them, as suggested in the psychological safety literature (cf. Kahn, 1999). The specific antecedents to psychological safety are not coherently theorized in psychological safety theory. In the literature, psychological safety in teams is an optional benefit to enhancing team and organizational performance (Edmonson, 1999). By contrast, psychosocial safety climate, like safety climate, may well be mandated legally, under duty of care provisions (See & Jhinku, 2002).

By defining a new psychosocial safety climate construct, we build on the foundational work of psychological safety and the safety climate literature, and hone in on the features of climate specifically expected to affect psychological health. We argue that psychosocial safety climate flows principally from the priority given by senior management to the balance of production imperatives versus concern given to the psychological health of the workers (Dollard & Bakker, in press).

According to Zohar and Luria (2005), even though organizations have formal policies, practices, and procedures, the best indicators of an organization's true priorities are the enacted counterparts. In the case study presented here, we examine how changes to policies, practices, and procedures implemented in work groups within schools as part of an organizational intervention affect work-related stress. We expect that perceptions of these activities at a group level and the perceptions of the process and progress of the implementation may be good indicators of an emerging psychosocial safety climate at the group or team level. This is the focus of the intervention evaluation. To provide the context, next we describe how PSC may be built at the organizational level.

How to Build PSC—A Multilevel Socially Coordinated Response

Recent research has emphasized a hierarchy of causes in relation to occupational health (Sauter et al., 2002). Efforts to build PSC within organizations could feasibly come from sources external to the organization, from the organizational level, or the team level. Theoretical and empirical research in the work-related stress literature has mainly focused on individual or job task domain causes of work-related stress (Kang, Staniford, Dollard, & Kompier, 2008). Accordingly, interventions are also pitched at these levels. However according to the logic of a hierarchy of causes, the "causes of the causes" (Marmot, 2008), the greatest impact should arise from targeting more distal causes. Therefore, building an intervention at an organizational level seems a promising option. An intervention at an organizational level may include monitoring and modifying working conditions and funneling resources where needed, filtering or gate-keeping overwhelming and unpredictable demands, and in turn building conditions that are conducive to healthy production.

In his treatise regarding the "associationist" Demand–Control model, Karasek (2008) argues that contemporary forms of economic and social organization may be associated with evidence of the increasing prevalence of chronic disease problems that may potentially be stress-related such as cardiovascular disease, mental disorders, and musculoskeletal problems. The reason given is that, very possibly, the work- and economic-system burdens may potentiate low control in social organizations (Karasek, 2008). Intervention is therefore required to coordinate or implement control at a higher level, so that it can have effects at a lower level.

Most of the traditional models of work-related stress posit a load-response pathway to describe the development of stress related illness. However the idea behind the "associationist" Demand–Control model is that the impact of the burden results from the lack of control an individual has over the complex physiological coordination required in response to increasing demands. According to Karasek (2008), physiological coordination has been pushed to extremes because of long-term exposure to stressors in the current global economy. The social policy implication is that diminished capacity for physiological coordination finally leads to chronic disease. The stress-disequilibrium component of the "associationist" demand–control perspective as applied here describes how development of higher levels of internal organizational order allows the organism to effectively deal with environmental demands—without damaging the "health" and stability of the lower level systems. Employees, work groups, and so on, can maintain their health in the face of strong external demands, e.g., competitive global markets or demanding parents within schools.

Using the same principles, we argue that at a higher level within the organization, a lack of coordination and resourcing of incoming demands could in turn lead to threats to individual workers' stable self-regulation—interfering with coordination of tasks, personal development, job stability, and work/family life at the individual level. Our proposed alternative is that a social collective structure at the organizational level ought to be created to control and coordinate incoming demands to help to build external social control, and theoretically to facilitate worker control and internal capacity for self-regulation without the worker being overwhelmed.

Perhaps more so than ever before, the platforms of stability outside an organization are being eroded or undermined by global economic phenomena (e.g., breakdown of the family) (Karasek, 2008). Therefore, it is argued that internal organizational level regulatory structures are required. Such systems have the potential to produce order in the environment, through the coordination of responses to demands, and thus decrease entropy in the environment (ibid.).

Karasek (2008) views the individual in the organization and in the environment as an energy based system, a series of flows. The theory draws on the second law of thermodynamics which asserts that all order in complex structures runs

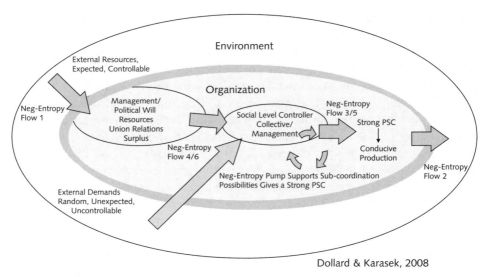

Dollard & Karasek, 2008

Figure 11.1   Healthy Conducive Production Model

downhill, so called increasing entropy. "Thermodynamic work is ordered energy with few degrees of freedom" (p. 121). To perform work an individual needs to convert disorganized energy into "structured responses." According to Karasek, "at work there are constant flows of energy or inputs that are constantly transformed into ordered action (work)" (ibid). Work is defined as "the purposeful and precise organization of the actions of the organism to meet unpredictable demands for action from the environment (external work)" (ibid).

In this chapter we argue that the effect of demands at the task level would be reduced if a social level controller was introduced into the system – with the goal of supporting a positive psychosocial safety climate (see Figure 11.1.). The idea is that foundational resources may become available from the external and internal environment, stemming, for example, from management political will, employee good will, financial surpluses, union support, trust, and other resources. These inputs need to be transformed from their uncoordinated form, through work, to outputs in terms of effective organizational performance, and especially in terms of the "state" of employees internal work environments. This could be achieved through a committee that is, for example, responsible for constraining the degrees of freedom of the disorganized energy, by designing specific sets of well-coordinated policies across levels and between departments, as well as practices and procedures to protect the psychological well-being of workers. These policies could relate to workload, profits, health programs, and return to work. In turn, these policies and ensuing procedures and practices reduce the chaos of disorganized and overwhelming demands (see bottom arrow, Figure 11.1), and actually create a reasonable number of feasible, alternative (and now well-supported) approaches. Participative democratic discussion at this point can ensure that the final multilevel solutions integrate worker contributions—and are consistent with moral goals for democratic engagement.

We see social coordination as an opportunity structure for social dialogue between competing interest groups (e.g., employers and employee representatives), and for providing political empowerment and voice particularly for those with the least power in organizations (e.g., those working at the coal face). Leka and Cox (2008) argue the urgent need for stronger social dialogue structures given the global market pressures for organizations to meet competing demands by adopting short-term economic goals, rather than longer-term sustainable work systems, that balance competitiveness with quality of work life. Social dialogue in this context is necessary for the development, implementation, and sustainability of stress prevention initiatives (developed in the social structure).

In accordance with Karasek's theory, the social structure acts as a negative entropy (NegEntropy) pump acting to create ordering capacity from random energy or "cheap" available disordered energy in the environment. As shown in Figure 11.1., when a higher social level controller is developed it can support a NegEntropy flow, which allows new action alternatives at the higher level, which in turn can be supportive of lower-level contribution. This implies that a new high-level structure is created which can support "stable function"—safe work environments—at sublevels. Subcoordination of demands at an individual level is possible because strong PSC is built through social coordination. Workers are freer to utilize their decision making authority which can then potentially directly affect psychological health or moderate the impact of demands (Karasek & Theorell, 1990). In turn, the efforts of the committee and the workers produce a NegEntropy flow to the environment, e.g., a new product or improved teaching, within the context of sustained well-being.

The notion that job demands can overtax or exhaust one's energy supplies is also discussed in other work-related stress theories, such as Job Demands–Resource (JD–R) theory. In JD–R theory the health impairment/erosion process is hypothesized when high or unfavourable job demands drain employees' energy resources and may lead to burnout *and in turn* to health problems (Schaufeli & Bakker, 2004). We argue that healthy conducive work means that performance must be maintained at humanely sustainable levels. Given the seemingly inevitable negative consequences of unremitting high demands, consideration must be given to the social regulation of demands, and the facilitation of control at higher levels in the organization.

Case Study

The aim of this case study is to describe the establishment of social structures that enabled the facilitation, development, and implementation of a participatory action research–risk management (PAR–RM) intervention to reduce stress. The intervention was based on a number of best practice principles identified as underlying successful work-related stress interventions and psychosocial risk management including: (1) a stepwise method; (2) the participation of workers; (3) risk assessment and task analysis; (4) context-specific interventions based on an accurate assessment of both individual and organizational factors rather than relying on pre-packaged, context-independent programs, and; (5) (top) management support (Cox et al., 2000; Jordan et al., 2003; Kompier & Cooper, 1999).

The intervention also used a participatory action research (PAR) approach. Applied to work stress prevention, PAR involves workers in a cyclic risk management process (PAR-RM) concerned with: (1) defining the issues or problems/ psychosocial risks; (2) developing the methodology and data collection to inform the problem (risk assessment); (3) making sense of the data; (4) defining interventions (risk controls); (5) helping to implement interventions, and; (6) evaluating the results (Wadsworth, 1998). PAR approaches involve active participation, collaboration, employee empowerment, and increased local knowledge (Dollard, le Blanc, & Cotton, 2008).

The second aim is to evaluate the impact of the intervention. Although we do not supply evidence to test explicitly this proposition, we argue that first and foremost the impact of an intervention is dependent on the social structures that enable it to occur (see Figure 11.2.). Thus, if an intervention is successful, by implication the social structures must have been conducive to the development of an effective intervention. Then the impact of the intervention itself could theoretically be due to the intervention having a specific effect on risk factors or stress outcome factors. Additionally, a net or global effect of a large-scale intervention involving employees, unions, managers, and facilitators may occur due to changes in the overall *climate* of psychosocial care as indicated by actions taken to modify policies, practices, and procedures that may relate to psychological well-being: observed changes; whether plans were being implemented; whether one's voice was listened to; and the extent to which trust was developed. In this chapter we focus on these *global* effects of the intervention, and argue that these are the fundamental components of PSC.

We view PSC as an organizational level resource (Dollard & Bakker, in press). As mentioned, the best indicators of PSC will be policies, procedures, and practices that are actually implemented. Therefore, the wider the spread of genuinely crafted actions implemented to address stress risk factors, the greater the evidence of the true priorities of the organization; in this case, its concern for the psychological well-being of the individual, thus PSC, should increase. We expect that over a 12-month period, distress and exhaustion would reduce for those who experience greater exposure to the intervention (more specific details of the intervention are provided below), because of the broad exposure to a range of new policies, practices, and procedures to reduce distress, as well as the reassurance of genuine care provided by the organization. We expect that workers operating in such a resource-rich climate characterized through the intervention process as "responsive", "listening", and "enabling trust to be developed" (Nielsen, Randall, & Albertsen, 2007), may be better able to offset or cope with the negative impact of core job demands articulated in Job Demand–Control theory (Karasek & Theorell, 2001). Two demands commonly identified as having a detrimental effect on psychological well-being are work pressure (Stansfeld & Candy, 2007) and emotional demands (Dollard, Skinner, Tuckey, & Bailey, 2007). These demands were key psychological distress risk factors identified in interviews with employees, and were subsequently used in the study. We hypothesized that:

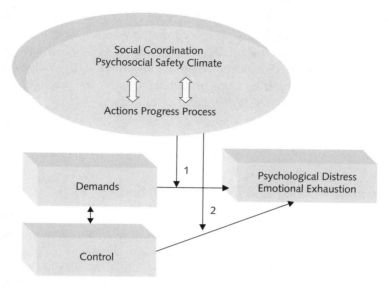

Figure 11.2   Study Model

Hypothesis 1. The positive relationship between high job demands and psychological distress/emotional exhaustion will be moderated by high levels of PSC (see Figure 11.2., path 1).

Specifically, we predicted that under conditions of low PSC the positive relationship will prevail whereas under conditions of high PSC the positive relationship will be significantly reduced. In a separate study of education workers we found that PSC, when operationalized explicitly, moderated the relationship between job demands and psychological distress (Dollard & Bakker, in press). In a second study of customer service interactions involving 46 German service employees of car dealers including 233 interactions, Zimmermann, Dormann, and Dollard, (2009) found that the positive relationship between negative customer behavior and employee well-being was moderated by PSC: when PSC was low, employees' negative affect increased more steeply when customers' behavior was negative compared to under high PSC conditions.

Participation in decision making has been commonly shown to be beneficial in reducing psychological distress (Dollard, et al., 2007; Mikkelsen, Saksvik, Erikesen, & Ursin, 1998). Yet in an environment characterized by a lack of care, workers may feel a level of risk in utilizing their resources fully. Specifically, when workers do not feel safe or protected, as in low-PSC contexts, they may be less willing to make decisions or exercise control (see also Edmonson, 1999). PSC may create an environment conducive to taking full advantage of job control characteristics available to workers. In conditions of high PSC, decision authority opportunities would be fully grasped. Thus we predict:

Hypothesis 2. The negative (beneficial) relationship between job control and psychological distress/emotional exhaustion will be evident under conditions of high PSC, but not under conditions of low PSC (see Figure 11.2., path 2).

In summary, this chapter theorizes that a higher level of social coordination of psychosocial risks may prove beneficial to worker psychological health. Specifically, it tests whether an intervention theorized to build PSC could reduce psychological health problems in Australian public sector education workers. We extend the results of a study reported by Dollard, Zapf, Dormann, Cox, and Petkov (forthcoming) that found support for the direct impact of exposure to actions on psychological health problems via job resources using a similar data set. Here we test possible multi-level moderation effects (Mathieu & Taylor, 2007).

Method

Organizational context and social coordination

The study was undertaken in an Australian state government Department of Education (DE). Work-related stress compensation claims in state public sector agencies accounted for approximately 20% of all claims between 2002 and 2003, and 23% between 2004 and 2005. In 2003, stress was identified as a key health and safety priority by a state government Occupational Health and Safety (OHS) Roundtable, which comprises senior executives of state government departments and agencies, unions, and the state government OHS regulator. The Roundtable initiated and provided resources for a primary stress prevention study in the DE which delivers both primary and secondary education.

A new social coordination and tripartite (employee, employer, regulator) structure was established for the project. Figure 11.3. outlines five social layers, the interrelationship between them, and the frequency of meetings. The five layers were: (1) the OHS Roundtable; (2) the Stress Stakeholder Committee (SSC), comprising senior representatives of the DE and unions, and the state government OHS regulator, that oversaw the implementation of the study and reported directly to the Roundtable; (3) the Stress Working Group, comprising representatives of the DE head office and regional department, unions, the state government OHS regulator, and the lead researcher and was responsible for implementing the study and reporting developments to the SSC; (4) the Regional Steering Committee (see below), and; (5) the Work Groups (intervention groups). Each social structure represented worker and management interests. The Regional Steering Committee (RSC) was established within DE and met bimonthly to oversee the implementation of the intervention within the DE organization. The committee assisted with local administration and communication, monitored and supported the implementation of actions, and helped resolve issues that were escalated from the workgroups (see below). The chair of the committee provided regular emails to staff in the intervention schools about the progress of action plans and overall progress of the project. The implementation of intervention actions by workgroups was monitored by the RSC and reported to the Stress Working Group over a 10-month period. In sum, the level of stakeholder participation was extensive, and involved all levels of the organization, employee representatives, and high levels of government. Social coordination took roughly 18 months of development before the baseline T1 survey was implemented.

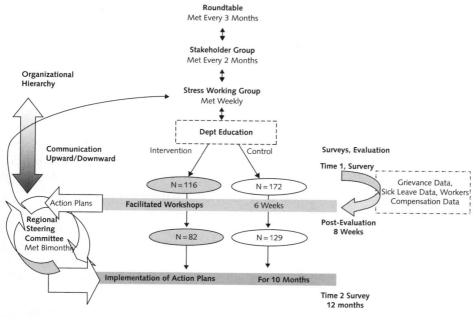

Figure 11.3   New Social Coordination-Tripartite Development

Participants

The study comprised a baseline ($n = 288$) and a postintervention measure ($n = 212$) 12 months later in a sample of DE workers in 18 different schools, within two geographical regions in an Australian state. Two separate geographic regions that could be matched in terms of the socio-economics of the student population were randomly selected as the experimental/intervention or the control region. Schools within regions were then matched as far as possible by their size and nature (e.g., high school, primary school). Volunteers were recruited as below, and were DE staff members, comprising teachers (80%) at all levels, e.g., principal, assistant principal, leading teacher, classroom teacher; and administrators (20%), e.g., school support officers, from 18 schools; 11 primary schools, 1 high school, 3 secondary colleges, 1 preparation to year 12 college, and 2 special schools. The number of participants in each school ranged from 6 to 24 in the intervention groups and 6 to 25 in the control groups. In total 9 intervention groups and 9 control groups from 18 different schools, representing a population of 1,342 employees in participating schools ($n = 655$ intervention; $n = 688$ control) participated in the study. Participants at Time 1 were: intervention ($n = 116$); control ($n = 172$); and at Time 2 were: intervention ($n = 83$) and control ($n = 129$). At Time 1, 74% of volunteers in both the control and intervention group, for whom consent forms were received, responded to the survey. At Time 2, 53% of volunteers in the intervention group, and 55% of the volunteers in the control group responded. There was no difference between the intervention and control group by employment classification.

As reported by Dollard et al., (forthcoming) gender proportions (80% female, 20% male) and age range 45–54 (50% intervention, 40% control) were representative of the DE&T, thus providing evidence of nonbiased sampling.

Design and procedure

Middle-level management support is a key ingredient for success in work-related stress management interventions (Kompier & Cooper, 1999). Therefore, seminars were convened for principals in participating schools to explain the study and seek their support and involvement. Volunteers were recruited via briefing sessions held throughout the two regions. Full ethics approval was obtained and confidentiality was assured. Volunteers were sent surveys, one prior to the intervention and one after the intervention, and the data was matched via identifiers. Next, some volunteers from the intervention groups participated in the intervention workshop process.

The intervention component of the study comprised two parts: (1) workshops, followed by (2) the implementation of actions incorporating changes to policies, practices, and procedures designed to target key psychosocial risks/issues identified by the participants.

Workshops. Workshops as described in Dollard et al., (forthcoming) were conducted within schools during the first 8 weeks of the project, and involved training participants in psychosocial risk management. An external professional facilitator with expertise in organizational psychology, or a related area, led these workshops. Each workgroup comprised study volunteers, managers, supervisors, teachers, and administrators. Within their schools, participants attended a maximum of 16 workshop hours (usually 4×4 hour sessions) within the 6-week period. Precise numbers of participants are not known, but estimates suggest that in excess of 55% of those in the intervention group ($n = 116$) participated. The interactive group sessions had the following output goals: to develop an action plan of practical measures to reduce identified risks; to specify reasonable time frames for actions to be put in place; and to identify the person/s responsible for ensuring actions were implemented to reduce risks. In the workshops, participants then triangulated data from a range of sources (e.g., aggregated grievance data, absenteeism records, and baseline Time 1 survey data) to identify potential school and organizational psychosocial risks of local significance.

Intervention. For the intervention, participants were asked to focus mainly on work and organizational psychosocial risks, rather than individual risks. Then they considered risks in the context of current management systems and employee support mechanisms available to them, and determined after accounting for these if there was any residual risk. This was done qualitatively by group consensus. To tackle work-related stress effectively a wide variety of interventions were implemented and these varied by group, according to the school action plans developed by school based work groups (Nielsen et al., 2007). Evaluation information was obtained from 63 participants immediately following the workshops (at eight weeks) and showed that participants agreed or strongly agreed with the following: 87% ($n = 52$, two missing) that the sessions were worthwhile; 89% ($n = 56$) that workshops improved their understanding of stress; and 82% ($n = 50$, two missing) that their understanding of risk management had improved. In survey two (post intervention at 12 months), 77% ($n = 43$) agreed that their workgroup was able to determine actions to address stress factors in the workplace. Note that it was *not* compulsory to attend the workshops to be able to participate in the baseline and postintervention surveys. The main intervention was assessed as exposure to actions, the progress, and process of the intervention, which we interpret as building PSC, not participation in workshops.

During the second phase of the intervention, the 10 months following the workshop, action plans developed by the nine intervention work groups were implemented. Actions were mainly implemented at the school level. All action plans were presented to the organizational Regional Steering Committee (RSC) by a liaison person nominated by each workgroup (see Figure 11.3.).

Prior to the Time 2 survey at 12 months, the Regional Steering Committee was asked to categorize or cluster all activities in the action plans into groups of related activities (see also Nielsen et al., 2007). Nine key "theme areas" were identified by content analysis of action plans by the PSC. For example, according to the RSC a key issue of concern was school discipline and standards. According to the RSC this issue was tackled by eight intervention schools as indicated in their action plans. Actions or changes to policy, practices, and procedures taken in relation to this issue of concern included: involving parents in the school; developing a code of conduct; conflict resolution training; staff safety; critical incident management; and identifying community-based supports. The nine key theme activity areas were: school discipline and standards, interpersonal demands, student welfare, role clarity, learning/professional development, workload/work organization, resources and facilities, health and well-being, and communication and consultation. These activity areas were included in the Time 2 survey so that exposure to these clusters of policy, practice, and procedure changes could be assessed.

In sum, using a PAR-RM approach, intervention groups participated in workshops to design and plan an intervention over a two month period. The content of the intervention was designed by participants themselves and targeted towards nine activity or cluster areas and was implemented over the following 10 months. The fundamental elements of PSC, operationalized here as exposure to the actions, the progress, and process of the intervention, was implemented in the nine areas and was evaluated at Time 2. In composite, this exposure, with three components, constituted the intervention. The control groups were not exposed to the intervention. Realistically in organizations the "intervention" is not even across the intervention groups. Some in the intervention group may not even receive the intervention, and therefore significant effects could be diminished because of this (for a discussion on this issue see the chapter by Nielsen, Randall, & Christensen in this volume). Consistent with organizational intervention analysis approaches that assess exposure rather than merely control versus intervention group effects (Randall, Griffiths, & Cox, 2005) we progressed using PSC gradient measures rather than the control versus intervention dichotomy measure.

Measures

As mentioned previously, the survey was used to assess key risks. Subscales of the Copenhagen Psychosocial Questionnaire (COPSOQ) were used for the psychosocial factors (Kristensen, Hannerz, Høgh, & Borg, 2005).

Work pressure was assessed using the 4-item subscale (e.g., "I have to work very fast"). Responses were on a 5-point scale, 1 (*strongly disagree*) to 5 (*strongly agree*) (Time 1, α = .75; Time 2, α = .77). Stability was r = .59, p < .01.

Emotional demands were assessed using the 4-item subscale (Time 1, α = .75; Time 2, α = .79). An example item is, "Does your work put you in emotionally demanding situations?" (= .73). Responses were on a 5-point scale, 0 (*very rarely / never*) to 4 (*very often / always*). Stability was r = .68, p < .01.

Decision influence was assessed using a 3-item subscale such as "Do you have any influence in deciding how to do your work?" Responses were on a 5-point scale, from 0 (*very rarely / never*) to 4 (*very often / always*) (Time 1, α = .62; Time 2, α = .68). Stability was r = .55, p < .01.

Psychological well-being. We used the GHQ-12 (Goldberg, 1978) (e.g., "Have you recently felt you couldn't overcome your difficulties?"). Typical responses were: 0 = *not at all*; 1 = *no more than usual*; 2 = *rather more than usual*; and 3 = *much more than usual* (Time 1, α = .78; Time 2, α = .79). The GHQ-12 is generally accepted as a valid and reliable measure of psychological impairment (Andrews, Hall, Teeson, & Henderson, 1999). Stability was r = .33, p < .01.

Emotional exhaustion. The MBI-exhaustion subscale was used (Schaufeli, Leiter, Maslach, & Jackson, 1996). We used two items from the 5-item scale (i.e., "I feel emotionally drained from my work"; and "I feel used up at the end of the work day"). Responses were scored on a 7-point scale, 0 (*never*) to 6 (*always, every day*). Inter-item correlations were: Time 1, r = .73; Time 3, r = .79. Good reliability and validity of the 2 items scale is reported in Dollard and Bakker (in press). Stability was r = .56, p < .01.

Psychosocial Safety Climate indicators. Three indicators of PSC were assessed only at Time 2.

1.   *PSC – Action exposure – continuous measure.* As mentioned, prior to the Time 2 survey the organizational working committee (RSC) reviewed all action plans to determine cluster activity areas where actions had been implemented by the work groups. Nine possible cluster themes were pre-identified by the commit-tee as outlined earlier. At the follow up Time 2 survey, participants were asked to tick activity theme areas where they perceived actions had been implemented in their workplace (more than one theme was allowed) (yes = 1, no = 0). We added eight items together (see Dollard et al., forthcoming) as a PSC indicator (action exposure scale). The control group was assigned to 0 on this scale. Responses ranged from 0 to 8.

2.   *Progress of implementation.* Two items were used to assess the extent of the implementation of the intervention: "To what extent are actions from your work group action plans being addressed in your workplace?"; "Based on your experience to what

extent has the stress study process led to change in your work environment?" Responses were given on a 6-point scale 0 (*not at all*) to 5 (*to a large extent*). The control group was assigned to 0 on this scale (Time 2, α = .75, inter-item correlation, r = .61).

3. *Process of implementation.* Two additional indicators were used: "To what extent have you been listened to in the stress project process?", and "To what extent has trust within the organization been built as a result of the stress project process?" Both were answered on 5 point scale, 0 (*to a very small extent*), to 4 (*to a large extent*). The control group was assigned to 0 on this scale (Time 2, α = .81, inter-item correlation, r = .70).

These 3 factors were considered as fundamental indicators of PSC.

Statistical Analyses

At Time 1 there were 288 participants and at Time 2 there were 212. To assess whether missing data gave rise to any bias in responses, we devised a dichotomous measure with 0 = participated at Time 1 only (n = 77), and 1 = participated at both Time 1, and Time 2 (n = 212). We regressed this on to the outcome measures of interest— psychological distress and emotional exhaustion at both Time 1 and Time 2. The results showed that at Time 1 F (2, 278) = .01, p =.99, and at Time 2 F (2, 207) = .84, p = .43, indicating that missing data was not due to psychological health status. Missing data was not related to gender or age (chi-square tests). In aggregate, the results suggest that the retained samples for Time 1 and Time 2 were not systematically biased in such a way as to affect the findings of our study. However the sizeable dropout rate and multilevel data, discussed next, indicated hierarchical linear modeling (HLM) as the most appropriate technique for data analysis. As HLM does not require listwise deletion of missing data as is required, for example, in repeated measures analysis of variance, it is a useful method to maximize utilization of data (Le Blanc, Hox, Schaufeli, Taris, & Peeters, 2007).

Our data was nested and evident at 2 levels; individuals were nested within schools. We used multilevel modeling (HLM) and the computer program HLM 6.06 (Raudenbush, Bryk, Cheong, Congdon, & Du Toit, 2004) to analyze all hypotheses. Dependent measures (psychological distress and emotional exhaustion), along with demands and control were at Level 1. Actions, progress, and process were aggregated at the school level and assessed at Level 2.

To test the hypotheses we first determined if sufficient between-group variance existed for cross-level moderation testing. We assessed the variation in the level 1 criterion variables, using analysis of variance and the intra-class correlation coefficient ICC (Bliese, 2000). For psychological distress at Time 1, F_{III} (17, 264) = 2.36, p < .05, and at Time 2, F_{III} (17, 192) = 2.02, p < .05, schools accounted for 9% of the variance, suggesting sufficient variance to proceed with multi-level analyses. For emotional exhaustion at Time 1, F_{III} (17, 264) = 1.98, p < .05, school variance was 5% and at Time 2, F_{III} (17, 192) = 2.37, p < .01, school variance was 10%, suggesting sufficient variance in emotional exhaustion to proceed with multilevel analyses.

Aggregation procedures

To assess whether perceptions of PSC actions could be meaningfully aggregated to the school level we used the James, Demaree, and Wolf (1984) mean $r_{(WG)(j)}$ agreement index to assess homogeneity of the global action measure at the group level. The mean $r_{(WG)(j)}$ was .81(SD = .37) representing adequate levels of agreement within schools and justification for aggregation. One-way random effects ANOVA, F_{III} (17,163) = 26.10, $p < .001$ was significant, indicating significant between group variance. Intra-class coefficient, ICC(1) was .7144 indicating 71.44% of the variance in actions could be explained by differences between schools. These results provide justification for aggregating the action exposure measure to the school level (Bliese, 2000) and potential support for the notion of action exposure as a climate effect.

To test the reliability and validity of this group-level action exposure measure we assessed the correlation between this self-reported exposure measure and evidence provided independently from the RSC that identified schools and actual actions implemented. When actions were aggregated to a school level and correlated with the RSC objective ratings of actions implemented in the school there was high concordance between measures, r (17) = .96, $p < .01$. In sum, the self report measures of actions implemented accords very highly with objective assessments of the intervention by the RSC.

For PSC progress, one-way random effects ANOVA, F_{III} (16, 81) = 2.59, $p < .01$ was significant, indicating significant between group variance. Intra-class coefficient, ICC(1) was .2036 indicating 20% of the variance in progress could be explained by differences between schools. For PSC process, one-way random effects ANOVA, F_{III} (16, 81) = 2.09, $p < .05$ was significant, indicating significant between group variance. Intra-class coefficient, ICC(1) was .2066 indicating 21% of the variance in process could be explained by differences between schools. Note, we did not estimate mean $r_{(WG)(j)}$ for PSC process and progress as values are largely dependent on the number of items, and each of these scales had only 2 items (Cohen, Doveh, & Eick, 2001).

The correlation between the aggregated measures of PSC were: actions with process, r (18) = .85, $p < .01$; actions with progress, r (18) = .92, $p < .01$; and process with progress r (18) = .39, $p = .06$ (1 tailed).

Results

The results in Table 11.1 show that at Time 1 the experimental group had higher levels of demands than the control group, and this was also the case at Time 2. This indicated that levels of demands did not change relative to the group (intervention versus control) over time. Levels of decision influence did not differ by group on either occasion. For GHQ and emotional exhaustion, at Time 1 the intervention group was significantly higher but at Time 2 there was no difference between groups. This suggested an intervention effect. Paired samples t-tests showed that there was a

Table 11.1   Means and Standard Deviations of Study Variables at Time 1 and Time 2

	Intervention		Control		
	M	SD	M	SD	t
Demands Time 1	11.95	3.10	11.08	3.62	2.11*
Emotional Demands Time 1	10.62	2.83	9.63	2.42	3.14**
Decision Influence Time 1	8.95	2.63	9.12	2.60	−.52
Psychological Distress Time 1	14.17	5.61	12.11	4.92	3.26**
Emotional Exhaustion	4.67	1.96	4.13	1.88	2.36*
Demands Time 2	11.58	2.56	10.83	2.68	2.01*
Emotional Demands Time 2	10.23	2.95	9.29	2.91	2.28*
Decision Influence Time 2	7.79	3.25	8.35	3.23	−1.29
Psychological Distress Time 2	12.31	6.99	11.95	5.80	.41
Emotional Exhaustion Time 2	4.23	2.10	3.73	2.96	1.71

Note. $*, p < .05$; $**, p < .01$, $n = 212$.

significant reduction in GHQ in the intervention ($p < .05$) but not the control group. For emotional exhaustion there was a significant reduction for the intervention group ($p < .05$) and for the control group ($p < .05$). Using GLM we confirmed that there was a Time X Group effect for GHQ, $F (1, 205) = 4.79, p < .05$ consistent with a significant intervention effect but not for emotional exhaustion.

Table 11.2. shows inter-correlations between variables at Time 1 and Time 2. Each work environment measure was significantly correlated with psychological health problems at either Time 1 or Time 2 confirming its status as a stress risk factor. Finally, there were few associations between the demographics (age, gender) and either the risk factors or stress outcomes so these are not reported further.

We tested Hypothesis 1, the two-way interaction effect of job demands X PSC indicators on Time 2 psychological health outcomes, controlling for Time 1 psychological health outcomes. No significant interactions were found. Therefore Hypothesis 1 was not supported.

We found conclusive evidence in support of Hypothesis 2. As shown in Table 11.3. (see also Figure 11.4.a–e), the relationship between decision influence at Time 2 and emotional exhaustion at Time 2, controlling for Time 1 emotional exhaustion, was significant and negative at high levels of action, high levels of progress and high levels of process. Alternatively, when actions were low, progress was low, or process was low the relationship between decision influence and emotional exhaustion was not as strong. In other words the intervention facilitated the beneficial impact of high levels of decision influence on psychological health. The interactions were also significant, and in the expected direction but not when the outcome was psychological distress, and the independent measure was actions.

In sum, the results indicate that PSC fundamental components facilitated the positive influence of decision influence in reducing psychological distress, and emotional exhaustion over time.

Table 11.2 Inter-Correlations

	1	2	3	4	5	6	7	8	9	10	11	12
1. Decision influence T1												
2. Work pressure T1	-.21**											
3. Emotional demands T1	-.07	.45**										
4. Psychological distress T1	-.21**	.37**	.32**									
5. Emotional exhaustion T1	-.12*	.49**	.48**	.57**								
6. Decision influence T2	.55**	.02	-.00	-.23**	-.03							
7. Work pressure T2	-.15*	.59**	.43**	.29**	.35**	-.18**						
8. Emotional demands T2	.01	.36**	.68**	.30**	.41**	-.03	.55**					
9. Psychological distress T2	-.27**	.14*	.17*	.33**	.24**	-.44**	.33**	.29**				
10. Emotional Exhaustion T2	-.08	.34**	.41**	.49**	.56**	-.26**	.54**	.57**	.44**			
11. Actions T2	-.04	.08	.16*	.23**	.09	-.01	.22*	.11	-.06	.05		
12. Progress T2	-.06	.10	.15*	.21**	.11	-.01	.16*	.11*	-.05	.09	.87**	
13. Process T2	-.02	.13*	.18**	.22**	.12	.00	.13	.18**	-.05	.09	.75**	.91**

Note. *, p < .05; **, p < .01, n = 212.

Table 11.3 Longitudinal Multilevel Random Coefficient Model of Main and Interaction Effects of School Actions, Process, and Progress with Decision Influence on Psychological Distress and Emotional Exhaustion

Actions	Psychological Distress T3	Emotional Exhaustion T3
Intercept	12.35 (.49)***	3.96 (.13)***
Dependent T1	1.79 (.43)***	1.20 (.15)
Actions X Dependent T1	−0.34 (.36)	−0.22 (.15)
Decision Influence T3	−2.42 (.39)***	−0.53 (.11)
Actions T3	−0.60 (.44)	−0.02 (.13)
Actions X Decision Influence T3	−0.55 (.37)	−0.27 (.15)*^

Progress	Psychological Distress T3	Emotional Exhaustion T3
Intercept	12.38 (.49)***	3.95 (.13)***
Dependent T1	1.80 (.41)***	1.20 (.11)
Progress X Dependent T1	−0.61 (.40)	−0.21 (.12)
Decision Influence T3	−2.43 (.39)***	−0.51 (.11)
Progress T3	−0.53 (.48)	−0.02 (.13)
Progress X Decision Influence T3	−0.85 (.43)*^	−0.34 (.12)**

Process	Psychological Distress T3	Emotional Exhaustion T3
Intercept	12.30 (.50)***	3.95 (.14)***
Dependent T1	1.70 (.42)**	1.19 (.11)***
Process X Dependent T1	−0.49 (.41)	−0.19 (.12)
Decision Influence T3	−2.45 (.39)***	−0.51 (.11)***
Process T3	−0.31 (.50)	−0.02 (.13)
Process X Decision Influence T3	−0.94 (.44)*	−0.33 (.12)*

Note. *^, $p < .10$; *$p < .05$; **, $p < .01$; ***, $p < .001$. The first value is the parameter estimate and the value in parentheses is the standard error. Actions, progress and process, all assessed at the School level.

Discussion

The aims of this chapter were to argue, theoretically, that: (1) a socially coordinated PAR-RM organizational approach provides the mechanism (structure and process) to reduce work-related stress and (2) the global impacts of a work-related stress intervention, the actions, process, and progress may provide fundamental elements of psychosocial safety climate. We tested empirically the moderating impact of PSC on the relationship between demands/ control on psychological health outcomes using a longitudinal exposure design.

We outlined how an intervention could be developed by applying Karasek's (2008) "associationist" Demand–Control Stress Disequilibrium theory for the first time to the level of the organization, and described and outlined a process about how an organization can organize itself into higher levels of coordination through the development of a social level collective, build a strong PSC and, in turn, build conditions that are conducive to healthy production. Then we looked at how resources from the

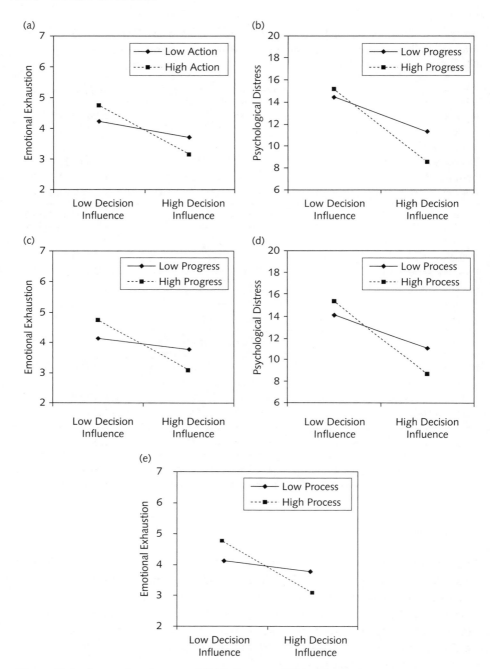

Figure 11.4   Interactions between PSC Indicators and Decision Influence

external environment could combine with those available internally and through a socially coordinated process develop a higher level of complexity and provide new options for the reduction of stress at work. These inputs and processes are encapsulated in the Health Conducive Production Model. Finally we provided a case study that illustrates how a social structure can theoretically stimulate changes to policies, procedures, and practice in relation to psychological health (so called psychosocial safety climate) and result in reduced psychological distress.

The socially coordinated PAR-RM intervention was intended to emulate best practice intervention principles and elements identified as essential ingredients for successful change (Kompier & Cooper, 1999). These elements we similarly identify as essential to build a strong PSC in organizations at all times.

We theorized that the mechanism through which to build psychosocial safety climate in an organization and reduce work stress ought to involve a socially coordinated structure. In this project such a mechanism involved the cooperation and participation of government, employers, unions, OHS regulators, and employees. Each of the five layers of coordination required specific inputs, monetary and time resources, political will, and good will. Through this social coordination, actions, progress, and process reflecting changes to policies, practices, and procedures were the outputs that potentially could reduce work-related stress. By definition, these outputs are the foundations for building a psychosocial safety climate. Theoretically, PSC can arise from the actions (what), progress (extent), and the process (how) of an organizational stress intervention. We believe that the socially coordinated structure provided an opportunity structure and mechanism through which the coordination of resources available internally and externally was created at a higher level of control (organization and school level), this then facilitated control at the task or individual level.

We showed, for instance, that the intervention effects worked by moderating the job characteristics—stress outcome relationship. Specifically we showed that high PSC (exposure to high actions, progress, and process) enabled the expected beneficial effects of the control—decision influence—to be realized. Note that the intervention did not increase levels of control, but rather facilitated its utilization. By contrast, when PSC was low the positive effects of high control levels were nullified. Therefore, changes in relevant practices, policies, and procedures may be particularly helpful in surfacing and facilitating the positive benefit of job control.

In sum, the results support the conclusion that when stress interventions are implemented using the principles of a PAR-RM approach significant change in stress outcomes may be achieved (see also Bond & Bunce, 2001; Landsbergis & Vivona-Vaughan, 1995; Saksvik, Nytro, Dahl-Jorgensen, & Mikkelsen, 2002). Our study, however, emphasizes the socially coordinated elements of the approach. We also add to the literature by verifying through objective RSC ratings that the intervention was actually implemented but noted that the extent of the intervention itself within intervention groups was variable. This justified looking at an exposure effect rather than assessing control versus intervention group effects.

Theoretical implications

We argued that the global effect of the PAR-RM intervention could be due to the development of a psychosocial safety climate, resulting from perceptions of actual evidence of psychosocial care provided by the organization to the employees, through concerted action, extent of actions, and the process utilized to tackle work-related stress and reduce worker psychological distress. Some evidence to suggest a climate effect of the intervention can be derived by: (1) noting that the global actions, progress, and process in this study all worked similarly and had a moderating impact on control when operationalized at a group level; and (2) the observation that numbers of actions implemented and the extent of the intervention were associated with qualitative components, specifically increased trust. This attests to the importance of the opportunity for upward communication in the organization and participation as key components in the socially coordinated intervention process (Jordan et al., 2003). The development of trust through the intervention process was reported by nearly 62% of participants in the original intervention group. This is an extremely important outcome of the intervention especially as in many large (Australian) bureaucracies trust between management and workers is severely lacking. Finally, top management support was evident in both supporting the research design and supporting the comprehensive participative intervention, another key ingredient of psychosocial safety climate.

Theoretically the study adds to our knowledge of intervention research, design and implementation, and risk management. By linking the theory of social coordination, risk management and PAR intervention (building trust and participation) to psychosocial safety climate we bring some theoretical coherence in relation to the intervention processes required and expected outcomes. Finally we bring this all together in the Model of Healthy Conducive Production.

Practical implications

The socially coordinated structure and process articulated here, enabling the PAR-RM approach, was evident in five layers. While some of the layers were time-limited and related to the project objectives, the organizational level structures continued as did the external Roundtable after the project finished. Research suggests that participatory work improvement methods need to be integrated to have long lasting effects (Mikkelsen, Saksvik, & Landsbergis, 2000). As such, the DE worked towards the integration of the work PAR-RM process for the prevention of stress into their occupational health and safety management practices. In other organizations similar structures may be identified that could be used for social coordination, for example, extant OHS committees, or the enterprise bargaining structure, or new structures could be built. The main starting ingredients are political will and a balance of ideals regarding productivity and psychological health. Then the social coordination of activities towards these goals could offset unexpected assaults to the system, and provide an organizational level control of these demands rather than expecting the individual to cope in isolation, leading to stronger PSC and healthy production. The principles of building PSC are also described in the chapter by Brooks, Staniford, Dollard, and Wiseman (this volume). In composite, what is built is a resilient system, able to adapt to or resist system challenges, that fosters resilience at both an organizational and individual level. Additionally, the outputs could unfreeze the potential to use job control at an individual level more effectively. Within the social structure at the group level, work teams with some education, training, and facilitation are capable of identifying and implementing actions to target risks and reduce work stress. Through the socially coordinated structures and processes they are able to communicate concerns, so that the voice of those in the front line may be heard at higher levels in the organization. Currently in many Australian workplaces the only way for workers to communicate about stress is through a formal legal workers compensation stress claim process.

Limitations and future research

There are some limitations in the study. The timing for evaluation was dictated by project resources; as such the evaluation may have been too early (10 months of actions). Problem-solving interventions may require 12 months or longer to show effects (Landsbergis & Vivona-Vaughan, 1995).

We did not directly assess PSC development as a result of the intervention, rather we inferred it from fundamental components, actions, progress, and process. Since Dollard and Bakker (in press), and Zimmermann et al., (2009) have shown moderating effects of PSC on the relationship between emotional demands and psychological distress we suggest that this hypothesis needs retesting. Specific before and after measures pertaining to psychosocial safety climate, its evolution, and change, and links with genuine attempts to address work-related stress issues would be beneficial in advancing the theory of PSC and stress intervention.

PSC could lead to direct changes in psychosocial risk factors. This was shown in the Dollard and Bakker (in press) paper: the relationship between PSC and psychological health problems was fully mediated by job demands and PSC also moderated the demands-psychological health relationship consistent with Hypothesis 1 in this study. As reported, Dollard, Zapf, Dormann, Cox, and Petkov, (forthcoming) found that the direct impact of exposure to actions on psychological health problems was via job resources. This latter effect could have been due to the substantive effects of actions or to a global effect resembling PSC. To disentangle the effects, future research should measure PSC as well as the impact of separate actions. One possibility that could reconcile the results of the studies is that extant PSC may have substantive effects through impacts on job demands, whereas change in PSC via an intervention may have more immediate effects on resources, both as a main and moderator effect.

Additionally, future research may evaluate whether participants have knowledge about the social structures (e.g., committees, specific policies) established for stress prevention. Participants' perceptions of committee achievements would also be of interest. In addition, it would be interesting to explore whether social dialogue regarding the stress problem leads to increases in understanding between committee members with diverse perspectives on the issue (see Ertel, Stilijanow, Cvitkovic, & Lenhardt, 2008). We know, for example, from the workshop participants that understanding of work-related stress and the risk management process improved and that their workgroups were able to determine actions to address stress factors in the workplace. Finally, we can conclude that the social structure of this intervention was successful, but we cannot draw conclusions about the most effective kind of social structure.

Conclusions

Our study adds to the literature by demonstrating the beneficial effect of a socially coordinated PAR-RM approach particularly by facilitating the positive benefits of decision making influence on psychological health outcomes. It adds to the results of a few studies conducted using longitudinal designs (e.g., Bond & Bunce, 2001) which show that participative work reorganization can lead to significant improvements in work-related psychological health outcomes. Few studies describe the social coordination underpinning the intervention. Second, it adds to a limited number of previous studies that demonstrate the *way* the intervention may work through PSC. Third the research is innovative in that it emphasizes organizational social coordination, and fundamental aspects of PSC. Fourth, it addresses a lack of organizational studies on work-focused interventions (primary prevention), and illuminates the quantitative and qualitative elements of the intervention (Mikkelsen & Gundersen, 2003; Randall et al., 2005).

The research enhances our understanding of the elements of the PAR-RM process that may lead to psychosocial safety climate phenomenon. These include management priority, communication, voice, participation, and trust. It shows that workers and managers can prevent work-related stress within the context of international best practice standards using PAR-RM techniques, and exemplifies the social coordination context. Finally we developed a new model, the Healthy Conducive Production model to illustrate the ingredients, and process required for sustainable production.

Acknowledgement

This research was funded by WorkSafe Victoria, Australia

References

Andrews, G., Hall, W., Teeson, M., & Henderson, S. (1999). *Mental health of Australians.* Commonwealth Department of Health and Aged Care: Canberra.

Bliese, P.D. (2000). Within-group agreement, non-dependence, and reliability: Implications for data aggregation and analyses. In K. J. Klein, & S. W. J. Kozlowski (Eds.), *Multilevel theory research and methods in organizations: Foundations, extensions, and new directions* (pp. 349–381). San Francisco CA: Jossey-Bass.

Bond, F. W. & Bunce, D. (2001). Job control mediates change in a work reorganization intervention for stress reduction. *Journal of Occupational Health Psychology, 6*, 290–302.

Carr, J. Z., Schmidt, A. M., Ford, K., & DeShon, R. P. (2003). Climate perceptions matter: A meta-analytic path analysis relating molar climate, cognitive and affective states and individual level work outcomes. *Journal of Applied Psychology, 4*, 605–619.

Cohen, A., Doveh, E., & Eick, U. (2001). Statistical properties of the rwg(j) index of agreement. *Psychological Methods, 6*, 297–310.

Coyle, I.R., Sleeman, S.D., & Adams, N., (1995). Safety climate. *Journal of Safety Research, 26*, 247–254.

Cox, T., Griffiths, A., Barlow, C., Randall, R., Thomson, L. & Rial González, E. (2000). *Organisational interventions for work stress: A risk management approach.* Sudbury: HSE Books.

Dollard, M. F. (2007a). Necrocapitalism: Throwing away workers in the race for global capital. In J. Houdmont & S. McIntyre (Eds.), *Occupational health psychology: European perspectives on research, education and practice* (Vol. 2) (pp. 169–193). Maia, Portugal: ISMAI Publishers.

Dollard, M. F. (2007b). *Psychosocial safety culture and climate; Definition of a new construct.* Work & Stress Research Group, University of South Australia, Adelaide.

Dollard, M. F., & Bakker, A. B. (in press). Psychosocial Safety Climate as a precursor to conducive work environments, psychological health problems, and employee engagement. *Journal of Occupational and Organizational Psychology.* doi:10.1348/096317909X470690

Dollard, M. F., le Blanc, P., & Cotton, S. (2008). Participatory action research as work stress intervention. In K. Näswall, J. Hellgren, & M. Sverke (Eds.), *Balancing work and wellbeing: The individual in the changing working life* (pp. 351–353). Cambridge: Cambridge University Press.

Dollard, M. F., Skinner, N., Tuckey, M. R., & Bailey, T. (2007). National surveillance of psychosocial risk factors in the workplace: An international overview. *Work & Stress, 21, 1–29.*

Dollard, M. F., Zapf, D., Dormann, C., Cox, T., & Petkov, J. (forthcoming). An exposure evaluation of a longitudinal PAR risk management stress prevention study.

Edmonson, A. (1999). Psychological safety and learning behavior in work teams. *Administrative Science Quarterly, 44*, 350–383.

Ertel, M., Stilijanow, U., Cvitkovic, J., & Lenhardt, U. (2008). Social policies, infrastructure and social dialogue in relation to psychosocial risk management. In S. Leka, & T. Cox (Eds.), *The European Framework for Psychosocial Risk Management* (pp. 60–79). Nottingham: I-WHO.

EU-OSHA (European Agency for Safety and Health at Work). (2002). *Systems and programmes: How to tackle psychosocial issues and reduce work-related stress.* Luxembourg: Office for the Publications of the European Communities.

Goldberg, D. (1978). *Manual of the General Health Questionnaire.* London: Oxford University Press.

James, L.R., Demaree, R.G., & Wolf, G. (1984). Estimating within-group interrater reliability with and without response bias. *Journal of Applied Psychology, 69*, 85–98.

Johnson, J. (2008). Globalization, workers' power and the psychosocial work environment—is the demand–control–support model still useful in a neoliberal era?, *Scandinavian Journal Work Environment and Health, Supplements, 6*, 15–21.

Jordan, J., Gurr, E., Tinline, G., Giga, S.I., Faragher, B., & Cooper, C.L. (2003). *Beacons of excellence in stress prevention.* Manchester: Robertson Cooper & UMIST.

Kahn, W. A. (1990). Psychological conditions of personal engagement and disengagement at work. *Academy of Management Journal, 33*, 692–724.

Kang, S. Y., Staniford, A., Dollard, M. F., & Kompier, M. (2008). Knowledge development and content in occupational health psychology: A systematic analysis of the *Journal of Occupational Health Psychology*, and *Work & Stress*, 1996–2006. In J. Houdmont & S. McIntyre (Eds.), *Occupational health psychology: European perspectives on research, education and practice* (Vol. 3) (pp. 27–62), Maia, Portugal: ISMAI Publishers.

Karasek, R.A., & Theorell, T. (1990). *Healthy work: Stress, productivity and the reconstruction of working life.* New York: Basic Books.

Karasek, R. A. (2008). Low social control and physiological deregulation – the stress-disequilibrium theory, towards a new demand-control model. *Scandinavian Journal of Work Environment and Health, 6*, 117–135.

Kompier, M. A. J., & Cooper, C. (Eds.) (1999). *Preventing stress, improving productivity: European case studies in the workplace.* London: Routledge.

Kristensen, T. S., Hannerz, H., Høgh A., & Borg, V. B. (2005). The Copenhagen Psychosocial Questionnaire–A tool for the assessment and improvement of the psychosocial work environment. *Scandinavian Journal of Work Environment and Health, 31*, 438–449.

Landsbergis, P. A., & Vivona-Vaughan, E. (1995). Evaluation of an occupational stress intervention in a public agency. *Journal of Organizational Behavior, 16*, 29–48.

Le Blanc, P. M., Hox, J. J., Schaufeli, W. B., Taris, T. (2007). Take care! The evaluation of a team based burnout intervention program for oncology providers. *Journal of Applied Psychology, 92*, 213–227.

Leka, S., & Cox, T. (2008). The future of psychosocial risk management and the promotion of well-being at work in the EU: A PRIMA time for action. In S. Leka, & T. Cox (Eds.). *The European Framework for Psychosocial Risk Management* (pp. 174–184), Nottingham: I-WHO.

Marmot, M. (2009, March). *Social inequalities in a globalising world of work.* Paper presented at the 29th International Congress of Occupational Health conference, Cape Town.

Mathieu, J., & Taylor, S. (2007). Framework for testing meso-mediational relationships in organizational behavior. *Journal of Organizational Behavior, 28*, 141–172.

Mikkelsen, A., & Gundersen, M. (2003). The effect of a participatory organizational intervention on work environment, job stress, and subjective health complaints. *International Journal of Stress Management, 10*, 91–110.

Mikkelsen, A., Saksvik, P. Ø., Eriksen, H. R., & Ursin, H. (1999). The impact of learning opportunities and decision authority on occupational health. *Work & Stress, 13*, 20–31.

Mikkelsen, A., Saksvik, P. Ø., & Landsbergis, P. (2000). The impact of a participatory organizational intervention on job stress in community health care institutions. *Work & Stress, 14*, 156–170.

Nielsen, K., Randall, R., & Albertsen, K. (2007). Participants' appraisal of process issues and the effects of stress management interventions. *Journal of Organizational Behavior, 28*, 793–810.

Randall, R., Griffiths, A., & Cox, T. (2005). Evaluating organisational stress-management interventions using adapted study designs. *European Journal of Work and Organizational Psychology, 14*, 23–41.

Raudenbush, S.W., Bryk A.S., Cheong Y.F., & Congdon, R. (2005). HLM6.01: Hierarchical Linear and Nonlinear Modeling [software]. Lincolnwood, Ill: Scientific Software International.

Reichers, A.E., & Schneider, B. (1990). Climate and culture: An evolution of constructs. In Schneider B. (Ed.). *Organizational climate and culture* (pp. 5–39). San Francisco: Jossey-Bass.

Saksvik, P. Ø., Nytro, K., Dahl-Jorgensen, C., & Mikkelsen, A. (2002). A process evaluation of individual and organizational occupational stress and health interventions. *Work & Stress, 16*, 37–57.

Sauter, S. L., Brightwell, W. S., Colligan, M. J., Hurrell, J. J., Jr., Katz, T. M., LeGrande, D. E., ... Tetrick, L. E. (2002). *The changing organization of work and the safety and health of working people* (DHHS [NIOSH] Publication No. 2002–116). Cincinnati, OH: National Institute for Occupational Safety and Health.

Schaufeli, W. B., & Bakker, A. B. (2004). Job demands, job resources, and their relationship with burnout and engagement: A multi-sample study. *Journal of Organizational Behavior, 25*, 293–315.

Schaufeli, W. B., Leiter, M. P., Maslach, C., & Jackson, S. E. (1996). *The Maslach Burnout Inventory—General survey test manual.* Palo Alto, CA: Consulting Psychologists Press.

Schneider, B. (2000). The psychological life of organizations. In N. M. Ashkanasy, C. P. M. Widerom, & M. F. Peterson (Eds.), *Handbook of organizational culture and climate* (pp. 7–21). Thousand Oaks, CA: Sage.

See, A., & Jhinku, S. (2003). Duty of care: Obligations of employers and others. In CCH Australia Ltd. (Ed.) Australian master OHS and environment guide (p. 118). Sydney: McPherson's Printing Group.

Silva, S., Lima, M. L., & Baptista, C. (2004). OSCI: An organisational and safety climate inventory. *Safety Science, 42*, 205–220.

Stansfeld, S., & Candy, B. (2006). Psychosocial work environment and mental health. A meta-analytic review. *Scandinavian Journal of Work and Environmental Health, 32*, 443–462.

Wadsworth, Y. (1998) *What is Action Research?* Action Research International, November 1998. Retrieved from www.scu.edu.au/schools/sawd/ari/ari-wadsworth.html

Zimmermann, B., Dormann, C., & Dollard, M.F. (2009). Reciprocity and stress in service interactions; Main and moderating effects of psychosocial safety climate. In P. H. Langford, N. J. Reynolds, & J. E. Kehoe (Eds.), *Meeting the future: Promoting sustainable organisational growth, 8th Industrial and Organisational Psychology Conference proceedings* (pp.150–155). Sydney: APS.

Zohar, D. (1980). Safety climate in industrial organizations: Theoretical and applied implications. *Journal of Applied Psychology, 65*, 96–102.

Zohar, D., & Luria, G. (2005). A multilevel model of safety climate: Cross-level relationships between organization and group-level climates. *Journal of Applied Psychology, 90*, 616–628.

12

Internet Addiction and the Workplace

Noreen Tehrani
Child Exploitation and Online Protection Centre, U.K.

This chapter looks at misuse of the internet in the workplace and identifies how using the internet has become one of the most powerful addictive activities to be found in the working environment. Whilst most people use the internet in moderation for business or personal ends, other people become totally preoccupied by its use. The breadth of information and material available on the internet is constantly growing, and what may begin as harmless fascination can become total dependence, with serious implications for individual and organizational health. The power of the internet to create behaviors, symptoms, and responses which are indistinguishable from those found in addicts of alcohol and drugs suggests that there may be a single addiction syndrome which links substance abuse to behavioral addictions such as excessive exercise, gambling, and internet usage. In the workplace, substance abuse is commonly treated as an illness, with employees who admit to becoming addicted to drugs or alcohol being offered an opportunity to seek treatment and support rather than a summary dismissal (CIPD, 2007). Employees addicted to the internet are generally treated differently, with organizations failing to recognize or respond to evidence that their workers are becoming addicted to social chat rooms, playing fantasy games, shopping, gambling, viewing pornography—or summarily dismissing them (CIPD, 2003). Whilst most internet addictive activities are within the law, an increasing number of employees are seeking illegal sexual contact with children or creating and viewing images involving the sexual exploitation of children on their employer's computers or storage equipment.

Occupational health psychologists have a role in the identification and treatment of emerging risks within the workplace. The dramatic growth of internet addiction suggests that this is an important area to understand if they are to provide useful support and guidance for organizations and employees who may find themselves affected by this phenomenon. This chapter provides some background information, describes interventions which may be utilized by occupational health psychologists when advising organizations on how to deal with internet addictions, and discusses how this information can be used by employees and organizations.

Background

The growth in use of the internet has been exponential. In 1989 there were around 500,000 internet users (Morahan-Martin, 2005), whereas today there are over 1.5 billion (IWS, 2008). Although the internet was originally designed to facilitate the communication of information within academia and the military (Young, 2004), the technology has received wide usage in the business and leisure domains. Today the internet is accessed by wide sections of the world's population: nationally the highest percentages of people using the internet come from North America (74%), Australasia (60%), and Europe (48%) (IWS, 2008). This rapid growth in the availability of the internet is encouraged by politicians and health workers across the world. Within the UK, for example, the government has made £300m available to provide free computers and internet access to children from low income families (BBC, 2008). Middle-aged and older people are encouraged to use the internet as a means of boosting brain power and counteracting dementia (Small & Vorgan, 2008). Despite these significant benefits there is growing evidence that the internet is adversely affecting the mental health and well-being of a small proportion of users who spend excessive periods of time using the facility (Young, 2004). In the workplace an increasing proportion of employees have access to the internet. Whilst many organizations have software to monitor and block internet access, many find that their workers are spending excessive periods of time browsing the web or accessing dubious or illegal websites thereby placing themselves and their organizations at risk. In the UK, nearly a third of organizations have dismissed staff for excessive or inappropriate use of e-mail or the internet (CIPD, 2003); however, a survey of firms undertaken by the Internet Watch Foundation (IWF, 2005) found that 74% of IT managers would not report staff guilty of accessing child sex abuse images to the police and 40% would not take steps to discipline or dismiss them. The ability of the internet to provide easy access to information, amusement, and social contact has proven irresistible to many people who find that they are spending the majority of their waking hours in this virtual world. This behavior has led to the view that some employees may have developed an addiction to their use of the web.

One of the tasks for the occupational health psychologist is to help organizations to identify the best way to train and educate its employees on the dangers of excessive internet usage, to recognize those employees who may become addicted to the internet and to provide counseling and support for employees wishing to deal with their internet addiction. To carry out their responsibilities, information technology and human resource managers need to understand the full implications of internet addiction and to develop clear policies and guidance on what constitutes acceptable use of the internet in the workplace. Perhaps more controversial is the need to consider whether internet addition should be regarded in a similar way to alcohol or drug addiction where the employee is likely to be offered therapy and support rather than automatic dismissal (Beard, 2005; Griffiths, 2000). However, organizations and therapists need to be aware that, when an employee's internet behavior involves child sex abuse, the organization has a duty to recognize its legal and moral responsibility towards the abused child by reporting this crime to the police. Signs of internet addiction can be difficult to recognize with the addict using a range of masking techniques to avoid detection. However, where the occupational health psychologist is aware of the possibility of this risk to employees and organizations, it becomes easier to introduce appropriate organizational and individual tools and interventions.

Internet Addiction

Around 20 years ago a researcher in the UK recognized that some, mainly male students, were becoming obsessively engaged with their computers (Shotton, 1989). Seven years later the concept of internet addiction was presented to a meeting of the American Psychiatric Association (Young, 1998). At that time the notion that people could become addicted to the internet was controversial (Morahan-Martin, 2005). Today there are some researchers who do not recognize the existence of a specific diagnosis of internet addiction as a psychiatric disorder in its own right (Yellowlees & Marks, 2007). Other researchers maintain the view that any extension of a diagnosis of addiction from one relating purely to the abuse of drugs and alcohol to a group of obsessive behaviors such as eating disorders, exercising, shopping, playing computer games, gambling, and viewing pornographic images trivializes the condition (Jaffe, 1990). Jaffe argues that use of the term "addiction" in relation to internet usage is not only inappropriate but also harmful in that it provides an opportunity for people to interpret their lack of behavioral control as a disease about which they can do nothing; in this way it may bring about an increase in the incidence of so-called addictive behaviors. Despite these reservations, there has been a call for internet addiction to be recognized as a psychiatric disorder (Block, 2008). There is also some evidence to support a biological basis to behavioral addictions. Neurological studies have found that the maintenance of substance addiction and behavioral addiction involves stimulation of the same systems in the brain (Albrecht, Kirschner, & Grusser, 2007), supporting the view that there is a common addictive syndrome. Within internet addiction a number of different types of addiction have been identified, based on (1) sex (addiction to pornography, pedophilia and adult chat rooms); (2) social relationships (online friendships, social networking, chatrooms); (3) gambling or trading (compulsive gambling, day trading or auction shopping); (4) information seeking (compulsive searching of the web or databases); or (5) compulsive games playing (Soule, Shell, & Kleen, 2003). However, internet users tend to adopt more than one of the internet addiction types (Song, Larose, Eastin, & Lin, 2004).

A meta-synthesis of research published between 1996 and 2006 (Douglas et al., 2008) identified several constructs associated with internet addiction including antecedents, addict profile, pull and push factors, negative effects, deviant behaviors, and control strategies. Douglas and colleagues identified a need for more practical research in the development of internet addiction theory. In order to understand internet addiction it is important to establish a criterion that differentiates between normal and pathological use of the internet. Of the diagnoses found in DSM IV (APA, 2000) it has been suggested that the one most appropriate to internet addictive behavior is the Impulse-Control Disorder (Young, 1998). This diagnosis covers a number of other behavioral addictions including psychological gambling, pyromania, and kleptomania. Using Young's criterion it has been estimated that between 6–10% of internet users exhibit symptoms consistent with a pathological use of the internet (Greenfield, 1999; Soule et al., 2003).

On this basis, psychological internet addiction would consist in persistent and recurrent nonessential computer/internet behaviors as indicated by five or more of the following during a 6-month period (Young, 1998):

- preoccupation with the internet (e.g. preoccupation with reliving past on-line activity or planning the next on-line session)
- needing to use the internet for an increasing amount of time to achieve satisfaction
- repeating unsuccessful attempts to control, cutback, or stop internet use
- becoming restless, moody, depressed or irritable when attempting to cut down or stop internet use
- staying on the internet as a way of escaping problems or of relieving a dysphoric mood (e.g. feelings of helplessness, guilt, anxiety or depression)
- staying on the internet longer than originally intended
- lying to family members, therapist or others to conceal the extent of the involvement with the internet
- breaking the Law or organizational requirement, regulation or procedures to engage with the internet
- jeopardizing or losing a significant relationship, job, or educational or career opportunity because of the internet.

The Internet Addict

A typical internet addict spends between 40 and 80 hours a week on nonwork-related internet activity causing a disruption to their sleep patterns, relationships, and physical well-being, with addicts taking caffeine and other stimulants to keep themselves awake during extended internet sessions (Young, 2004). The attractiveness of the internet to users has been increased by features inherent in the technology including the opportunity for personal anonymity, the possibility of creating and interacting as an "alter ego" freed from constraints of social or economic standing, age, gender, or culture, and the opportunity to communicate and form a relationship or community with likeminded people with the convenience of being able to log onto the internet at any time or location (Davies, Flett, & Besser, 2002). Addicted internet users have been found more likely to take emotional risks, be flirtatious, give positive and negative feedback to each other, to express ideas and take risks which they would be unable or unwilling to express in the real world (Greenfield,

1999; Niemz, Griffiths, & Banyard 2005). There have been attempts to identify vulnerability factors that are involved in the development of an internet addictive behavior. Grohol (2005) argues that many of those who spend excessive time on the internet do so to escape from life problems; he goes on to suggest that internet over-use typically follows a three-stage pattern: enchantment, disillusion, and balance, with a number of people becoming stuck in the first stage resulting in the development of an obsessional engagement or fixation. A study looking at the demographic characteristics of heavy internet users found that those who spend most time online were not married, were younger than other users, and there were no significant differences between the usage levels of men and women (Soule et al., 2003). Nevertheless, it is suggested that the way men and woman use the internet may differ, with women being more likely to spend time forming relationships in adult chat rooms whilst men prefer the visual stimuli of pornography websites (Cooper, Delmonico, & Burg, 2000). Excessive internet users have been found to experience problems in their academic, social, or personal relationships (Niemz et al., 2005) and to have lower self-esteem and be more socially inhibited. Chak and Leung (2004) found that heavy internet users tended to be shy with a strong external locus of control. This evidence suggests that people with a higher level of social confidence and a belief in having control over their lives are less likely to become addicted to the internet. One of the problems with current research is that of causal relationships: are people who are shy and isolated more likely to be attracted to the internet or does excessive internet activity cause people to become shy and withdrawn?

Criminal Internet Behavior

Interpol (2008) maintains a database of legislation enacted by member countries relating to the use of the internet for the purpose of sexual grooming, procuring or inciting a child to display him or herself sexually. In most countries these behaviors are against the law, as is the accessing, transmission, and downloading of sexual images of children. In March 2009, the European Commission adopted a proposal to protect children from grooming over the internet (see EU, 2009). In England, The Sex Offences Act (2003) updated previous sexual offences legislation by introducing the new offence of sexual grooming which made it a crime for an adult to befriend a child on the internet with the intent of sexually abusing them online or through facilitating physical contact. This amendment to the law also extended the age of protection for children from 15 to 17. The law defines making an indecent image as taking and transmitting photographs or films as well as the downloading of pictures or films made by others onto a computer hard drive or other data storage tool. People who engage in these activities, with the exception of those employed by a recognized organization such as the Child Exploitation and Online Protection Centre (CEOP), or specialist police units, break the law. In certain circumstances, IT managers are also allowed to copy images as evidence of illegal activity prior to informing the police. In the late 1990s credit card evidence was used for the first time to identify people who had downloaded child sex abuse images from a pedophile site. In the UK the tracking of these people was named Operation Ore (BBC, 2003); over 7,000 people were identified as having downloaded images involving the sexual abuse of children; those arrested included judges, magistrates, teachers, IT professionals, community workers, and police officers (O'Brian & Webster, 2007). The majority of those charged with sexually abusing children were British, white, well-educated men, mainly employed in nonmanual roles, with no previous criminal records. Whilst much of this activity took place in the privacy of the abuser's home it has been suggested (Gamble, 2005) that the viewing and downloading of internet child sex abuse images was increasingly taking place in the workplace with employees sexually grooming children, taking or obtaining images of child sex abuse on a work computer or laptop. Gamble suggests that the motivation for this is a fear of family members coming across evidence of child sex abuse activity on the home computer, together with the relative ease of engaging in these activities outside the home. Gamble further suggests that many people involved in the online abuse of children believed that the police are more likely to raid their homes to look for evidence of child sex abuse than to seize their company computer. The increasing potential to use organizational property in this criminal activity makes it more important for organizations to be aware of their responsibilities to monitor the way in which equipment is used by workers.

There is little research into whether someone who engages in viewing sexually abusive images of children is likely to progress to commit contact sexual offences against children. In a study of 201 men convicted of possessing, distributing, or producing child pornography (Seto & Eke, 2005) it was found that within 2½ years 17% of the men had reoffended and 4% had committed a sexual contact crime. The research found that men most likely to reoffend were those who had previously committed a sexual contact crime. In addition to viewing child sex abuse images, a significant number of people use the internet as a means of contacting children with the intention of grooming them to become available for online or contact sexual encounters. These offenders use a range of internet communication methods including instant messaging, email, and chatrooms to develop intimate relationships with children (Wolak, Finkelhor, & Mitchell, 2008). In many cases children are aware that they are conversing online with adults. Wolak and colleagues also suggest that as few as 5% of offenders pretend to be in their teens. In the UK it has been found that the likelihood of a child being contacted by an adult seeking sexual contact is high with around a third of children experiencing sexually explicit approaches from people online and one in twelve agreeing to meet a stranger following online contact (Livingstone & Haddon, 2007).

Assessment Tools

There are a number of assessment tools designed to assess problematic internet usage. One of the first was developed by Young (1998): the Internet Addiction Test (IAT), which is designed to help to identify internet addicts, assess the impact of the addiction on life, and to educate the public to recognize internet addiction in others.

Caplan (2002) created the Generalized Problematic Use Scale (GPUS), which was developed through a process of factor analysis, and includes seven dimensions that were then found to be highly correlated with psychosocial health including depression, loneliness, shyness, and self-esteem. Davis, Flett, and Besser (2002) developed the Online Cognition Scale (OCS) which measures procrastination, rejection, sensitivity, loneliness, depression, and impulsivity from which four factors emerge: diminished impulse control, loneliness, distraction, and social comfort. Davis and colleagues have proposed that their scale would be useful as part of a pre-employment screening program. An assessment tool has also been developed for assessing sexual offenders who access child sex abuse on the internet (O'Brian & Webster, 2007). The Internet Behaviors and Attitudes Questionnaire (IBAQ) has two factors: distorted thinking (e.g., I believe that all the children in the pictures I viewed enjoyed the experience) and problems in self-management (e.g., I feel panicky and anxious if I have not been able to view sexual pictures). O'Brian and Webster have used the IBAQ in the UK Prison Service to identify treatment approaches for convicted offenders. There has been little research into the pre-disposing factors leading to the use of the internet to abuse children. The evidence from Operation Ore and similar police investigations suggests that individuals engaging in the online abuse of children include successful business people and public servants rather than the socially inadequate loners predicted by researchers (e.g., Soule et al, 2003).

The Addiction Syndrome

Neurobiological evidence is growing to support the view that addictive disorders may not be independent but rather part of an underlying addictive syndrome (Shaffer & Hall, 2004). The same neurobiological systems are stimulated by both psychoactive drugs (e.g., alcohol, heroin) and behaviors (e.g., internet, gambling, sex), and are moderated by dopamine, a neurotransmitter linked to the brain's reward system (Betz, Mihalie, Pinto, & Raffa, 2000). This evidence suggests that regardless of the object of addiction the neurobiological circuitry is common. This finding is supported by evidence to show that the same genetic molecular mechanism is implicated in drug addiction and compulsive exercise (Werme, Lindholm, Thoren, Franck, & Brene, 2002). Twin studies have shown that there is no genetic evidence to indicate a specific genetic risk for a particular addiction but, rather, a general tendency towards addiction exists that can vary in its expression (Karkowski, Prescott, & Kendler, 2000).

Research has shown that circumstances play a much greater part in the choice of addiction than the addictive object itself (Shaffer & Hall, 2002). Hopping between addiction objects has been demonstrated in drug users, alcoholics, obsessive shoppers, gamblers, and internet users. Frequently an addict will appear to be recovering from an addiction only to be found engaging in another addictive behavior, activity, or substance. Figure 12.1. illustrates this tendency in a model of multiple addictions. At the centre of the model is the individual's pre-existing vulnerability to addictive

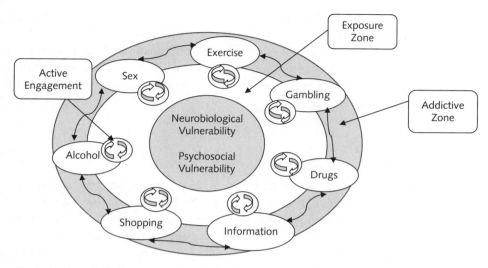

Figure 12.1   A Model of Multiple Addictions

behavior that is determined by two kinds of factor: (1) physically determined neu-robiological factors, and (2) environmentally determined psychosocial factors. It is possible that these two factors interact; recent findings demonstrate the plasticity of gene expression occurring in individuals who have experienced sexual or physical abuse in their early life (McGowan et al., 2009). However, not everyone with a pre-disposition to addiction becomes addicted; the addictive behavior requires a second stage to occur in which the individual actively engages with a particular addictive source responsible for creating the addictive behavior. Depending upon the nature of the source of the addiction, a number of barriers or detractors may become involved. These can include a range of fears such as that of detection or ridicule. In addition, there may be emotional barriers such as guilt and shame. These detractors will need to be counterbalanced by motivators such as personal or sexual gratifica-tion, together with the experience of power and excitement. For many addictions the entry is relatively easy as the barriers are relatively low. For example, in the case of internet shopping the activity can be justified on the basis of convenience or choice before it develops into an expensive and time consuming obsession. On the other hand, illegal addictions such as viewing child sex abuse images typically involve a more difficult entry with the individual having to deal with feelings of guilt and fear of detection. These powerful detractors require a much higher level of motiva-tion to allow the initial exposure to develop into a desire which is strong enough to facilitate progression into a full blown addiction.

The multiple addiction phenomena has an important role in reducing entry bar-riers because established addictive behaviors can act as the mechanism for introduc-ing or developing other addictions. For example, an addiction to alcohol or drugs can reduce the sensitivity to guilt or fear, thus allowing the individual to engage in risky levels of gambling or shopping or even in criminal acts. Multiple addictions can also be seen as ways of "managing" addictions with addicts switching between addictions, combining addictions to intensify gratification, or masking one addiction with a more socially acceptable alternative. For occupational health psychologists and organizations it is important to recognize the possibility of multiple addictions with, for example, the alcoholic or gambler becoming addicted to other, perhaps more serious, addictions.

Crime or Illness?

Whilst there is recognition of the need to provide treatment, support, and counseling for people with alcohol or drug addictions this is not always the case for people with more complex behavioral addictions where the impact of the addiction on the individual and relationships can be equally damaging. It is generally recognized that excessive exercise, shopping, social networking, drinking, and gambling can be bad for health and that taking hard drugs, drink-driving, and viewing child sex abuse images constitute a breaking of the law. Is there a point at which people should be regarded as sick rather than wicked, criminal, or feckless? It would seem that some addictions are more socially acceptable than others and that the focus on substance abuse as the only credible addiction stands in the way of the development of integrated programs to educate and treat the underlying addictive condition. Much of this argument is being carried out in the courts of law. For example, in the UK, a man fired by IBM for logging onto an adult chat room sued his employer for £2.6m on the basis that he deserved treatment and sympathy rather than dismissal (*The Times*, 2007). The claimant argued that IBM workers with an alcohol or drug problem would be able to enter a substance abuse recovery program to help them, and he thought that he deserved to have the same level of support. However, in order to provide support for addicted employees it is important to know what is happening regarding their internet usage and to be able to monitor that usage. Unless this is clearly spelt out in an organizational internet policy, these preventative measures can be challenged, as occurred in a case involving an employee of Carmarthenshire College, Wales, who was awarded £9,000 damages and costs by the European Union Court of Human Rights because her emails and internet usage had been monitored by the vice-principal who believed that she had been excessively using college resources for personal reasons (Out-Law, 2007). Equally, organizations with monitoring capacity within their internet policy need to undertake an appropriate level of monitoring. In the case of a New Jersey (USA) employer, the court ruled that organizations have a duty to investigate employee internet activities and take prompt action when the organization's policy is breached. The case involved an employee who was using his company computer to access pornography. The employee was arrested in 2001 and when his computer was investigated it was found to contain sex abuse pictures of his stepdaughter which he had been secretly filming and placing on the internet. The child's mother sued the organization for the harm caused to her daughter. The Judge found that because the organization had an internet policy which provided it with the right to monitor employees' internet activities and clearly stated that employees were only permitted to access sites which were of a business nature, they had failed in their duty to apply their own policy that would have prevented the downloading of child sex abuse images.

The Internet and the Workplace

The internet has revolutionized business, and the rapid increase in its use has taken some organizations by surprise. Whilst the internet provides important benefits it also creates major challenges for unwary employers. Addicted employees become increasingly impulsive and prone to taking excessive risks (Potenza, 2007). Employees addicted to substances or behaviors including excessive internet usage are liable to behave in ways that can put the organization, themselves, and others at risk. Therefore, it is important to make sure that wherever possible vulnerable employees are identified and the harmful aspects of their addiction addressed.

A survey of 305 employees (Hyman, 2002) showed that 24% of workers used the internet during their working hours for shopping, 18% for accessing pornography, 8% for gambling, and 6% for buying and selling on e-bay. A survey of companies (Clearswift, 2007) found that social media sites were widely used, especially by younger employees, with 71% of 18–29-year-old office workers in the UK accessing social media sites from work a few times a week, 39% accessing these sites several times a day, and up to 27% spending half a working day a week on these sites. However, it is possible that, with the increasing popularity of social networking sites over the past 2 years, these estimates fail to provide an accurate indication of the scale of usage. In addition, almost a third of UK workers have been found to discuss work-related issues on a social networking site. The amount of time that employees spend accessing these sites has a significant impact on productivity and may lead to the accidental or intentional disclosure of company information. The Clearswift survey also found that although companies were aware of the popularity of social media sites, a substantial number (19.5%) were not taking any action to protect themselves by educating their workers, or by maintaining a best practice policy with written guidelines on using the internet, including the social networking sites. Although many companies have the capacity to monitor employee internet usage, over a third with this capacity do not do so. The result is that they have no knowledge of whether they have lost confidential corporate information. The Clearswift survey found the top five computer security concerns reported by IT managers in the UK were: (1) the introduction of computer viruses, (2) loss of confidential corporate information, (3) damage to the organization's reputation, (4) harassment of colleagues, and (5) downloading of pornography. It is interesting to note that loss of productivity was not mentioned, suggesting that many IT managers and organizations are unaware of the loss of time due to personal internet activities.

Online pornography was one of the first industries to take advantage of the internet and has been shown to account for around 70% of the time spent online. Most of the internet pornography traffic occurs during working hours, suggesting that people are likely to be accessing these sites at work (Griffiths, 2003). Internet gambling has gained popularity with a rapid growth in opportunities for gambling in the workplace with a large number of internet sites dedicated to the activity. Gambling sites make it easy for customers to pay for their services by credit card; as a result many people find themselves with massive debts. A survey in the UK by the CIPD (2004) found that 71% of organizations had dealt with an employee who had downloaded child sex abuse images in the previous 2 years and 54% of managers were unaware of their legal responsibilities for dealing with illegal images. With the increase in sex-related internet crime, organizations need to be aware that there is a legal requirement to report any employee suspected of engaging in any aspect of sex-related internet crime, particularly when it involves young people and children. The CIPD survey found that most large organizations have the technology to prevent child sex abuse images being downloaded via the web or attached to emails, however nearly 70% had not installed technology to prevent child sex abuse images being downloaded or accessed from memory sticks or DVDs. One of the important provisions within the Sexual Offences Act 2003 (retrievable from www.opsi.gov.uk/ACTS/acts2003/en/ukpgaen_20030042) involved the protection that it provides for IT managers. As mentioned previously, the Act introduced a conditional defense which protects IT professionals who, as part of their day to day management of electronic networks and services, may need to make or download and store potentially illegal child sex abuse images as evidence to be assessed by the police or a body such as CEOP. This defense was included in the Act as a means of reassuring IT professionals, who may need to identify and secure such data for evidential and investigative purposes, that they can do so without the fear of prosecution. However, IT professionals would not be protected should they engage in random, casual or deliberate viewing of child sex abuse images. This could lead to a prison sentence of up to 10 years (IWF, 2004). The prosecution of an employee is also likely to have a significant impact on the employer. This would be particularly true where the employee's role gave access to children. In a British case, a swimming instructor was jailed after he had been found to have downloaded hundreds of child sex abuse images onto his work computer (Journal Live, 2006). Similarly, an IT specialist working for an insurance company was found to have viewed abusive images of young girls in his place of work (*The Argus*, 2008). In both cases wide press coverage caused significant damage to the reputation of the employer.

Writing a Policy

A good starting point for any organization is to have a comprehensive internet policy that includes a statement on the purpose and role of the policy, i.e., to (1) protect the organization and the workforce from misuse of the internet, and (2) ensure that maximum value and benefit can be derived from use of the internet. It is essential that any restrictions to internet use and sanctions that apply as a result of improper usage are clearly communicated so that there can be no misunderstanding in regard to what would happen if an employee breached any of those restrictions or requirements. Table 12.1

identifies the areas that an organization should consider when developing a policy. The establishment of an internet acceptable use policy provides a framework which deters employees from using the internet inappropriately (Ugrin & Pearson, 2008).

Table 12.1   Internet Acceptable Use Policy—Areas for Consideration

Area	Areas for consideration
Policy	Purpose of Policy • What values does the policy support? • Why is it important to the organization? • What would the organization like to achieve?
Monitoring	Is the policy consistent with the Data Protection Act 1998? (or equivalent) • What is the purpose of monitoring? • What are the benefits of monitoring? • How will the monitoring be undertaken? • How will the confidentiality of personal information be maintained?
Pre-employment screening	Is there a need to screen your employees prior to employment in a sensitive area? • What tools will you use? • Who will do the screening? • Are they competent? • What will you do if someone fails the screening?
Network security	How will you protect your company security? • What rules do you have on downloading software or other files? • How do you ensure individual security through passwords? • How safe is your information?
Using the Web	What do you want to allow and what will be restricted? • Only business sites? • Which sites are you blocking? • Are you able to block unauthorized sites?
Downloading illegal images	Are you blocking inappropriate text and images? • How will you deal with employee with illegal images on his/her computer? • Will you report employees to the police for breaking the law? • Do you have ways of checking laptops and data storage equipment for illegal images?
Copyright laws	Preventing any breaches of copyright laws • How do you make sure that there are no illegal copies of programs on computers? • How do you prevent downloading copyright material? • What are you going to do if you find breaches of copyright law?
Introducing viruses	How do you prevent the introduction of viruses • What are your rules on opening attachments or downloading programs?
Time wasting	How do you deal with employees who spend too much time on personal web browsing?

Table 12.1   (*Cont'd*)

Area	Areas for consideration
	• How much time is allowed for personal e-mails, instant messaging or browsing? • When can the employees use the internet? • What happens if they exceed their allocation of time?
Keeping a blog	Blogs are becoming increasingly popular • What are the company's views on blogs? • What will you do if an employee breaches company confidentiality? • What happens if that blog is maintained from a personal computer?
E-mails & instant messaging	Etiquette on using the email • Can employees use the email for personal use? • Respecting other email users
Education	The importance of understanding the way the internet is used • Raise awareness of internet abuse and addiction • Recognition of vulnerabilities to overuse/addiction • Responsibilities to behave courteously to others and respect the organization
Training	Manager training • Monitoring usage • Handling internet abuses • Maintaining security • How to identify and support internet addicted employees
Counseling & support	Support for employees in dealing with internet addictions • Help available to employees with personal issues • Provide employees with addiction awareness tools • Opportunities for employee screening for high-risk roles • Do you want to introduce addiction counseling and support for employees?

Prevention and Treatment

The most effective way to deal with internet addiction is through prevention. One of the most important tools involves education of the organization and the workforce in how to recognize and reduce the likelihood of anyone becoming overly dependent on the internet for relaxation and stimulation. It is also important that the well-being of the workforce is considered; organizations ought to adopt strategies designed to help employees enhance their personal well-being through the establishment of a healthy lifestyle and good work–life balance. If an employee lacks basic relationship skills, opportunities should be made available to help in the development of these skills. This is not only a good way to reduce internet dependence, it also improves the employee's effectiveness (Mangrum, Fairley, & Wieder, 2001). If an individual has been identified as having an internet addiction problem, the organization needs to consider providing appropriate counseling and support. Whilst there are a wide range of treatments for people with substance abuse addictions, no preferred methodology has been established for dealing with behavioral addictions. Young (2007), who has been running a treatment centre for internet addiction since 1995, proposes a model of therapy which uses Cognitive Behavioral Therapy (CBT) to address the compulsive internet behavior. CBT is based on the notion that thoughts determine feelings. During the CBT process addicted employees are taught to monitor their thoughts and identify those that trigger addictive feelings at the same time as learning new coping skills and mechanisms to prevent relapse. An alternative treatment involves motivational interviewing to help the addict change their addictive behavior (Miller & Rollnick, 1991). The approach involves a number of stages that begin with the employee building commitment to reach a decision to make a change. This approach draws on a number of strategies taken from client-centered counseling, cognitive therapy, systems theory, and social psychology.

The organization also has an important role in supporting the recovering internet addict. Organizations often create an environment in which workers are encouraged to be constantly available via email and the internet through the use of handheld smart phones with the possibility of creating a culture in which addictions are easier to establish and more acceptable to colleagues and families. Organizations need to set an example by establishing clear boundaries to the working day, and to recognize that, whilst the internet can be damaging, if used appropriately it can provide valuable personal and business opportunities. If problems related to internet addiction are to be solved, then organizations and workers need to work together to establish a balanced approach to internet usage.

Illustrative Cases

Working in organizations provides occupational health psychologists with an opportunity to observe the impact of internet abuse at first hand. The following examples taken from the author's own experiences as an occupational health psychologist show how internet addiction can play a role in causing problems in the workplace.

A senior probation officer had done well in his career. He had worked exceptionally hard and had passed through the ranks very quickly. He spent most of his free time studying for exams. His marital relationship began to suffer and he began to abuse alcohol. He was referred for counseling and immediately cut out all alcohol and attended an alcohol treatment center. He appeared to be recovering from his alcohol addiction when he became obsessed with playing fantasy games on the internet.

The officer had been referred for counseling for his marital problems and alcohol abuse; however, these were treated independently. When he was eventually referred for a psychological assessment it was found that he had an underlying obsessive-compulsive personality and this pattern of addictive behaviors had been evident for most of his life. He had learnt to hide less acceptable addictive behaviors behind those which were generally seen as worthwhile. His workaholic tendencies had hidden a compulsive use of pornography and his use of exercise became part of his attraction for an extreme form of fantasy role playing.

> An IT consultant found his personal and working life collapsing. He had a good job delivering IT solutions to blue-chip customers. However, he found that he was constantly leaving work to the last minute. Generally he was able to handle things, although he knew that there were occasions where he let the company down. He spent most of his free time playing fantasy games and in online chat rooms. At the end of an eight to ten hour session he would feel guilty and angry about the waste of time.

This consultant came for counseling when his relationship was breaking down and he was about to lose his job. His employer had received a complaint from one of the company's major customers about the way that the consultant was handling a project. This consultant was highly imaginative and, when not exhausted by his all-night fantasy role-playing sessions, was a creative member of the team. The consultant had developed a fascination for the high risks he engaged with in his fantasy roles and found that by comparison real life was dull. He then began to adopt his fantasy behaviors in his real life with major repercussions for his job and personal relationships. He refused to accept that he had a problem and continued this pattern of behavior, which resulted in him being sacked from his job and his partner leaving him.

> A small children's charity was shocked when it was visited by the police investigating a report that one of their employees had been downloading child sex abuse images. The person identified was a valued and hardworking member of the team who seemed to get on with everyone. The investigation showed that he had downloaded several thousand child sex abuse images.

The organization had never considered that any of its employees would have been involved in downloading anything inappropriate. Everyone was extremely shocked, particularly as the employee involved had always seemed so dedicated. He had a young family and appeared devoted to his wife and children. The case was reported in the local press and the charity found it very difficult to continue with its work. Several years later the scandal still affected the ability of the charity to operate.

Discussion

Internet addiction is a new and often unrecognized issue for organizations. Understanding the nature of the condition can help in the identification of the most appropriate ways to reduce the incidence and treat outcomes. More research is required to focus on developing more accurate ways to identify and intervene when employees are having difficulties. However, it is essential that managers, supervisors, and occupational health psychologists become more aware of their role in raising awareness of potential problems relating to internet addiction and the harm that it can cause the employee and the organization. One of the first steps is to ensure that organizations have appropriate internet policies and procedures as well as effective screening software. Where possible, organizations should communicate clearly to their workforce what constitutes reasonable use of the internet and, conversely, what is unacceptable and liable to lead to disciplinary action with the possibility of more serious consequences. There is also a need for organizations to set an example by not expecting people to be constantly accessible by email and to limit the amount of work that is undertaken outside normal working hours.

While it is clear that internet addiction has the potential to become a health issue and needs to be taken seriously by employees and organizations, this should be balanced against the significant personal and business benefits, not to mention enjoyment, the internet can provide when used appropriately.

References

Albrecht, U., Kirschner, N., & Grusser, S. (2007). Diagnostic instruments for behavioral addiction: an overview. *GMS Psycho-Social-Medicine*, 4. Retrieved from www.ncbi.nlm.nih.gov/pmc/articles/PMC2736529/

American Psychiatric Association (2000). *DSM-IV (TR) Diagnostic and statistical manual of Mental Disorders* (4th edition). Washington, DC: American Psychiatric Association.

BBC (2003). Operation Ore: Can the UK cope? Retrieved from news.bbc.co.uk/1/hi/uk/2652465.stm

BBC (2008). *No time for a novice says Brown*. Retrieved from http://news.bbc.co.uk/1/hi/uk_politics/7630567.stm

Beard, K. (2005) Internet addiction: A review of current assessment techniques and potential assessment questions, *Cyber Psychology & Behaviour, 8*, 7–14.

Betz, C., Mihalie, D., Pinto, M., & Raffa, R. (2000). Could a common biochemical mechanism underlie addictions? *Journal of Clinical Pharmacology Theory, 25*, 11–20.

Block, J. (2008). Issues for DSM-V: Internet addiction, *American Journal of Psychiatry, 165*, 306–307.

Caplan, S. (2002). Problematic internet use and psychological wellbeing: Development of theory based cognitive-behavioural measurement instrument. *Computers in Human Behaviour, 18*, 5553–5575.

Chak, K., & Leung, L. (2004). Shyness and locus of control as predictors of internet addiction and internet use, *CyberPsychology & Behviour, 7*, 559–570.

CIPD (2003). *E-mail and internet abuse survey*. Retrieved from www.cipd.co.uk/pressoffice/_articles/25062003144853.htm?IsSrchRes=1

CIPD (2004). UK Survey Highlights Problem of Illegal and inappropriate images in the workplace. Retrieved from www.cipd.co.uk/pressoffice/articles/1312200417381.htm

CIPD (2007). *Managing drug and alcohol misuse at work—A guide for people management professionals*. London: CIPD.

Clearswift (2007). Content security 2.0: the impact of Web 2.0 on corporate security. Retrieved from, http://i.i.com/cnwk.1d/html/itp/clearswift_SurveyReport_US_07.PDF

Cooper A., Delmonico, D., & Burg, R. (2000). Sexual addiction and compulsion. *Journal of Treatment and Prevention, 7*, 5–30.

Davies, R., Flett, G., & Besser, A. (2002). Validation of a new scale for measuring problematic internet use: implications for pre-employment screening. *CyberPsychology & Behaviour, 5*, 331–345.

Douglas, A., Mills, J., Niang, M., Stepchenkova, S., Byun, S., Ruffini, C., Lee, S., Loutfi, J., Lee, J., Atallah, M., & Blanton, M. (2008). Internet addiction: Meta-analysis of qualitative research for the decade 1996–2006, *Computers in Human Behaviour, 24*, 3027–3044.

EU (2009). *The EU commission cracks down on modern slavery and child sexual abuse*. Retrieved from, http://gozonews.com/item/eu-commission-cracks-down-on-modern-slavery-and-child-sexual-abuse/

Gamble, J. (2005). *Wipe it out campaign conference*. Retrieved from www.iwf.org.uk/media/page.157.htm

Greenfield, D. (1999). *Virtual addiction: Help for netheads, cyberfreaks, and those who love them*. Oakland, CA: New Harbinger.

Griffiths, M. (2000). Excessive internet use: Implications for sexual behavior. *CyberPsychology & Behaviour, 3*, 537–552.

Griffiths, M. (2003). Internet abuse in the workplace: issues and concerns for employers and employment counselors. *Journal of Employment Counselling, 40*, 87–96.

Grohol, J. (2005). *Internet addiction guide*. Retrieved from http:/psychcentral.com/netaddiction/

Hyman, G. (2002). *Web addiction on the rise*. Retrieved from www.clickz.com/1450371

Interpol (2008). *Legislation of INTERPOL member states on sexual offences against children*. Retrieved from www.interpol.int/public/children/sexualabuse/nationallaws/default/asp

IWF (2004). *87% of managers not aware of changes to the law*. Retrieved from www.iwf.org.uk/media/news.archive-2004.83.htm

IWF (2005). *Wipe it out campaign*. Retrieved from www.iwf.org.uk/media/page.157.htm

IWS (2008). *Internet usage statistics: the internet big picture*. Retrieved from www.internet-worldstats.com

Jaffe, J. (1990). Trivialising addiction. *British Journal of Addictions, 85*, 1425–1427.

Journal Live (2006). *Northumberland swimming Instructor faces Jail.* Retrieved from www. journallive.co.uk/north-east-news/uk

Karkowski, L., Prescott, C., & Kendler, K. (2007). Multivariate assessment of factors influencing illicit substance use in twins from female–female pairs. *American Journal of Medical Genetics, 96*, 665–70.

Livingstone, S., & Haddon, L. (2007). *What do we know about children's use of on-line technologies? A report on data availability and research gaps in Europe*, London: LSE.

McGowan, P., Sasaki, A., D'Alessio, A., Dymov, S., Labonte, B., Szyf, M., Turecki, G., & Meaney, M. (2009). Epigenetic regulation of the glucocorticoid receptor in human brain associates with childhood abuse. *Nature Neuroscience, 12*, 342–348.

Miller, W., & Rollnick, S. (1991). *Motivational interviewing.* New York: Guildford Press.

Morahan-Martin, J. (2005). Internet abuse: Addiction? Symptom? Alternative Explanations? *Social Science Computer Review, 2*, 39–48.

Mangrum, F., Fairley, M., & Wieder, D. (2001). Informal problem solving in technology-mediated work place. *Journal of Business Communication, 38*, 315–336.

Niemz, K., Griffiths, M., & Banyard, P. (2005). Prevalence of pathological internet use among university students and correlations with self-esteem and the General Health Questionnaire (GHQ) and disihition. *CyberPsychology & Behaviour, 8*, 562–570.

O'Brian, M., & Webster, S. (2007). The construction and preliminary validation of the Internet Behaviours & Attitudes Questionnaire. *Sex Abuse, 19*, 237–256.

Out-Law (2007). *EU court rules monitoring of employee breached human rights.* Retrieved from, www.theregister.co.uk/2007/04/05/monitoring_breached_human_rights/

Potenza, M. (2007). To do or not do? The complexities of addiction, motivation, self-control and impulsivity. *American Journal of Psychiatry, 164*, 4–6.

Seto, M., & Eke, A. (2005). The criminal histories and later offending of child pornography offenders. *Sexual Abuse, 17*, 201–210.

Shaffer, H., & Hall, M. (2002). The natural history of gabling and drinking problems among casino employees. *Journal of Social Psychology, 142*, 405–424.

Shotton, M. (1989). *Computer addiction.* New York: Taylor Francis.

Small, G., & Vorgan, G. (2008). *iBrain: Surviving the technological alteration of the modern mind.* New York: Harper Collins.

Song I., Larose, R., Eastin, M., & Lin, C. (2004). Internet gratification and internet addiction: on the uses and abuses of new media. *CyberPsychology and Behaviour, 7*, 384–394.

Soule, L., Shell, L., & Kleen, B. (2003). Exploring internet addiction: Demographic characteristics and stereotypes of heavy internet users. *Journal of Computer Information Systems, 41*, 64–73.

The Argus (2008). *Paedophile downloaded porn at Legal & General*, Retrieved from, http://www.theargus.co.uk/news/3696494.print/

The Times (2007). Fired worker sues IBM over internet addiction, Retrieved from, http://business.timesonline.co.uk/tol/business/law/article1406502.ece

Ugrin, J., & Pearson, J. (2008). Exploring internet abuse in the workplace: How can we maximize deterrence efforts? *Review of Business, 28*, 29–40.

Werme, M., Lindholm, S., Thoren, P., Franck, J., & Brene, S. (2002). Running increases ethanol preference. *Behavioural Brain Research, 133*, 301–308.

Wolak, J., Finkelhor, D., & Mitchell, K. (2004). Internet-initiated sex crimes against minors: Implications for prevention based on findings from a national study. *Journal of Adloescent Health, 35,* 11–20.

Young, K. (1998). Internet addictions: the emergence of a new clinical disorder. *CyberPsychology and Behaviour, 3,* 237–244.

Young, K. (2004). Internet addiction: A new phenomenon and its consequences. *American Behavioural Scientist,* 48, 402–415.

Young, K. (2007). Cognitive behavioural therapy with internet addicts: Treatment outcomes and implications. *CyberPsychology & Behaviour, 10,* 671–679.

13

Organizational Culture and Knowledge Management Systems for Promoting Organizational Health and Safety

Dolores Díaz-Cabrera, Estefanía Hernández-Fernaud, Yeray Ramos-Sapena, and Sara Casenave
University of La Laguna, Spain

This chapter provides an introduction to the role of organizational culture in the implementation of knowledge management systems in health and safety promotion. The first section introduces the notion of health in organizations and its relationship with occupational health psychology. Subsequent sections discuss the role of organizational culture as a potential enabler or barrier in the implementation of knowledge management systems. Finally, we put forward a proposal in regard to the role of cultural barriers and enablers in the development of a specific knowledge management system within the framework of a research project conducted by the authors.

Intervention-focused research on the promotion of organizational health and safety is significant both socially and scientifically. Intervention research within occupational health psychology has highlighted the need for a multilevel approach that combines individual, social, and organizational perspectives. This procedure calls for a comprehensive and holistic modus operandi that is capable of facilitating high-level information processing which, in itself, is a prerequisite for the maintenance of a healthy organization. To this end, knowledge management systems can provide a useful working philosophy.

The incorporation of such systems into organizations frequently involves a process of organizational change in which culture plays a critical role as a barrier or enabler. Even when a process of change is not required, the organizational culture must be consistent with the underlying objectives of the system that is to be implemented. Likewise, the organization's practices and values must be oriented to organizational learning and to health and safety promotion, in order that both the knowledge management system and health and safety promotion activities form part of its day-to-day operations. These notions underpin the development of the following sections of this chapter.

Health within Organizations

Interest in health and safety in the workplace is not new. During the First World War, studies were performed to investigate how working hours and resting times affect worker fatigue and performance. Shortly thereafter, Elton Mayo (1933, 1945) scrutinized work environment factors that affected workers' well-being. This concern for the well-being of the workforce is reflected today in the existence of numerous public bodies whose activities are dedicated to the study and monitoring of working conditions and a wealth of scientific research that aims to define factors that are beneficial or detrimental to workers' quality of life.

Changes in the nature of work that have taken place during the last 30 years have contributed to professionals having increasingly focused their attention on the management of occupational health. Companies have reduced personnel and modified their management policies and production processes. In many organizations the number of middle managers has dwindled, giving workers more responsibility and control over their work. The competences required for many jobs have gradually increased; workers must be increasingly flexible and capable of multitasking, and prepared to change jobs several times in their working lives. Jobs increasingly require higher-level cognitive and knowledge management skills. These changes may be linked to both positive outcomes, such as greater worker satisfaction through enhanced responsibility, and to negative outcomes including work-related stress (Sauter et al., 2002; Sauter & Hurrell, 1999).

According to the Fourth European Working Conditions Survey, the intensification of work is one of the most significant workplace trends in recent years (Parent-Thirion, Macías, Hurley, & Vermeylen, 2007). This trend affects all countries, sectors, and professional categories, and is directly related to stress outcomes and musculoskeletal disorders. Furthermore, temporary work, which often involves the poorest working conditions, has increased: by 2002, 15% of workers in Europe were on temporary contracts (European Foundation for the Improvement of Living and Working Conditions, 2002).

Most people consider good health to be a key factor when defining quality of life (Delhey, 2004). Work plays a major role in the maintenance of not only physical health, but also psychological well-being, since it can contribute to a sense of identity and social benefit, and occupies a large part of a person's time. Therefore, working conditions and their impact on health and safety play an important role in quality of life. The Fourth European Working Conditions Survey (Parent-Thirion et al., 2007) revealed that the level of physical and psychological work factors associated with a risk to health have remained largely unchanged over the preceding 15 years. The survey showed that health problems most often linked to the working environment include musculoskeletal disorders, fatigue, strain, headaches, and irritability.

The Annual Review of Working Conditions in the European Union 2007–2008 (European Foundation for the Improvement of Living and Working Conditions, 2008) demonstrated that musculoskeletal disorders related to physical work have declined, while those related to stress and overload have increased. In 2007, the European Agency for Safety and Health at Work (EU-OSHA) published a report on psychosocial risks related to health at work that identified five core emerging risks: new forms of employment contracts and job insecurity, an aging workforce, work intensification, high emotional demands at work, and poor work-life balance (EU-OSHA, 2007a). Although many health and safety risks have continued over time or have been replaced by others, it is true that both serious and fatal accidents have declined significantly since 2001 (EU-OSHA, 2007b).

Changes to the content and context of work that have taken place in recent decades highlight the imperative need for a multidisciplinary approach to the management of occupational safety and health. That multidisciplinary perspective must include a contribution from psychology. From its early days, psychology has informed occupational health and safety, although, arguably, a clear definition of the role of psychology in occupational health protection and promotion has only emerged in recent times with the advent of occupational health psychology. The emergence of this discipline can be attributed, in part, to the recognition of stress-related psychological disorders as a costly occupational health problem and the growing importance attributed to psychosocial factors in organizational health and safety (Barling & Griffiths, 2002; Sauter & Hurrell, 1999).

The U.S. National Institute for Occupational Safety and Health defines occupational health psychology as concerning "the application of psychology to improving the quality of worklife, and to protecting and promoting the safety, health, and well-being of workers" (NIOSH, 2008). NIOSH asserts that health, safety, and worker well-being are directly or indirectly influenced by three levels or groups of factors: (1) the external context, including economic, political, legal, technological, social, and demographic factors, (2) the organizational context, which refers to management, supervision, production methods, and human resources policies, and (3) the work context or work station design.

Schaufeli (2004) delves further into the definition of occupational health psychology by highlighting several aspects. First, the term health, as conceptualized from an occupational health psychology perspective, is a positive term which accords with that posited by the World Health Organization whereby health is not merely the absence of disease. Occupational health psychology employs a broad conceptualization of mental health that includes cognitive, motivational, and behavioral aspects, as well as the emotional well-being of the worker. Second, occupational health psychology does not restrict its study population to large organizations, but also includes the unemployed. Moreover, it studies the effects of work or unemployment on health, as well as the impact of work on other areas of life and vice versa. Third, occupational health psychology is both a scientific discipline and an applied field. And, finally, the discipline examines worker health at four interrelated levels of analysis: the individual, the work environment, the organizational environment, and the external environment.

Although, in theory, these four levels of analysis are considered, a key line of work has concerned the advancement of primary prevention through the development of a greater understanding and control of organizational risk factors and their impact on disease and injuries. This is consistent with Sauter and Hurrell's (1999) assertion that the contribution of occupational health psychology should be: (1) to protect health by reducing exposure to risk factors by improving working conditions, and (2) to promote health by equipping workers with knowledge and resources that enable them to improve their health and resistance to occupational hazards.

In 1992, NIOSH and the American Psychological Association also suggested that while not neglecting individual-level risk factors, the discipline of occupational health psychology should focus primarily on improving our understanding of the influence of organizational factors—psychosocial hazards—on workers' health and safety. Sauter et al. (2002) proposed three avenues for activity: (1) research into the prevalence of organizational risk factors, (2) research to understand the health effects of organizational practices, and (3) intervention-focused research. Landsbergis (2003) added to the NIOSH proposals by suggesting a concomitant imperative to conduct research on vulnerable groups of workers, perform general studies on the identification of stressors, undertake work in multidisciplinary teams, and develop procedures to estimate the economic costs of occupational health and safety risks.

Although occupational health psychology attaches considerable importance to organizational context as it relates to health, the individual level has not been neglected (Arthur, 2006). Bennet, Cook, and Pelletier (2003) suggest three perspectives on practice and research in the discipline. The first is based on the concept of healthy environments, aspiring to a holistic view of the organization that learns, maintains, and improves health. The second involves the development of models oriented towards the practice of promoting organizational health. The third concerns the promotion of comprehensive or multifactorial health and the development of disease management programs. In our opinion, each of these perspectives can be addressed from different levels of analysis. For example, the first perspective—organizational learning—requires an individual, group, and organizational approach.

The ultimate aim of activities within disciplines involved in organizational health and safety promotion is to create healthy organizations. Wilson, DeJoy, Vandenberg, Richardson, and McGrath (2004) state that "A healthy organization is one characterized by intentional, systematic, and collaborative efforts to maximize employee well-being and productivity by providing well-designed and meaningful jobs, a supportive social–organizational environment, and accessible and equitable opportunities for career and work–life enhancement" (p. 567). Thus, healthy organizations are founded on explicit organizational and job design practices, and on specific relational dynamics between all members. In particular, they are based on aspects of the working environment that encourage the attainment of organizational objectives, which decrease the job demands resulting from physiological and/or psychosocial costs, and which stimulate personal growth, learning, and professional development (Demerouti, Bakker, Nachreiner, & Schaufeli, 2001).

Healthy organizations must accept that organizational health and safety is the responsibility of all. Consequently, organizational health and safety promotion must form an integral part of all organizational practices. Traditional approaches to health and safety have focused on reducing risk factors and disease, while contemporary models have complemented these by highlighting the role of employee resources in coping with multiple demands in the work environment.

Occupational health management concerns the optimization of organizational processes and structures that have a direct or indirect impact on workers' health. Dialogue and communication between all organizational units is essential for effective organizational health management. It also fosters an organization's capacity to be one that learns (Bauer & Jenny, 2007). In this respect, knowledge management systems (KMS) play a central role.

Knowledge Management Systems in Health and Safety Promotion

The Luxembourg Declaration on Workplace Health Promotion in the European Union (European Network for Workplace Health Promotion, 2005) proposes four factors as key to the development of a healthy organization. Firstly, all members of an organization must participate in health-promoting actions. Secondly, health promotion must be integrated in all important decisions and all areas of the organization. Thirdly, all actions to promote health and safety must follow a cycle: needs analysis, setting priorities, planning, implementation, continuous control, and evaluation. Finally, health promotion must combine risk reduction with the development of protection factors, and individual-directed and environment-directed measures.

Accordingly, optimum health and safety management calls for a holistic, comprehensive approach to processing information about health and safety that, in turn, can foster proactive interventions and organizational learning. Organizations can rely on a wide range of information about occupational risks and health problems. When all is said and done, health and safety promotion must be an activity that hinges on information and knowledge management. However, the fragmentation of information and information overload may occur often given that these activities can generate considerable data. As such, data may be inadequately processed within the organization, thus hindering organizational learning. The origin of this situation lies in the nature of intervention and evaluation, characterized, as both are, by multidimensional aspects of wellness including physical, psychological, and social health (Bennet et al., 2003), as well as by demands stemming from the need to integrate multiple data from evaluation and intervention programs.

The current development of the philosophy behind knowledge management systems, aided by the rapid development of information technologies, can benefit activities aimed at health and safety promotion, and the potential for organizational growth, to an extraordinary degree. In the last decade, KMS practices have gradually been put into effect in organizational processes in the health promotion sector.

An example of the linkage between health promotion in the workplace and knowledge management systems can be found in behavioral risk management. This combines evaluation and programming to reduce behavioral risk through a step-wise process. The process includes the auditing of behavioral risks and the integration of information through knowledge management systems with a view towards the identification of activities that have an impact on individual and organizational risks, and the development of appropriate intervention programs (Yandrick, 1996, cf. Bennet et al., 2003).

Knowledge management is an interdisciplinary action- and research-based field that involves the integration of knowledge from psychology, sociology, business administration, economics, computer science, and library and information studies, among others (García-Marco, 2003). Nicolini, Powell, Conville, and Martinez-Solano (2008) have proposed a definition of knowledge management systems within organizational health: "formal methodologies and techniques to facilitate the creation, identification, acquisition, development, preservation, dissemination and, finally, the utilization of the various facets of healthcare knowledge" (p.246). Knowledge management systems focus on improving knowledge creation and its use at group and organizational levels.

In short, this is an activity aimed at improving internal and external communication, utilizing data gathered from various programs, information handling and use, with a view towards the enhancement of individual, group, and organizational knowledge. End benefits include the optimization and integration of intervention programs through the conscious and systematic combination of several health and safety promotion activities and their full integration into the organizational and management processes of human resources (García-Marco, 2003).

Key Concepts in Knowledge Management Systems

Knowledge management systems feature a series of key concepts. In this section we provide a brief description of the concepts that are most central to the aim of this chapter. Thus, the focus is on social and organizational requirements, barriers, and enablers that are important to the successful implementation of knowledge management systems for managing health and organizational safety. The first issue is that of KMS classification. Based on the classification developed by Nicolini et al. (2008; see also Choy, Lee, & Cheung, 2005; Riege, 2005) three different initiatives are distinguished: (1) IT-based or technology-driven (electronic libraries, repositories of scientific information in the form of articles, guides, and clinical protocols, etc.); (2) socially based or people/culture-driven (communities of practice and network modes of organizing); and (3) human-resource-driven (development and professional training). This chapter centers on social learning or people-driven initiatives.

Moreover, a second question concerns the definition of the knowledge management and information management concepts. Knowledge is defined by García-Marco (2003) as:

> a collection of ways of thinking (some learnt, others improved or totally invented) that persons and organizations use to interpret this information. These ways of thinking then define their manner of reciprocally acting and of transforming the reality that informs them from outside. (p.159)

Knowledge management is on a higher level than information processing and integration and should not be limited to such information, despite being based on it. In our opinion, while information processing hinges on an IT-based activity, successful knowledge management depends on a suitable socially based or people-driven KMS.

The differences between the concepts of information management and knowledge management can also be seen in the sequence of KMS described by De Long and Fahey (2000) regarding the progression from data to information to knowledge. It is also important to acknowledge that knowledge can be explicit at a group or organizational level (Choy et al., 2005; De Long & Fahey, 2000; Riege, 2005).

De Long and Fahey (2000) suggest that there are at least three types of knowledge that are not generally differentiated in the literature: (1) human knowledge, which constitutes what humans know or know how to do; (2) social knowledge, which is shared in groups or teams; and (3) structured knowledge, which is embedded in organizational systems, processes, practices, and policies. A successful KMS needs to focus on all three types of knowledge. Structured knowledge is the final objective of KMS whereby health and safety promotion is integrated into daily life within organizations.

In recent years, research on information and knowledge management, particularly in the field of organizational safety, has focused on social and organizational activities that develop an organization's capacity for reflection and learning, or learning culture (e.g., Reason, 2003). Organizational requirements proposed for attaining this learning capacity include suitable systems of gathering and processing information about accidents and incidents to aid identification and analysis of risks or dangerous situations, feedback of such information, and the generation and ongoing review of control and intervention measures. These strategies also call for open and flexible communication channels that are not based on punishment for inappropriate performance, but which foster information exchange: a necessary condition for evolving a philosophy of innovation, development, and continuous learning within organizations (Moray, 2001; Vassie & Lucas, 2001). Along these lines, Reason (2003) proposes the coexistence of a just culture (as opposed to a punishment culture), a learning culture, and an information culture. Together these three elements aid the development of an organizational *report* that enables learning and risks to be faced through proactive and reactive measures. Proactivity, a questioning attitude, trust, and a permanent surveillance plan are essential features of research and intervention in modern-day organizational safety.

These contributions indicate that cultural aspects have made a powerful entry into the field of health and, in particular, organizational safety in the last few years (Bauer & Jenny, 2007; Guldenmund, 2007; Hale, 2000; Hopkins, 2006; Schaufeli, 2004; Wilson et al., 2004; Wren et al., 2006). This concept has experienced an increase in popularity in the scientific literature and has been closely linked to the development and implementation of knowledge management systems within organizations. However, though some research connects the fields of organizational culture and knowledge management systems, further development is still required. The following section deals with the links between these two areas of work.

Knowledge Management Systems and Organizational Culture

Knowledge management system implementation within organizations is a complex task that involves changes and/or adjustments to numerous activities and organizational processes. Bauer and Jenny (2007) consider that, depending on the organization, the implementation of occupational health management provision can lead to extensive reorganization due to the introduction of new processes, structures, and cultural change. However, the sociocultural aspects of evaluation processes and organizational change that may be required for KMS implementation, are often overlooked; attention tends to fall on technological aspects (Bennett et al., 2003; De Long & Fahey, 2000; Choy et al., 2005; Nicolini et al., 2008; Riege, 2005).

A key element of successful organizational change is the existence of an appropriate organizational culture. Accordingly, KMS implementation includes a process of cultural change and organizational learning in which cultural enablers and barriers to learning must be assessed. The complexity of KMS implementation calls for firm commitment from all members of the organization at all hierarchical levels, effective leadership, and an organizational culture coherent with the development of organizational knowledge. Individual, group, and organizational values, with their influence on behavior and organizational practices, must be congruent with the development of knowledge and learning. In particular, we refer to values that support the creation, dissemination, sharing, and storage of information throughout the organization.

An organization's learning capacity is based on the existence of a culture that supports learning (Beckhard & Pritchard, 1992; cf. Dibella, 2003; Easterby-Smith & Lyles, 2003). Schilling and Kluge (2008) have highlighted three categories of barrier to organizational learning: individual actions (individual thoughts, attitudes, and behaviors), organizational structures (strategies, technologies, culture, and regulations), and organizational environment (the social and material factors of the environment that the organization perceives as important for organizational activities, such as clients, suppliers, competitors, socio-political atmosphere, and technology).

Four ways in which culture influences knowledge sharing and use have been identified. First of all, culture determines the value of knowledge for an organization and its members. Second, it influences the degree to which knowledge is shared between individuals and departments. Third, culture affects the use given to knowledge in each situation. And last, it influences organizational processes in which knowledge is created and transmitted within and between organizations (De Long & Fahey, 2000).

Nevertheless, organizational culture is a polemic and complex concept that requires considerable theoretical and empirical clarification (see for a review Aaltio & Mills, 2002; Cooper, Cartwright, & Early, 2001; Díaz-Cabrera, Hernández-Fernaud, & Isla, 2007; Martin & Frost, 1996; Wilpert, 1995). In our opinion, the key divergences in perspective are as follows:

1.   Levels of organizational culture: organizational culture can be evaluated from various levels: (1) national culture (Hofstede, 1991, 2002; Hofstede & Peterson, 2000), (2) industrial or business sector (e.g. Gordon, 1991; cf. De Witte & Van

Muijen, 1999), (3) professional culture (McDonald, Corrigan, Daly, & Cromie, 2000), and (4) organizational subcultures. All these cultural levels play a significant part in research. However, it is essential to define clearly the level at which work is carried out, thereby avoiding confusion that may affect the interpretation of results and the development of theoretical models.

2. Concrete versus tacit aspects of culture: a key divergence—possibly with consequences for the empirical and intervention approach selected—concerns the distinction between obvious, concrete, visible, and conscious cultural aspects as opposed to tacit, hidden, and unconscious ones. The first approach accentuates organizational practices and behaviors, whereas the second highlights meanings and values. Theorists have attempted to find an intermediate approach that links both stances. Thus, Wilpert (2001; see also Hofstede, 2002; Reiman & Oedewald, 2007) points out that Schein's (1985) model integrates both perspectives and enables the development of a visible cultural indicator. This model proposes three cultural levels with indicators reflecting practically the whole organization. Accordingly, organizational culture can be construed as being manifested in shared values and meanings, and in particular organizational structures and processes, health and safety policies, strategies, goals, practices, and leadership styles. These components emanate from underlying patterns of shared meanings and beliefs, and can act as valid indicators in a culture evaluation process. This notion is closer to the vision of organization as *being culture* as opposed to *having culture*. In this respect, three alternative approaches for the development of analysis and intervention tools present themselves: (1) a focus on individual and organizational cultural values and meanings, (2) an emphasize on organizational policies and practices, and (3) consideration of both factors. The approach proposed in this chapter is related to the identification of cultural enablers and barriers in the development of knowledge management systems implied in both organizational practices and values. This presupposes that culture is manifested in specific organizational practices and policies, as well as in values and meanings.

3. Linking theoretical fields: KMS implementation, as considered above, involves a complex process of evaluation, change, and organizational learning to facilitate the realization of new procedures and systems. However, a theoretical review of the important aspects related to the effectiveness of an organizational change initiative shows multiple links between several research fields including organizational development, organizational change, organizational culture, culture change, organizational knowledge, and so on (Boonstra, 2004). A theoretical review of the literature from these fields indicates critical success factors for organizational change (e.g., Ashkanasy & Jackson, 2001; Choy, Lee, & Cheung, 2005; Rogers & Byham, 1994; Sinangil & Avallone, 2001; Van de Ven, 1995).

A group of factors related to the process of successful change has been proposed on the basis of the scientific literature drawn from several research fields. These factors include: (1) the establishment of a sense of urgency, (2) formation of powerful guiding conditions, (3) creation of a vision, (4) communication of that vision, (5) empowerment of others to act on the vision, (6) planning for and the creation of short-term gains, and (7) the consolidation of improvements. Furthermore, several key organizational characteristics have been highlighted. These include: (1) resources for innovation, (2) frequent communications across departments, (3) cohesive work groups with open conflict resolution mechanisms, (4) organizational and individual values that foster innovative behaviors and high involvement, (5) organizational climate, (6) motivating factors with a balance between intrinsic and extrinsic rewards for innovative behaviors, and (7) leadership styles or characteristics of the agents of change (e.g., interpersonal competences, problem-solving capacities, role as educator, self-awareness). However, despite this list of factors, there is a lack of clear orientation. Therefore, a priority task is to define a group of critical success factors in KMS implementation and to develop a model that enables the identification of relations among those factors. In the following section we provide a brief outline of leading enablers and barriers identified in a series of works.

Knowledge Management System Enablers and Barriers

At present, studies aimed at the identification of cultural aspects and other organizational features that enable the successful application of knowledge management systems are mainly limited to the field of health promotion. Nonetheless, some organizational resources that directly or indirectly affect health and safety, and may also influence knowledge management systems, have been put forward, including transparency, information and communication opportunities, task identification, opportunities for participation and decision making, feedback, time flexibility, opportunities for cooperation, social support, staff turnover, diversity, training opportunities, career development, and the meaning of work (Udris, 2006, cf. Bauer & Jenny, 2007).

Nicolini et al. (2008) have pinpointed a group of major enablers and barriers of KMS success in healthcare organizations, although they underline the fact that the enablers and barriers are generic, with certain exceptions. Specifically, these authors consider that, unlike other kinds of organizations, there are two important factors within the health sector that function as enablers: (1) the strong professionalization of the sector, and (2) the influence on other areas of society.

Table 13.1. shows the barriers and enablers proposed by Nicolini et al. (2008) applied to the healthcare sector. It also includes the components that facilitate KMS implementation in the aviation industry included by Choy et al (2005) in their KMCAT model (Knowledge Management Culture Assessment Tool). Also presented are the cultural characteristics outlined by De Long and Fahey (2000) that guide the diagnosis of cultural barriers to knowledge management. Finally, though not directly linked to the field of KMS, the barriers to effective pain management identified by Brockopp et al. (1998) are included.

Within the framework of the HILAS project (Human Integration into the Lifecycle of Aviation Systems 2005–2009) (www.hilas.info/mambo/), the authors of this chapter are currently participating in work to identify cultural characteristics in order to implement the HILAS KMS. The ultimate goal is the successful incorporation of these tools in participating organizations. HILAS is a European interdisciplinary

Table 13.1   Cultural Enablers and Barriers in Activities Directed at Organizational Health

Authors	Enablers	Barriers
Nicollini, Powell, Conville, & Martinez-Solano (2008)	Shared common values and culture	Over-management and interference from political sphere
	Minimizing concerns about power and status differences	Clinical managerial conflict
	Interdisciplinarity (broad-based membership)	Professional barriers
	Close proximity (operational)	Lack of trust
	Salient topics	Poor quality relationship
	Political commitment and endorsement	Insufficient technology skills
	Loose structure	Lack of strategic breadth and leadership
Choy, Lee & Cheung (2005)	*Coherence:* Mutual trust, competence development, delegation, and enhanced communication	
	Innovation: Creativity, flexibility, questionability, adaptability	
	Information & Collaboration: Information technology, collaboration technology, usefulness, effectiveness	
	Control: Supervision, rewards, recognition, evaluation	
	Alliance & Partnership: Integration, information sharing, competence broadening, continuous improvement	
De Long & Fahey (2000)	Discussibility of sensitive topics	
	Senior management's approachability	
	Frequency of interactions (horizontal and vertical	
	Collective responsibility for problem solving	
	Orientation to existing knowledge and expertise	
	Knowledge sharing (vs. accumulation)	
	Teaching	
	Learning from mistakes	

Table 13.1   (*Cont'd*)

Authors	Enablers	Barriers
Brockopp, Brockopp, Warden, Wilson, Carpenter, & Vandeveer (1998)		Lack of knowledge
		Nonfacilitative attitudes for effective pain management
		Inconsistent/nonexisting leadership
		Inability of nurses and physicians to work together
		Cultural/religious biases
		Physicians' fear of legal repercussions
		Lack of resources

research and intervention program. A total of 41 participating institutions are involved including airlines, aeronautical components manufacturers, universities, and research centers in 15 countries. The project is developed along four lines of work: (1) integration and management of knowledge about human factors, (2) assessment and improvement of performance in flight operations, (3) evaluation of new flight control technologies, and (4) evaluation and improvement of aircraft maintenance operations. The work will facilitate the development of a series of tools to help improve information management and use (see Figure 13.1.).

This program will facilitate the use and transmission of knowledge, as well as its transformation into organizational practices and policies, in and among HILAS companies and other relevant organizations. The HILAS project will develop a model of good practice for the integration of human factors across the life-cycle of aviation systems. The HILAS system will be directed at improving the safety and operations of airlines, maintenance repair organizations, and component manufacturers. The implementation of this system will involve processes of organizational change based on intra- and inter-organizational learning loops that facilitate an improved knowledge management system.

One of the principal objectives of our research is the identification of cultural enablers and barriers that may facilitate or, conversely, hinder KMS implementation and its successful development and integration into organizational policies and practices. The cultural approach for the implementation of the HILAS KMS proposed here has been developed from various sources including the relevant scientific literature on organizational culture and processes of change as well as knowledge management systems, input from partners in the knowledge integration strand, HILAS theoretical workshops, and interview data. The main objective of the interviews was to identify

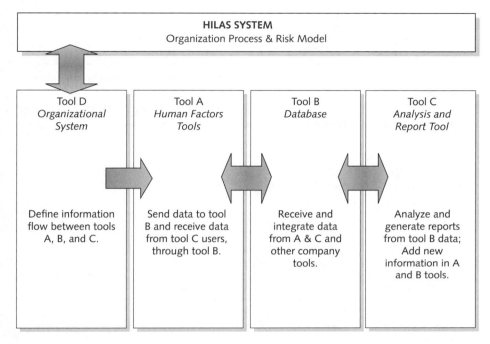

Figure 13.1   The HILAS Knowledge Management System

the cultural characteristics of organizations participating in the project that might facilitate or hinder the implementation of change.

A number of semi-structured exploratory interviews were designed and run between February 2006 and November 2007. Eighty-one workers from airlines, maintenance, and airport services from six companies in China, Ireland, Norway, and Spain participated in this study. The first set of interviews had fairly general objectives, and subsequent interviews focused on aspects that required more detailed information. Each interview protocol was therefore based on the findings of previous interviews, and the information resulting from this exploratory study is being used to develop standardized measures.

The information obtained in these interviews helped pinpoint a group of cultural characteristics that may act as barriers or enablers and may influence knowledge creation and sharing within and between relevant organizations, through the HILAS KMS (see Table13. 2.).

The central theoretical approach presented here is that organizations develop and assume a group of key values related to innovation and learning (Díaz-Cabrera, 2008). In our view, these values have considerable impact on organizations' capacity to implement new KMS tools and systems. Accordingly, we propose a range of values linked with organizational learning that foment information distribution and use. Thus, organizational values constitute the central dimension of this approach and include characteristics such as learning capacity value, and adaptability to change and innovation. The second dimension concerns organizational practices

Table 13.2   Core Implementation Cultural Dimensions

Organizational values	Organizational practices and policies
Communication and information processes	Information/communication/coordination systems
Learning capacity value	Information and communication about change
Adaptability to change and innovation	Organizational practices directed at changes and innovation
Degree of successful change	
Resistance to change	
Successful processes of change	
Sustainability of change initiatives	

Table 13.3   Modulatory Cultural Dimensions

Individual perceptions	Group perceptions
Individual values related to work	Group values related to work
Individual adaptability to change and innovation	Group adaptability to change and innovation
Individual resistance to change	Group resistance to change
Individual organizational commitment	Group organizational commitment
	Group pressure/cohesion
Trust	*Climate*
Trust in managers	Organizational Climate
Trust in organization	Proactive Climate

and policies related to innovation and learning that may facilitate knowledge management. This includes information, communication, and coordination systems, as well as organizational practices directed at change and innovation. The third dimension of this approach is the degree of successful change, which is specifically related to the development and degree of use of existing knowledge management practices and resistance to change. Organizational practices and policies related to innovation and learning will determine the end behaviors that evolve within organizations and, in this sense, organizational behaviors as well as individual behaviors (e.g., resistance to change) might also be considered. Where organizational behaviors are concerned, the central feature of the HILAS system is the capacity to transform HILAS data into knowledge (e.g., is knowledge transformed into organizational improvements?). Therefore, it is primarily a potential post-implementation measure.

Organizational values, practices, policies, and degree of successful change form the central sequence of this approach. However, it includes a group of dimensions that influence the above variables - individual and group perceptions, trust, and climate (Table 13.3.).

Individual and group perceptions include values of adaptation to change and organizational commitment. From surveys and input from other partners, a group of critical conditions has been identified for the variable "trust": (1) credibility: related to the existence of optimal two-way communication; (2) acknowledgement and respect: professional support, organizational and group collaboration, loss of pilots' status, motivational reinforcements; (3) pride/commitment: in the job, the team, the organization, as well as acknowledgement/identification with the management, department, organization and the system (i.e., common goals), and other organizations involved; (4) justice: equity and impartiality; and (5) fellowship: individuality and a welcoming atmosphere.

Another dimension is "proactive climate". Studies on proactive climate, or climate for innovation, have revealed that climates have the power to influence various processes through which organizations change (see, for a review, Evans, Glendon, & Creed, 2007; Fay, Lührmann, & Carsten, 2004). From Fay et al. we have selected two dimensions of proactive climate: (1) orientation towards work innovation; this implies being open to new approaches and practices, as well as being ready to try out new things and to initiate new working approaches, and (2) orientation towards error management. Error management climate is the collective tendency to discuss errors openly and to regard them as learning opportunities. Such an orientation should lead to organizational learning.

This group of barriers and enablers is based on studies undertaken to date. Following these lines of research, and within the framework of the HILAS project, we devised a questionnaire that included these cultural barriers and enablers. Our main objective was to undertake quantitative evaluations that would lead to more complex statistical analyses, thus allowing us to compare organizations and assess the relationship between the concepts outlined above.

Conclusions

The use of knowledge management systems in the field of health and safety promotion is highly beneficial for the organization and its members. It fosters information integration from several evaluations and intervention programs, leading to more efficient long-term management that pervades all organizational processes and practices. However, we are of the opinion that great inroads have been made into technology-driven knowledge management systems, while people/culture-driven knowledge management systems are still few. Specifically, as considered throughout this chapter, further theoretical and methodological study of social and cultural aspects is required.

The need for future development presents a considerable scientific challenge for the various disciplines involved. Health and safety promotion is an area noted for its high complexity that stems from, among other factors, the multidimensional aspects of well-being, the existence of numerous risks arising from the diverse nature of work, the different levels of analysis required, and individual ways of facing up to risk and its consequences.

Nevertheless, the scientific efforts and considerable progress made so far, and facilitated by the multidisciplinary nature of the field, have led to significant social improvements, the enhancement of the quality of life and wellness, and the development of healthy organizations.

Acknowledgement

This research has been undertaken within the 6th framework of the HILAS Project (Human Integration into the Lifecycle of Aviation Systems – AIP4-CT-2005-516181) supported by the European Union.

References

Aaltio, I., & Mills, A. (Eds.) (2002). *Gender, identity and the culture of organizations*. London: Routledge.

Arthur, A. R. (2006). Occupational health psychology in practice: The organisation, its employees and their mental health. In J. Houdmont & S. McIntyre (Eds.), *Occupational health psychology: European perspectives on research, education and practice*, Vol. I (pp. 155-176). Maia, Portugal: ISMAI Publishing.

Ashkanasy, N. M. & Jackson, C. R. A. (2001). Organizational culture and climate. In N. Anderson, D. S. Ones, & H. K. Sinangil (Eds.), *Industrial, work & organizational psychology*, Vol. II (pp. 398–415). London: Sage.

Barling, J., & Griffiths, A. (2002). A history of occupational health psychology. In J. C. Quick & L. E. Tetrick (Eds.), *Handbook of occupational health psychology* (pp. 19–33). Washington: APA.

Bauer, G. J. & Jenny, G. F. (2007). Development, implementation and dissemination of occupational health Management (OHM): Putting salutogenesis into practice. In J. Houdmont & S. McIntyre (Eds.), *Occupational health psychology: European perspectives on research, education and practice*, Vol. II (pp. 219–250). Maia, Portugal: ISMAI Publishing.

Beckhard, R. & Pritchard, W. (2002). *Changing the essence: The art of changing and leading fundamental change in organizations*. San Francisco: Jossey-Bass.

Bennett, J. B., Cook, R. F. & Pelletier, K. R. (2003). Toward an integrated framework for comprehensive organizational wellness: Concepts, practices and research in workplace health promotion. In J. C. Quick & L. E. Tetrick (Eds.), *Handbook of occupational health psychology*, (pp 69–95). Washington: APA.

Boonstra, J. J. (2004). *Dynamics of organizational change and learning*. Chichester: Wiley.

Brockopp, D. Y., Brockopp, G., Warden, S., Wilson, J., Carpenter, J. S., & Vandeveer, B. (1998). Barriers to change: A pain management project. *International Journal of Nursing Studies*, *35*, 226–232.

Choy, S. Y., Lee, W. B., & Cheung, C. F. (2005). Development of a knowledge management culture assessment tool with applications in aviation industry. *Journal of Information & Knowledge Management*, *4*, 179–189.

Cooper, C. L., Cartwright, S., & Early, P. (Eds.) (2001). *Handbook of organizational culture and climate*. New York: Wiley.

De Long, D., & Fahey, L. (2000). Diagnosing cultural barriers to knowledge management. *The Academy of Management Executive*, *14*, 113–127.

De Witte, K. & van Muijen, J. (1999). Organizational culture. *European Journal of Work and Organizational Psychology, 8*, 497–595.

Delhey, J. (2004). *Life satisfaction in an enlarged Europe.* Luxembourg: Office for Official Publications of the European Communities.

Demerouti, E., Bakker, A. B., Nachreiner, F., & Schaufeli, W. B. (2001). The job demands–resources model of burnout. *Journal of Applied Psychology, 86*, 499–512.

Díaz-Cabrera, D. (2008, November). *Safety and implementation culture developments in the framework of two European projects (Adams-2 & Hilas).* Paper presented at the eighth conference of the European Academy of Occupational Health Psychology, Valencia, Spain.

Díaz-Cabrera, D., Hernández-Fernaud, E., & Isla-Díaz, R. (2007). An evaluation of a new instrument to measure organisational safety culture values and practices. *Accident Analysis and Prevention, 39*, 1202–1211.

Dibella, A. J. (2003). Organizations as learning portfolios. In M. Easterby-Smith & M. A. Lyles (Eds.). *Handbook of organizational learning and knowledge management* (pp. 145–160). Oxford: Blackwell.

Easterby-Smith, M., & Lyles, M. A. (Eds.) (2003). *Handbook of organizational learning and knowledge management.* Oxford: Blackwell.

EU-OSHA – The European Agency for Safety and Health at Work. (2007a). *Expert forecast on emerging psychosocial risks related to occupational safety and health.* Retrieved from www.osha.europa.eu/en/publications/reports/7807118

EU-OSHA – The European Agency for Safety and Health at Work. (2007b). *OSH in figures: Young workers—Facts and figures.* Retrieved from www.osha.europa.eu/en/publications/reports/7606507/view

European Foundation for the Improvement of Living and Working Conditions. (2002). *Quality of work and employment in Europe: Issues and challenges.* Luxembourg: Office for Official Publications of the European Communities.

European Foundation for the Improvement of Living and Working Conditions. (2008). *Annual review of working conditions in the EU 2007–2008.* Luxembourg: Office for Official Publications of the European Communities.

European Network for Workplace Health Promotion. (1997). *Luxembourg declaration on workplace health promotion.* Luxembourg: European Network for Workplace Health Promotion.

Evans, B., Glendon, A. I., & Creed, P. A. (2007): Development and initial validation of an aviation safety climate scale. *Journal of Safety Research, 38*, 675–682.

Fay, D., Lührmann, H., & Kohl, C. (2004). Proactive climate in a post-reorganization setting: When staff compensate managers' weakness. *Journal of Work and Organisational Psychology, 13*, 241–267.

García-Marco, F. J. (2003). La gestión del conocimiento: aplicación a la promoción de la salud [Knowledge management: Its application to health promotion]. *Scire, 9*, 151–170.

Gordon, G. G. (1991). Industry determinants of organizational culture. *Academy of Management Review, 16*, 396–415.

Guldenmund, F. W. (2007). The use of questionnaires in safety culture research—an evaluation. *Safety Science, 45*, 723–743.

Hale, A. (2000). Culture's confusions. *Safety Science, 34*, 1–14.

Hofstede, G. (1991). *Cultures and organizations.* London: MacGraw-Hill.

Hofstede, G. (2002). Cultural constraints in management theories. In C. Cooper (Ed.), *Fundamentals of organizational behavior*, Vol. 3 (pp. 241–256). London: Sage.

Hofstede, G. & Peterson, M. F. (2000). Culture: National values and organizational practices. In N. M. Ashkanasy, C. P. Wilderom, & M. F. Peterson (Eds.), *Handbook of organizational culture and climate* (pp. 401–415). London: Sage.

Hopkins, A. (2006, May). *Studying organisational cultures and their effects on safety*. Paper presented at the International Conference on Occupational Risk Prevention, Seville, Spain.

Landsbergis, P. A. (2003). The changing organization of work and the safety and health of working people: A commentary. *Journal of Occupational and Environmental Medicine*, 45, 61–72.

Martin, J. & Frost, P. (1996). The organizational culture war games: A struggle for intellectual dominance. In S. R. Clegg, C. Hardy, & W. R. Nord (Eds.), *Handbook of organizational studies* (pp. 599–621). London: Sage.

Mayo, E. (1933). *The human problems of an industrial civilization*. New York: Macmillan.

Mayo, E. (1945). *The social problems of an industrial civilization*. Boston: Harvard University Press.

McDonald, N., Corrigan, S., Daly, C., & Cromie, S. (2000). Safety management systems and safety culture in aircraft maintenance organizations. *Safety Science*, 34, 151–176.

Moray, N. (2001). Cultural and national factors in nuclear safety. In B. Wilpert & N. Itoigawa (Eds.), *Safety culture in nuclear power operations* (pp. 37–59). London: Taylor & Francis.

Nicolini, D., Powell, J., Conville, P., & Martinez-Solano, L. (2008). Managing knowledge in the healthcare sector: A review. *International Journal of Management Reviews*, 10, 245–263.

NIOSH (2008). *NIOSH Safety and Health Topic: Occupational Health Psychology (OHP)*. Retrieved from www.cdc.gov/niosh/topics/stress/ohp/ohp.html

Parent-Thirion, A., Macías, E., Hurley, J., & Vermeylen, G. (2007). *Fourth European working conditions survey*. Luxembourg: Office for Official Publications of the European Communities.

Reason, J. (2003). *Managing maintenance error: a practical guide*. Aldershot: Ashgate.

Reiman, T. & Oedewald, P. (2007). Assessment of complex sociotechnical systems—Theoretical issues concerning the use of organizational culture and organizational core task concepts. *Safety Science*, 45, 745–768.

Riege, A. (2005). Three dozen knowledge-sharing barriers managers must consider. *Journal of Knowledge Management*, 9, 18–35.

Rogers, R. W. & Byham, W. C. (1994). Diagnosing organization cultures for realignment. In A. Howard (Ed.), *Diagnosis for organizational change* (pp. 179–209). New York: Guilford Press.

Sauter, S. & Hurrell, J. (1999). Occupational health psychology: Origins, content and direction. *Professional Psychology: Research and Practice*, 30, 117–122.

Sauter, S. L., Brightwell, W. S., Colligan, M. J., Hurrell, J. J., Jr., Katz, T. M., LeGrande, D. E., … Tetrick, L. E. (2002). *The changing organization of work and the safety and health of working people* (DHHS [NIOSH] Publication No. 2002–116). Cincinnati, OH: National Institute for Occupational Safety and Health.

Schaufeli, W. B. (2004). The future of occupational health psychology. *Applied Psychology: An International Review*, 53, 502–517.

Schein, E. H. (1985). *Organizational culture and leadership*. San Francisco: Jossey-Bass.

Schilling, J. & Kluge A. (2008). Barriers to organizational learning: An integration of theory and research. *International Journal of Management Reviews.* doi: 10.1111/j.1468-2370.2008.00242.x

Sinangil, H. K. & Avallone, F. (2001). Organizational development and change. In N. Anderson, D. S. Ones, & H. K. Sinangil (Eds.), *Industrial work & organizational psychology*, Vol. 2 (pp. 332–345). London: Sage.

Udris, I. (2006). Salutogenese in der Arbeit—ein Paradigmenwechsel? [Salutogenesis at work—a change of paradigm?]. *Wirtschaftspsychologie, Sonderheft zur Salutogenese in der Arbeit, 8*, 4–13.

Van de Ven, A. H. (1995). Innovation. In N. Nicholson (Ed.), *Encyclopedic dictionary of organizational behavior* (pp. 233–237). Oxford: Blackwell.

Vassie, L. H. & Lucas, W. R. (2001). An assessment of health and safety management within working groups in the UK manufacturing sector. *Journal of Safety Research, 32*, 479–490.

Wilpert, B. (1995). Organizational behavior. *Annual Review of Psychology, 46*, 59–90.

Wilpert, B. (2001). The relevance of safety culture for nuclear power operations. In B. Wilpert & N. Itoigawa (Eds.), *Safety culture in nuclear power operations* (pp. 5–18). London: Taylor & Francis.

Wilson, M., DeJoy, D., Vandenberg, R., Richardson, H., & McGrath, A. (2004). Work characteristics and employee health and well-being: Test of a model of healthy work organization. *Journal of Occupational and Organizational Psychology, 77*, 565–588.

Wren, B., Schwartz, A., Allen, C., Boyd, J., Gething, N., Hill-tout, J., Jennings, T., Morrison, L., & Pullen, A. (2006). Developing occupational health psychology services in healthcare settings. In J. Houdmont & S. McIntyre (Eds.), *Occupational health psychology: European perspectives on research, education and practice*, Vol. I (pp. 177–204), Maia, Portugal: ISMAI Publishing.

Yandrick, R. M. (1996). *Behavioral risk management: How to avoid preventable losses from mental health problems in the workplace.* Oxford: John Wiley & Sons.

14

Work–Family Positive Spillover
Where Have We Been and What Lies Ahead?

Kristi L. Zimmerman and Leslie B. Hammer
Portland State University, USA

Over the past fifteen years, work–family research has been established as a significant element of the field of occupational health psychology. However, as many researchers have observed, the majority of work–family research has focused solely on the conflict between the work and family domains, ignoring the idea that work and family roles may have beneficial and reciprocal effects on one another (Greenhaus & Parasuraman, 1999). This popular conflict perspective is guided by the scarcity hypothesis (Goode, 1960), which assumes individuals possess a fixed amount of time and human energy and that participation in multiple roles will result in more opportunity for conflict. More recently, there has been a call for research examining the positive effects of combining work and family roles. Ideas about the benefits of combining multiple roles originated in the early work of Sieber (1974) and others (e.g., Marks, 1977; Thoits, 1983), as arguments began to focus on the idea that participating in multiple roles could create energy rather than simply expend energy. Drawing on these early works, work–family researchers have begun to establish a body of research which focuses specifically the benefits of combining the work and family roles (e.g., Hanson, Hammer, & Colton, 2006; Greenhaus & Powell, 2006). With the expansion of this body of literature comes the need for a clarification and organization of the research, which is the overarching goal of the current chapter.

Research in the realm of work–family positive spillover has been evolving and has been focused on several developmental areas. First, research has concentrated on developing various constructs to measure the positive spillover phenomenon (e.g., facilitation, enhancement, enrichment). Second, researchers have voiced a need for theoretical models from which to study the process of work–family positive spillover and have begun to answer this call with the development of a few theories (Greenhaus & Powell, 2006; Wayne, Grzywacz, Carlson, & Kacmar, 2007). Finally, research has started to examine the antecedents and outcomes of positive spillover, with the majority of this research focusing on the outcomes (Stevens, Minnotte, Mannon, & Kiger, 2007).

The purpose of this chapter is to review these key research areas, to discuss where positive spillover literature has been in the past, and to suggest where we see this body of research going in the future. Thus, we begin by introducing the positive psychology movement, following this with a brief review of role theory and the work–family interface. Next, we provide an overview of the positive spillover construct and tease apart the various terms used to operationalize this phenomenon. We offer an explanation of the most current theoretical models of work–family positive spillover and review the body of research that has examined its antecedents and outcomes. Finally, we will put forward specific suggestions for the future of positive spillover research.

The Positive Psychology Movement

The positive psychology movement was strongly influenced by Martin Seligman and his seminal works in the area of optimism and happiness (Seligman, 1998; Seligman & Csikszentmihalyi, 2000). Positive Psychology is a branch of psychology that places emphasis on the study of positive emotions, strengths, character, virtues, and healthy institutions. It is the study of the conditions and processes that contribute to the flourishing or optimal functioning of people, groups, and institutions (Seligman & Csikszentmihalyi, 2000). The premise behind the positive psychology movement is the idea that the science of psychology has made great strides in understanding what goes wrong in individuals, families, groups, and institutions, but these advances have come at the cost of understanding what is right with people (Gable & Haidt, 2005). Thus, the focus of positive psychology is not just fixing what is broken but nurturing what is best (Seligman & Csikzentmihalyi, 2000). The first World Congress of Positive Psychology was held in June, 2009 and attracted an interdisciplinary group of psychologists from around the globe.

Consistent with the positive psychology movement, the idea of examining the positive side of work has recently come into play in organizational psychology research with regards to the study of work engagement (Schaufeli & Bakker, 2004; for a review of the positive psychology perspective and work engagement research in occupational health psychology see Bakker & Derks, 2010). Work engagement has been defined by researchers as a positive, fulfilling, work-related state of mind that is characterized by vigor, dedication, and absorption and is considered the "positive antipode" of burnout (Schaufeli & Bakker, 2004). Work engagement corresponds to optimal functioning and human strength, whereas burnout corresponds to what has been traditionally focused on in psychology—human weakness and malfunctioning in the form of disease, disability, disorder, and damage (Seligman & Csikszentmihalyi, 2000). Work engagement is not only a phenomenon studied in the research literature, but has also become a useful concept in organizational practice. Largely as a result of recent work published by the Gallup Organization (2008), employee engagement has become a buzz word in many organizations. Research published by Gallup and others has shown that engaged employees are more productive employees.

The research also proves that engaged employees are more profitable, more customer-focused, safer, and more likely to withstand temptations to leave (Gallup Research Institute, 2008). Thus, it is important to recognize this increasingly popular movement in both research and practice towards a better understanding of the positive aspects of the individual and the workplace.

Finally, in work–family research and practice, the concept of positive spillover also finds a place within the realm of positive psychology. With the work–family positive spillover construct, we narrow our focus to emphasize employee strengths that are explicitly obtained through resources which aid in the integration of work and family (Greenhaus & Powell, 2006). But before defining the concept of positive spillover and the various constructs used for its operationalization, it is important to review the theoretical roots underlying this concept.

Role Theory and the Work–Family Interface

Overview of role theory

A dominant theoretical perspective that has been used to explain the relationship between work and family is role theory (see Katz & Kahn, 1978). Kahn, Wolfe, Quinn, Snoek, and Rosenthal (1964) suggested that roles are the results of expectations that others hold about appropriate behavior in a particular situation. Role conflict is described as the psychological tension that is aroused by conflicting role pressures. According to role theory, inter-role conflict will occur when individuals engage in multiple roles that are incompatible (Katz & Kahn, 1978), and work–family conflict is a form of such inter-role conflict (Greenhaus & Beutell, 1985).

Multiple roles may also be beneficial and serve to enhance well-being (Thoits, 1983). Specifically, multiple roles can generate more resources and opportunity for energy to be recharged through enhanced self-esteem (Marks, 1977) and work–family positive spillover is one form of roles enhancing one another. Two role-related perspectives for describing the relationships between work and family are the scarcity hypothesis (Goode, 1960) and the enhancement hypothesis (Sieber, 1974).

The scarcity hypothesis and work–family conflict

The scarcity hypothesis assumes that human energy is a limited resource and that engaging in multiple roles will result in greater opportunity for conflict (i.e., work–family conflict). Research in the work–family domain has emphasized the importance of distinguishing between the two directions of spillover, either work-to-family (in which work interferes with or facilitates family) or family-to-work (in which family interferes with or facilitates with work) (Frone, Russell, & Cooper, 1992). Literature suggests that work-to-family conflict may have different antecedents and outcomes than family-to-work conflict (Frone, 2003). Frone et al. (1992) tested their model and demonstrated how work-related demands are most often associated with work-to-family conflict and family-related demands are most often associated with family-to-work conflict. That is, stressors in one domain are often related only to conflict originating in that same domain. For example, job stressors were predictive of work-to-family conflict, whereas family stressors and family involvement were predictive of family-to-work conflict (Frone et al, 1992, 1997). However, other researchers have demonstrated how the effects of the conflict can occur in the opposite domain from the originating stressor (e.g. Kossek & Ozeki, 1998). It is important to recognize that regardless of the direction of the interference, work–family conflict is triggered by simultaneous pressures or demands in both roles (Greenhaus, Allen, & Spector, 2006).

Enhancement hypothesis and work–family positive spillover

For roughly 30 years, theorists have recognized that positive spillover also occurs between work and family roles, in that one role can enhance the other. Dating back to the work of Marks (1977) and Sieber (1974), it has been argued that the benefits of occupying multiple roles outweigh the costs. Marks suggested that multiple role occupation could create energy rather than simply expend it. He argued that a theory involving multiple role occupation should not view energy as finite and should acknowledge the benefits as well as the drawbacks of multiple roles. In fact, he suggested that one role can create positive energy that carries over to other roles, thus energizing rather than draining the person.

Research has found that individuals report rewards and benefits of multiple role participation (e.g., Ingersoll-Dayton, Neal, & Hammer, 2001; Piotrkowski, 1979; Yogev, 1981). These benefits include reduced psychological distress (Pietromanoco, Manis, & Frohardt-Lane, 1986; Thoits, 1983), increased job satisfaction (Pietromanoco et al, 1986), improved work outcomes (Ingersoll-Dayton et al., 2001), and improved mental and physical health outcomes (Collijn, Appels, & Nijhuis, 1996; Crosby, 1991; Hammer, Cullen, Neal, Shafiro, & Sinclair, 2005; Repetti, Matthews, & Waldron, 1989). When comparing the scarcity and enhancement hypotheses, research has concluded that these two hypotheses are not mutually exclusive and that both stressors and rewards spill over from one role to another. As Friedman and Greenhaus (2000) put it, work and family are both "allies" and "enemies," in that resources and emotions can be shared across domains, but can also be depleted by an overdemanding role.

Most recently, Van Steenbergen, Ellemers, & Mooijaart (2007) demonstrated that work–family positive spillover contributes to the prediction of work and nonwork outcomes above and beyond work–family conflict. Specifically, they found that including four types of facilitation (energy-based, time-based, behavioral, and psychological) substantially improved the prediction of work outcomes (e.g., job performance, affective commitment, and work satisfaction) and nonwork outcomes (e.g., home performance, home commitment, home satisfaction, and global life satisfaction) above and beyond the effects of conflict. These results reveal the importance of viewing these constructs as distinct mechanisms rather than as existing along the same continuum.

The relationship between work–family positive spillover and work–family conflict

In the positive spillover literature, Carlson, Kacmar, Wayne, and Grzywacz (2006) offer a host of reasons as to why it is important to differentiate between work-to-family and family-to-work positive spillover. They suggest that the resources forged by one domain may be different from those initiated by another. For example, some of the benefits and privileges derived from involvement in one's work, such as income, may not be derived from involvement in one's family, and vice versa. Thus, different types of resource gains may or may not be equivalent across domains. They also note that positive spillover can occur bi-directionally such that work can provide resources that result in enhanced functioning in the family domain (work-to-family positive spillover) or family can provide resource gains that lead to enhanced individual functioning in the work domain (family-to-work positive spillover). In their review of the work–family enhancement literature, Greenhaus and Powell (2006) reported that the mean correlation between work–family conflict and work–family positive spillover ranged from a low of zero to a high of .35. The mean value of the 21 correlations reported by Greenhaus and Powell (2006) was only -.02. Thus, it is safe to conclude that these constructs are independent and not simply opposite ends of the same continuum. This review of role theory is central to understanding the historical roots of the positive spillover construct as well as the differentiation between the two directions of spillover.

Positive Spillover Construct Development

General construct development

A variety of construct names have been proposed to describe the benefits of participating in both work and family including *work–family positive spillover* (Edwards & Rothbard, 2000; Hanson et al., 2006), *work–family facilitation* (Grzywacz, 2002), *work–family enhancement* (Barnett & Baruch, 1985), and *work–family enrichment* (Greenhaus & Powell, 2006). As noted by Hanson et al. (2006) and others (e.g., Greenhaus & Powell, 2006), the distinction between these various terms is not well understood, and several different viewpoints can be taken on how these various operationalizations fit together. We propose work–family positive spillover as a meta-construct with the various operationalizations fitting within the overarching construct (e.g., facilitation, enrichment, and enhancement).

An early conception of the work–family interface was offered by Staines (1980) who proposed three mechanisms for understanding the relationship between work and family roles: segmentation, compensation, and spillover. The segmentation model postulates that work and family life represent independent domains that do not influence one another. The compensation model suggests a negative relationship between work and family. Specifically, it works on the assumption that increasing dissatisfaction in one life domain (e.g., the family) leads to a reduction of time and energy devoted to that role, which then leads to an increase in time and energy devoted to a second life domain (e.g., work) in an effort to compensate for the lack of rewards or for undesirable experiences in the first (Frone, 2003). Finally, the spillover model postulates a positive relationship between work and family such that a change in one domain leads to a related change in another domain. It became important to point out that spillover can be negative, such as bad experiences at work that lead to negative experiences at home or positive such that positive family experiences lead to positive work experiences. Thus, the concept of positive spillover emerged.

Crouter (1984) expanded on the work of previous researchers with the proposition that positive spillover is not limited to energy exchanges, arguing for two additional forms of positive spillover. The first is psychological spillover, in which positive mood or enhanced feelings of self-esteem from one role affect mood in another role. The second form is educational spillover, where skills gained and knowledge learned in one sphere can be used in the other. Examples of such skills include empathy, interpersonal skills, and time management. She argued that psychological spillover was much more transitory in nature, whereas educational spillover was more stable and occurred over longer periods of time (Crouter, 1984).

In addition, Crouter (1984) was one of the first researchers to examine positive family-to-work spillover. Crouter conducted interviews with 55 employees at a large manufacturing plant to identify themes associated with both positive and negative spillover. For positive spillover, two major themes emerged: (1) the supportive nature of family relationships, and (2) skills and attitudes acquired at home which could be useful in other settings, such as empathy or interpersonal skills. The researchers then compared overall spillover (negative spillover minus positive spillover) between groups of employees who had a variety of work and family situations (e.g., gender, parental status). Specifically, at the time there were suggestions in the literature that individuals may differ in their view of the work–family relationship based on factors such as gender, marital status, parental status and type of occupation. Thus, they selected a sample that had adequate variation along these dimensions. Mothers reported less positive spillover (i.e., more negative spillover) from family-to-work than fathers, but there was no significant gender difference between nonparents (Crouter, 1984).

At this point, the concept of positive spillover had been established in the work–family literature but there were many unanswered questions with regards to the predictors and outcomes of this construct. Further, research trends showed a peaked interest in the various ways of operationalizing the positive spillover meta-construct. Thus, with the popularity of this idea growing, research introduced several operationalizations of the positive spillover meta-construct including work–family positive spillover (e.g., Crouter, 1984, Edwards & Rothbard, 2000, Hanson et al., 2006), work–family facilitation (Grzywacz, 2002), work–family enhancement (Barnett & Baruch, 1985), and work–family enrichment (Greenhaus & Powell, 2006; Carlson et al., 2006) to describe the theoretical relationships and mechanisms that enable work and family to benefit one another.

Edwards and Rothbard (2000) contributed to the general understanding of positive spillover by offering four types of positive spillover and the processes by which these different types of spillover may occur. The four types of spillover include mood, values, skills, and behaviors and each of these occur from work to family and family to work. Mood spillover occurs when mood in one domain affects mood in the other domain. This can be in the form of positive mood spillover in which positive moods enhance cognitive functioning, increase task activity, and promote positive interactions with others, each of which facilitates role performance (Staw, Sutton, & Pelled, 1994). For example, a positive interaction that a mother has with her child in the morning can create a positive mood that transfers to an upbeat interaction with her client during a morning work meeting. This role performance brings intrinsic and extrinsic rewards which then enhance mood. The same process is true of the spillover of negative moods. In addition, positive affect also allows one to accumulate resources and enhance self-esteem and self-control. Edwards and Rothbard (2000) emphasize that mood spillover is largely unintentional and that intent regulates the degree to which the felt mood is manifested as expressed mood, and that people regulate expressed moods to fulfill role expectations, enhance role performance, and receive role rewards.

Another type of spillover offered by Edwards and Rothbard (2000) is value spillover, which suggests two causal structures. In the first, work and family are socializing forces that affect the values that are operative in an individual's life as a whole, and these general life values influence values specific to a domain. For example, values developed in the work domain, such as obedience, influence a particular person's general life values. Based on these general values, it is argued, this person will emphasize obedience in parenting techniques used in the family domain (Edwards & Rothbard, 2000). In the second, values acquired in one domain directly affect values in the other. Similarly, the spillover of work and family skills also implies two causal pathways. First, skills obtained in one domain influence one's general knowledge, which in turn influences family skills. For example, leadership skills obtained at work may enhance one's general knowledge of guidance which may, in turn, facilitate parental supervision skills. The second pathway for the spillover of skills is directly from one domain to the other, as when finance skills learnt for a work task become directly applicable to managing one's family finances. A final type of spillover offered by Edwards and Rothbard (2000) is behavioral spillover, which follows a two-part causal structure similar to that of values and skills. Specifically, behaviors developed in one domain either become ingrained as habits or styles that then influence the second domain or directly affect behaviors in the opposite domain.

Work–family facilitation

Another construct that has been used to measure the positive aspects of participating in both work and family roles is work–family facilitation (Grzywacz, 2002; Wayne, Musisca, & Fleeson 2004). Work–family facilitation is the notion that work and family are interdependent and complementary (Werbel & Walter, 2002). Grzywacz and colleagues define work–family facilitation as the extent to which an individual's engagement in one domain of life (e.g., work or family) is beneficial for the second domain and yields developmental, affective, capital or efficiency gains that result in enhanced functioning in another life domain (e.g., family or work). They argue that in contrast to positive spillover which involves the transfer of personal characteristics such as affect, skills, behaviors, and values from one domain to another, thus benefiting the second domain, facilitation is proposed to occur not just through personal gains but through capital gains as well (e.g., money, employment benefits, and social contacts; Hanson et al., 2006).

We now turn to the concept of work–family enrichment which has recently gained popularity due to Greenhaus and Powell's (2006) theory and Carlson et al.'s (2006) measure of enrichment.

Work–family enrichment

Work–family enrichment is said to occur when resources are generated in one role (e.g., family) that improve the quality of life in another role (e.g., work). Greenhaus and Powell (2006) define resources widely to include personal resources, similar to those in the definition of spillover, as well as social capital and material assets, which go beyond traditional definitions of positive spillover. Given this definition, some research proposes that constructs such as work–family positive spillover, and work–family facilitation can at times be broadly categorized under the rubric of work–family enrichment (Hanson et al., 2006). In addition, Greenhaus and Powell (2006) proposed a theoretical model which will be discussed in the next section as we highlight the most recent theoretical developments in the positive spillover literature.

Work–family enhancement

The construct of *enhancement* has also been introduced to measure the process of work–family positive spillover. The enhancement construct is conceptually very similar to the enhancement hypothesis discussed in the previous section on role theory. Specifically, work–family enhancement refers to the rewards that an employee accrues from simultaneously occupying roles in both the work and family arenas (Barnett & Baruch, 1985). It suggests that individual's personal resources are abundant and expandable and that activity in one domain may actually enrich experiences in the other domain rather than depleting energy. In other words, spillover from one role to another can be positive because participation in multiple domains can enrich the personal resources available for use in other domains (Kirchmeyer, 1992). According to Thompson and Bunderson (2001), from a time perspective, one role can positively affect another as long as the time spent in a particular one is meaningful to the individual and evokes a sense of personal satisfaction. They refer to this as "identity-affirming" time and propose that identify-affirming time spent in the work and family domains will result in a decreased perception of work–family conflict.

Measurement of Positive Spillover

General measurement

Early measurement of work–family positive spillover adapted more generic measures of spillover to capture the positive interdependencies between work and family. For example, facilitation has been measured using Kirchmeyer's (1992) scale, which presents 15 positive statements and asks participants to indicate the extent of their agreement. Sample items include "being involved with family life activities helps me to forget the problems at work" and "being involved in personal benefit activities provides me with the contacts that are helpful at work." Facilitation has also been assessed using measures that require individuals to reflect back on work–family experiences. For example, Grzywacz and Marks (2000a) measure facilitation using the following items: "How often have you experienced each of the following in the past year? (1) The things you do at work help you deal with personal and practical issues at home. (2) The things you do at work make you a more interesting person at home. (3) Having a good day on your job makes, you a better companion when you get home. (4) The skills you use on your job are useful for things you have to do at home." As positive spillover research started to flourish, researchers began to realize the need for measures designed specifically to capture the spillover relationship between work and family. The most popular of these measures are Hanson et al's (2006) measure of positive spillover and Carlson et al.'s (2006) measure of work–family enrichment. Thus, we turn to a review of these two measures.

Drawing on previous theoretical frameworks of positive spillover, Hanson et al. (2006) defined the construct of work–family positive spillover as the transfer of positively valenced affect, skills, behaviors, and values from the originating domain to the receiving domain, thus having beneficial effects on the receiving domain. Hanson et al. developed and assessed a multidimensional measure to capture these different facets of spillover based on the following six subdimensions: (1) work-to-family affective positive spillover, (2) work-to-family behavior-based instrumental spillover, (3) work-to-family value-based instrumental positive spillover, (4) family-to-work affective positive spillover, (5) family-to-work behavior-based instrumental spillover, (6) family-to-work value-based instrumental positive spillover. Instrumental spillover was defined as instances in which skills, abilities and values are applied effectively in another role, and affective spillover as instances in which affect or emotion is carried over from one role to another (Hanson et al., 2006). Sample items include, "Being in a positive mood at work helps me to be in a positive mood at home" (affective work-to-family positive spillover), "Values developed in my family make me a better employee" (value-based family-to-work positive spillover), "Skills developed in my family life help me in my job" (behavior-based family-to-work positive spillover).

With regards to the measurement of enrichment, Carlson et al. (2006) developed a multi-dimensional measure of work–family enrichment that involves resources gains. The measure consists of three dimensions from the work to family direction (development, affect, and capital) and three dimensions from the family to work direction (development, affect, and efficiency). The items in this scale were developed to capture the true essence of the definition of enrichment by incorporating the transfer of resource gains into the other domain in ways that enhance functioning for the individual. Sample items include, "My involvement in work helps me to gain knowledge and this helps me to be a better family member," (work-to-family development), "My involvement in my family puts me in a good mood and helps me to be a better worker" (family-to-work affect), "My involvement in my family encourages me to use my work time in a focused manner and then helps me to be a better worker" (family-to-work efficiency). With regards to measurement, in comparison to spillover and facilitation, this measure of enrichment adds the idea of efficiency gains to the affective, instrument and capital gains introduced by the measures of facilitation and positive spillover. A problem with this measure, however, is that the items appear to contain two phrases, and thus one person could reasonably agree with the first phrase while disagreeing with the second, while another person might do the opposite. Thus, interpretability may be compromised. We now turn to a discussion of the measurement of work–family enhancement which has received less attention in the literature than facilitation and enrichment.

With regard to the measurement of enhancement, there does not appear to be one consistent "work–family enhancement scale" that is used when hypothesizing relationships with enhancement. For example, Gordon, Whelan-Berry, and Hamilton (2007) examined the relationships between conflict, enhancement and work–family culture using a measure drawn from the Midlife Development Inventory, Part 2 (e.g., "What you do at work helps you deal with personal and practical issues at home"; "Your home life helps you relax and feel ready for the next day's work"). In another case, Tiedje et al. (1990) examined role-compatibility perceptions, satisfaction, and mental health and measured work–family enhancement using measures developed specifically for this study (e.g., "Having a career often helps me to better appreciate the time I spend with my children"). Finally, Ruderman, Ohlott, Panzer, and King (2002) conducted a qualitative study examining the benefits of multiple roles for managerial women. To measure enhancement, they asked a series of questions about the various roles participants were engaged in and developed several enhancement themes from this qualitative data such as, "opportunities to enrich interpersonal skills," "psychological benefits," "emotional support and advice." Drawing on the previous examples, there does not appear to be a consistent form of measurement for the construct of work–family enhancement. Taking into consideration this inconsistency in measurement and a vague definition that fails to differentiate this construct from that of enrichment or facilitation, we suggest that enhancement is not a unique process but is simply another term used to describe the positive spillover phenomenon. In conjunction with a focus on measurement, researchers have also taken interest in developing specific theories of positive spillover which will be reviewed in the next section.

Theories of Positive Spillover

Greenhaus & Powell's (2006) theory of work–family enrichment

In 2006, Greenhaus and Powell answered a call for the development of a theoretical model of work–family positive spillover with their influential article entitled "When work and family are allies: A theory of work–family enrichment." There are three main components in Greenhaus and Powell's theoretical framework of work–family enrichment: First, they conceptualize work–family enrichment as being bidirectional. That is, work can provide resource gains that enhance performance in the family domain, or family can provide resource gains that improve performance in the work domain. Second, their framework defines a resource as "an asset that may be drawn on when needed to solve a problem or cope with a challenging situation" (p. 80). Along with this definition, Greenhaus and Powell identify five types of resources that can be generated in a role (work or family). They proposed that these resources generated in one domain (work or family) will promote high performance and positive affect in the opposite domain. The five types comprise (1) flexibility resources, (2) material resources, (3) skills and perspectives, (5) psychological and physical resources, and (5) social capital resources.

A third component of their framework rests on the idea that resources promote work–family enrichment primarily through two different paths: instrumental and affective. The instrumental pathway suggests that employees believe their family or work involvement has increased their ability to perform in the opposite role. For example, family-domain support may provide individuals with resources necessary to handle coworkers or beneficial to their ability to perform on the job. The affective path promotes work–family enrichment indirectly through influence on moods and emotions resulting from role participation. Specifically, as individuals gain greater resources through participation in one role (work or family), their positive mood in that role will increase and then aid their performance in the other role (Greenhaus & Powell, 2006). Finally, they propose the salience of role B (work or family) to moderate both the relationship between role A resources and role B performance as well as the relationship between positive affect in role A and role B performance.

Resource–gain–development theory
(Wayne, Grzywacz, Carlson, & Kacmar, 2007)

In conjunction with the empirical research examining the concept of positive spillover, there has been a recent call for the development of a theoretical framework from which to examine this construct (Frone, 2003). Wayne, Grzywacz, Carlson, and Kacmar (2007) offer a theoretical explanation and model of the antecedents and outcomes of positive spillover based on the concepts of positive organizational scholarship (Cameron, Dutton, & Quinn, 2003), ecological systems theory (Bronfenbrenner, 1979), and conservation of resources theory (Hobfoll, 1989).

They suggest that personal characteristics (e.g., positive affectivity, self-efficacy, work identity) and environmental resources in the form of energy resources, support resources, and condition resources would enable work–family facilitation. They propose that this facilitation will then promote positive system functioning as reported by other system members. As for work, this would involve ratings from coworkers on work group cohesion or perceived unit effectiveness. At home, this would involve family ratings of marital quality, parent–child interactions or family well-being. Finally they propose that demand characteristics will directly influence the availability of environmental resources and also moderate the relationship between environmental resources and facilitation. For example, they suggest gender as a demand characteristic such that women may be more likely to use family supportive resources than men, thus resulting in a greater likelihood of facilitation.

As noted previously, research has given more attention to the outcomes of positive spillover and we suggest these two theoretical models will provide avenues for additional research on both the antecedents and outcomes of positive spillover. Thus, with these theoretical models in mind, we now turn to a discussion of the antecedents and outcomes of positive spillover.

Antecedents and Outcomes of Positive Spillover

Antecedents

As mentioned previously, little research has examined the predictors of work–family positive spillover. In early research on predictors of spillover, Kirchmeyer (1992; 1993) examined positive spillover from nonwork roles including parenting, community work, and recreation, to the role of the employee. Results showed that the resource of psychological parent involvement was positively related to spillover between parenting and work roles, whereas the demand of actual time spent parenting was negatively related to positive spillover (Kirchmeyer, 1992). In 1993, Kirchmeyer found higher levels of positive spillover reported by individuals who used certain coping strategies such as role redefinition. We suggest that a useful framework for understanding the antecedents of positive spillover involves categorizing predictors as either work-related resources, family-related resources or personal characteristics. Thus, we will begin with a review of predictors originating in the work domain followed by those originating in the family domain and conclude with a those antecedents that are not specific to the work or family domains (e.g., personality traits, health).

Work-domain resources

Grzywacz and Marks (2000a) offered a comprehensive examination of the antecedents of positive spillover. Using data from the National Survey of Midlife Development in the United States (MIDUS), with a sample of 1,986 employed adults, the researchers examined the relationships of work and family antecedents to both work-to-family and family-to-work positive spillover. As regards work-related antecedents, the resource of decision latitude had a positive relationship with both work-to-family and family-to-work positive spillover whereas the demand of pressure at work was negatively related to both directions of spillover. Although the previous findings have laid the ground work for establishing the antecedents of work–family positive spillover, the authors recognize that the cross-sectional nature of these studies does not allow us to draw causal inferences with regards to the direction of this relationship and suggest that longitudinal research is needed to fully understand the determinants of positive spillover (Grzywacz & Marks, 2000a).

Thompson and Prottas (2006) examined supervisor support, coworker support and supportive culture as antecedents to positive spillover and found that supervisor and coworker support were significantly related to positive spillover. This finding emphasizes that supervisors and coworkers, who are key in establishing a family-supportive culture, act as resources in the work domain to influence positive outcomes in the family domain. Similarly, Wayne, Randel, and Stevens (2006) used Greenhaus and Powell's (2006) theoretical framework to examine both formal family-friendly policy use and informal family-supportive culture as predictors of work–family enrichment. Similar to the previous work–family research, they found that informal workplace practices, particularly having a family-supportive culture, were more important to the work–family experience than formal organizational practices. They suggest that informal practices may be more relevant to enrichment than formal approaches because they provide a more flexible, personalized response to individual work–family needs. As a result, employees more readily experience positive affect to transfer to the family domain.

Other work domain resources include energy resources as proposed by Wayne et al. (2007). They suggest that enriched jobs and developmental opportunities are resources that create energy and enable work–family facilitation. For example, they suggest that working on a complex project may require the use of routine and new skills that allow individuals to experience a combination of learning and competence, providing energy gains to the family domain. Similarly, developmental opportunities such as workplace training are suggested to provide skills that transfer to the family domain. For example, Voydanoff (2007) found that self-reported learning opportunities on the job were associated with more work–family enrichment.

In a recent study conducted by Zimmerman, Hammer, and Kossek (2009), Greenhaus and Powell's (2006) theoretical framework was used to test the antecedents of work–family positive spillover. Specifically, the five types of resources proposed by Greenhaus and Powell (e.g., skills and perspectives, material, physical and psychological, flexibility, and social capital resources) were operationalized using constructs from the work and family domains and tested as longitudinal and cross-sectional predictors of work-to-family and family-to-work positive spillover. For example, decision latitude and family supportive culture were used to operationalize flexibility resources. Results showed that income adequacy acts as a material work-domain resource facilitating positive affective outcomes in the family domain. In addition to these findings, Zimmerman et al. (2009) were able to draw several conclusions about the sample selection and the measurement of predictors to work–family positive spillover. With regards to sample selection, the current study found that in a sample of low-income grocery employees, very few of the proposed resources were significantly related to spillover due to low means and lack of variables. For example, decision latitude was modeled as a predictor of work-to-family positive spillover but with a mean of 2.64, it was concluded that this job was characterized by low levels of decision latitude and it could not, in turn, be modeled as a resource. Thus, when modeling work-domain resources as predictors of positive spillover, we suggest taking the characteristics of the job into consideration.

Family-domain resources

Kinnunen, Feldt, Geurts, and Pulkkinen (2006) posit that having a supportive partner and the opportunity to talk through difficulties at work may help individuals to recover from stressful days and that spouse support is an important buffer for job-related stress. Grzywacz and Marks (2000b) explored the relationship between family factors and negative and positive spillover from family to work. They found a positive relationship between affectual support from family such that less affectual support from both spouse and other family members was associated with less positive spillover from family to work.

Further, Aryee, Srivivas, and Tan (2005) found that family support was significantly related to family-to-work facilitation. They suggested that supportive family experiences may allow individuals to work longer hours and gain development opportunities. Similarly, Barnett (1994) found that the relationship between work experiences and psychological distress was moderated by experiences in the family for both men and women and that when relationships between wives and husbands were good, a poor job had little effect on people's psychological distress. Finally, Zimmerman, Hammer, & Kossek (2009) found that the presence of children under the age of 18 in the household acts as a social capital, family-domain resource facilitating positive affective outcomes in the work domain. The finding mentioned earlier with regards to income adequacy predicting work-to-family spillover may also be interpreted as a family-domain resource as a household measure of income adequacy was used to test this hypothesis.

Personal resources

Although the research has primarily focused on environmental antecedents of work–family positive spillover, the importance of understanding individual characteristics that influence one's ability to experience spillover has been recognized as well (Eby, Casper, Lockwood, Bordeaux, & Brinley, 2005).

Individual differences. Wayne, Musisca, and Fleeson (2004) explored the relationship between each of the Big Five personality traits and work–family facilitation and found that as a set, the Big Five explained 7% of the variance in work-to-family positive spillover and 8% of the variance in family-to-work positive spillover. They found extraversion to be predictive of both work-to-family and family-to-work positive spillover and found conscientiousness and openness to experience to be positively related to work-to-family positive spillover but unrelated to family-to-work positive spillover. Further, those individuals high on agreeableness reported greater family-to-work positive spillover but not work-to-family positive spillover. Similarly, Grzywacz and Marks (2000a) found that high levels of extraversion were associated with high levels of both work-to-family and family-to-work facilitation, whereas low levels of neuroticism were related to both types of work–family facilitation. In addition, Wayne et al. (2007) suggest that positive affectivity and self-efficacy are personal characteristics that enable work–family facilitation. In addition to personality characteristics, research has also examined gender as an individual difference variable related to positive spillover and shows that men and women may differ on levels of positive spillover. Specifically, Powell & Greenhaus (2009) found that women reported higher levels of femininity, a construct that was positively related to positive spillover and thus reported higher levels of positive spillover than men.

Health. While most research on positive spillover and health investigates health as an outcome of spillover, Hill et al., (2007) conducted a qualitative study with data from the IBM 2004 Global Work and Life Issues Survey and examined mental and physical health as predictors of positive spillover. Respondents reported that physical and psychological health resulting from work benefits were features that positively influenced home life. For example, one mother reported that a benefit of working at home was her ability to get more sleep in the morning. This work benefit improves her physical health and allows her to feel less stressed and less tired when performing work and family domain tasks. Respondents in this study also identified physical and psychological resources as aspects of home that positively influence work life. Specifically, a young father spoke of home as, "a place of physical renewal where he released work pressure by exercising every week and eating healthy." Further, a middle-aged women spoke about home as "a place of psychological renewal…a good home life provides emotional support to help relieve and regulate the work pressure." This qualitative study lends further support to the idea that physical and psychological health act as resources in both the work and home domains.

Outcomes

Drawing on the few established theoretical models of work–family enrichment, we see that work–family positive spillover is most often predictive of cross-domain role performance outcomes or individual well-being (Greenhaus & Powell, 2006). The majority of research has focused on individual outcomes such as well-being with a few recent studies focusing on outcomes in the work and family domains.

Work-domain outcomes

With regards to family facilitating work domain outcomes, research has suggested that involvement in family roles such as parenting can enrich personal resources such as self-esteem and competences which then carry over into the job and increase one's potential to meet his or her work demands (Kirchmeyer, 1992). In addition, Wayne et al. (2007) suggest that it is important to examine the effects of work–family facilitation from a systems perspective. As the cross-over literature suggests, work–family experiences of one system member are likely to influence the attitudes, behaviors, and work–family experiences of other members (Hammer, Allen, & Grigsby, 1997). Thus, they suggest that facilitation promotes positive system functioning as reported by other system members. For example, they suggest that as individuals report high levels of work–family facilitation, other members of the receiving system should report enhanced functioning in that system. They suggest that facilitation relates to system ratings from system members in the work domain such as supervisor and coworker ratings of OCBs, cohesion, group effectiveness, etc.

Family-domain outcomes

With regards to work facilitating family-domain outcomes, we have seen less research. In a longitudinal, multisource, multimethod study conducted by Ilies, Wilson & Wagner (2009) results showed the main effects of daily job satisfaction on daily marital satisfaction and affect at home. Drawing on their systems framework discussed above, Wayne et al. (2007) suggest that work-to-family facilitation would relate positively relate to system members' evaluation of functioning in the family domain, such as ratings of marital quality, parent–child interactions and overall family well-being.

Personal outcomes

Health. Several studies have found relationships between positive spillover (work-to-family and family-to-work) and individual health (mental and physical). Positive work–family spillover has been linked to outcomes such as health and role satisfaction (e.g., Crouter, 1984; Grzywacz & Marks, 2000a; Hammer et al., 2005a; Kirchmeyer, 1992; Pavalko & Smith, 1999; Wayne et al., 2004). Gryzwacz and Marks (2000a, 2000b) examined positive spillover outcomes in their MIDUS study and found that positive work-to-family spillover resulted in better physical and mental health, whereas positive family-to-work spillover was related to fewer chronic conditions, better overall well-being (Gryzwacz, 2002), and decreased likelihood of problem drinking (Gryzawacz & Marks, 2000b). In addition, Hammer et al. (2005a) demonstrated significant longitudinal crossover relationships between work–family positive spillover experienced by a spouse and a decrease in an individual's experience of depressive symptoms one year later. Barnett and Hyde (2001) found that engaging in multiple roles benefits both mental and physical health. Similarly, Grzywacz and Bass (2003) found that work–family facilitation was associated with lower risk of mental illness, depression, and problem drinking. Specifically, each unit increase in family-to-work facilitation was associated with a 15% decrease of reported depression and a 38% decrease in reported problem drinking. In addition, Hanson et al. (2006) found that the more resources available to individuals at home, the higher their level of mental health. In a recent study of sleep quality, Williams, Franche, Ibrahim, Mustard, and Layton (2006) found that family-to-work positive spillover was associated with better sleep quality after controlling for a number of health-related factors. Stoddard and Madsen (2007) found a relationship between enrichment and health such that overall health and mental-emotional health were strongly correlated with enrichment in the family-to-work direction, suggesting that family participation supports the mental-emotional and overall health of an individual.

Where to Go from Here?

This chapter has offered a review of positive spillover including a discussion of various constructs used to operationalize the concept as well as the most recent theoretical models designed to further research on the antecedents and outcomes of positive spillover. Based on this review, we now turn to our suggestions for future work–family positive spillover research.

Consistency in operationalization

Suggestion 1: Clarify the differences between the various constructs used to measure work–family positive spillover and provide direction on how the research question should guide measure selection.

As mentioned previously, we suggest that all of the constructs presented fall under the meta-construct of work–family positive spillover. However, the choice of measurement may depend on the research question and future research should attempt to clarify when each measure may be most appropriate. For example, if we are simply interested in affective spillover, we may choose to use Hanson et al.'s (2006) or Carlson et al.'s (2006) affective subscale rather than the entire measure of positive spillover or enrichment. Thus, future research can help to identify and guide work–family researchers towards the most appropriate measures.

Developing a broader understanding of antecedents and outcomes

Suggestion 2: Test further antecedents and outcomes of work–family positive spillover using Greenhaus and Powell's (2006) theory of enrichment and Wayne et al.'s (2007) resource-gain-development theory.

As mentioned previously, much of the research in work–family positive spillover has been focused on construct development and theoretical models. At this point, we encourage research to use these constructs and theories to learn more about the resources that predict positive spillover and the outcomes that result in the work and family domains.

Occupational differences

Suggestion 3: Examine how resources as predictors of positive spillover manifest themselves differently in the work and family domains depending on the type of occupation (e.g., hourly workers, white collar workers, etc.).

As mentioned in the section reviewing the antecedents of positive spillover, Zimmerman Hammer, and Kossek (2009) conducted a study of resources predicting positive spillover and found that the low levels of resources in the hourly workforce made it difficult to establish a relationship between these predictors and the outcome of positive spillover. Unlike the concept of work–family conflict, which assumes demands exist in and spill over between the work and family domains, we cannot assume that resources exist in these domains. For example, Zimmerman et al. (2009) hypothesized that decision latitude would be predictive of work-to-family positive spillover in a sample of hourly grocery store employees. However, due to the low levels of decision latitude reported by the workers, this could not be established as a resource present in this particular sample. Thus, we encourage future research to consider the work and home environments when hypothesizing predictors of positive spillover.

Longitudinal assessments

Suggestion 4: Examine the longitudinal relationships between predictors and outcomes of positive spillover.

   In their study examining the antecedents of positive spillover, Zimmerman et al. (2009) found the model hypothesizing resources as longitudinal predictors of positive spillover to fit the data better than the cross-sectional model. In addition, income adequacy was significantly predictive of work-to-family spillover both cross-sectionally and longitudinally, but parental status was predictive of family-to-work positive spillover only when tested in the cross-sectional structural equation model. Thus, we learned that resources as predictors of positive spillover may manifest themselves differently over time, and we encourage future research to continue testing predictors and outcomes using longitudinal research design in order to understand more about these relationships. In addition, resources may be changing or manifesting at different rates over time. For example, the interactions someone experiences with his or her children may vary from day to day, whereas income adequacy may be more a more stable resource. We therefore suggest that daily longitudinal assessments may be more appropriate when examining dynamic resources.

Ecological systems theory

Suggestion 5: Future research should consider the broader family and work systems in the examination of positive spillover.

   In addition to role theory, ecological systems theory provides a useful framework for understanding the integration of work and family. Specifically, with the introduction of Ecological Systems Theory, Bronfenbrenner (1977) argued that human development could be examined within four interrelated systems. The first is the *microsystem*, which includes the individual and his or her immediate settings, such as home, school, or work. According to systems theory, the interrelationship between microsystems yields another level called a *mesosystem*. The interactions between work and family settings would be an example of a mesosystem and, as a result, the majority of work–family research is focused primarily on this level. The next level is the *exosystem*, which expands upon the mesosystem by including other social structures which influence behavior. These structures can be both formal (e.g., government, the corporate world) or informal (e.g., social networks, media influences). The *macrosystem*, encompasses the economic, social, educational, political, and other systems that influence interactions in all of the other subsystems. These are societal-level patterns that reflect the values of a particular culture and thereby exert influence on the lower-level systems. For example, in the United States value is placed on an organization's or person's monetary worth. Thus, in our society, the importance and esteem of a business executive is often placed above that of a teacher or caregiver. These social values influence the behaviors and decisions of individuals, families, and organizations. In his later work, Bronfenbrenner (1986) introduced a fifth system, the *chronosystem*, which is the idea that there is an evolution of the external systems over time.

By making these five levels explicit, researchers can examine the system level that most appropriately fits their own field. Psychologists, who are generally more interested in individual outcomes, tend to focus more on the micro- and mesosystems. Sociologists may be more inclined to examine exosystem influences, whereas economists and public policy makers may be more concerned with the macrosystem. This is not to say, however, that a researcher will study only one system. Due to the fact that systems are interrelated, understanding is enhanced when all systems are given due consideration.

Grzywacz and Marks (2000a) used Bronfenbrenner's (1977) ecological systems theory as a framework to examine correlates of positive and negative spillover within the work–family microsystem. Specifically, using Bronfenbrenner's theory, they suggest that the work–family experience is a joint function of process, person, context, and time characteristics and that each type of characteristic exerts an additive, and potentially interactive, effect on an individual's work–family experience (Grzywacz & Marks, 2000a). They found that individual and contextual factors interact to influence the amount of work–family spillover that individuals experience. Some studies (e.g., Hammer et al., 1997) have used certain systems principles by including couple-level data, but did not use family systems theory as a basis for the study.

Family systems theory provides a model for understanding the organizational complexity of families, as well as the interactions among family members (Anderson & Sabatelli 1999). Westman, Etzion, and Danon (2001) used a systems perspective when examining the reciprocal effects that marital partners have on one another. Other studies (e.g. Berry and Rao, 1997) utilized a systems framework to examine work–family stress in fathers, but neglected to include data from the partners of the fathers. Similarly, Wayne et al. (2007) used ecological systems theory as a piece in the development of their Resource-Gain-Development perspective to understanding the antecedents and outcomes of positive spillover.

Finally, Voydanoff (2007) used ecological systems theory to examine work, family and community as microsystems consisting of networks of face-to-face relationships. She suggested that relationships among microsystems may operate through linking mechanisms and proposed a conceptual framework for the differential salience of within-domain demands and resources. She proposed that within-domain demands and resources are differentially salient in relation to work–family conflict and facilitation. The framework posits that within-domain demands are positively related to work–family conflict, whereas within-domain resources are positively associated with work–family facilitation. Specifically, within-domain work resources are positively associated with work-to-family facilitation and within-domain family resources are positively associated with family-to-work facilitation. Within-domain demands are salient for work–family conflict because they are associated with processes that limit the ability of individuals to meet obligations in another domain. Within-domain resources are relatively salient for work–family facilitation because they engender processes that improve one's ability to participate in other domains.

Conclusion

The goal of this chapter was to provide a review and organization of the positive spillover research and to use this review to develop suggestions for the future of this field. We began with a discussion of positive psychology and role theory, areas of research which were very influential in developing the positive spillover construct. We reviewed the different constructs that have been used to operationalize the concept of positive spillover and singled out two measures (Hanson et al., 2006; Carlson et al., 2006) and two theories (Greenhaus & Powell, 2006, Wayne et al., 2007) that are currently playing a predominant role in the emergence of this body of research. These theoretical models provide structure for the examination of the antecedents and outcomes of positive spillover and we reviewed the literature that has started to establish resources as predictors of spillover and various health related outcomes. Finally, we offer our suggestions for the future of positive spillover research and urge researchers to consider these ideas as we continue to grow this body of research.

References

Anderson, S., & Sabatelli, R. (1999). *Family interaction: A multigenerational developmental perspective* (2nd ed.). Needham Heights, MA: Allyn & Bacon.

Aryee, S., Srinivas, E. S., & Tan, H. H. (2005). Rhythms of life: Antecedents and outcomes of work–family balance among employed parents. *Journal of Applied Psychology, 90*, 132–146.

Bakker, A., & Derks, D. (2010). Positive occupational health psychology. In S. Leka, & J. Houdmont (Eds.), *A textbook of occupational health psychology*, Chichester, United Kingdom: Wiley-Blackwell.

Barnett, R. C. (1994). Home-to-work spillover revisited. A study of full-time employed women in dual-earner couples. *Journal of Marriage and the Family, 56*, 647–656.

Barnett, R. C., & Baruch, G. K. (1985). Women's involvement in multiple roles and psychological distress. *Journal of Personality and Social Psychology, 49*, 135–145.

Barnett, R. C., & Hyde, J. S. (2001). Women, men, work and family: An expansionist theory. *The American Psychologist, 56,* 781–796.

Berry, J. O., & Rao, J. M. (1997). Balancing employment and fatherhood: A systems perspective. *Journal of Family Issues, 18,* 386–402.

Bronfenbrenner, U. (1977). Toward an experimental ecology of human development. *American Psychologist, 32,* 513–530.

Bronfenbrenner, U. (1986). Ecology of the family as a context for human development: Research perspectives. *Developmental Psychology, 22,* 723–742.

Cameron, K. J. Dutton, J. E., & Quinn, R. E. (2003). Foundations of positive organizational scholarship. In K. Cameron, J. Dutton, & R. E. Quinn (Eds.), *Positive organizational scholarship* (pp. 3–13). San Francisco: Berrett-Koehler Publishers.

Carlson, D. S., Kacmar, K. M., Wayne, J. H., & Grzywacz, J. G. (2006). Measuring the positive side of the work–family interface: Development and validation of a work family enrichment scale. *Journal of Vocational Behavior, 68,* 131–164.

Collijn, D. H., Appels, A., & Nijuis, F. (1996). Are multiple roles a risk factor for myocardial infarction for women? *Journal of Psychosomatic Research, 40,* 271–279.

Crosby, F. J. (1991) *Juggling: The unexpected advantages of balancing career and home for women and their families.* New York: Free Press.

Crouter, A. C. (1984). Spillover from family to work: The neglected side of the work–family interface. *Human Relations, 37*(6), 425–442.

Eby, L. T., Casper, W. J., Lockwood, A., Bordeaux, C., & Brinley, A. (2005). Work and family research in IO/OB: content analysis and review of the literature (1980-2002). *Journal of Vocational Behavior, 66,* 124–97.

Edwards, J. R., & Rothbard, N. P. (2000). Mechanisms linking work and family: Specifying the relationships between work and family constructs. *Academy of Management Review, 25,* 178–199.

Friedman, S. D., & Greenhaus, J. H. (2000). *Work and family—Allies or enemies? What happens when business professionals confront life choices.* New York: Oxford University Press.

Frone, M. R. (2003). Work–family balance. In J. C. Quick & L. E.Tetrick (Eds.), *Handbook of occupational health psychology* (pp. 143–162). Washington, DC: American Psychological Association.

Frone, M. R., Russell, M., & Cooper, M. L. (1992). Antecedents and outcomes of work–family conflict: Testing a model of the work–family interface. *Journal of Applied Psychology, 77,* 65–78.

Gable, S., & Haidt, J. (2005). Positive psychology. *Review of General Psychology, 9,* 1089–2680.

Goode, W. J. (1960). A theory of role strain. *American Sociological Review, 25,* 483–496.

Gallup Research Institute (2008). *Employee engagement: The employee side of the human sigma equation.* Retrieved from www.gallup.com/consulting/52/Employee-Engagement.aspx.

Gordon, J. R., Whelan-Berry, K. S., & Hamilton, E. H. (2007). The relationship among work–family conflict and enhancement, organizational work–family culture, and work outcomes for older working women. *Journal of Occupational Health Psychology, 12*(4), 350–364.

Greenhaus, J. H., Allen, T. D., & Spector, P. E. (2006). Health consequences of work–family conflict: The dark side of the work–family interface. In P. L. Perrewe, & D. C. Ganster (Eds.). *Research in occupational stress and well being.* Amsterdam: JAI Press/Elsevier.

Greenhaus, J. H., & Beutell, N. J. (1985). Sources of conflict between work and family roles. *Academy of Management Review, 10,* 76–88.

Greenhaus, J. H., & Parasuraman, S. (1999). Research on work, family, and gender: Current status and future directions. In Powell, G. N. (Ed.), *Handbook of gender and work* (pp. 391-412). Newbury Park, CA: Sage.

Grzywacz, J. G. (2002). *Toward a theory of work–family facilitation.* Paper presented at the 34th Annual Theory Construction and Research Methodology Workshop, Houston, TX.

Grzywacz, J. G., & Bass, B. L. (2003). Work, family, and mental health: Testing different models of work–family fit. *Journal of Marriage and Family, 65,* 248–262.

Grzywacz, J. G., & Marks, N. F. (2000a). Reconceptualizing the work–family interface: An ecological perspective on the correlates of positive and negative spillover between work and family. *Journal of Occupational Health Psychology, 5,* 111–126.

Grzywacz, J. G., & Marks, N. F. (2000b). Family, work, work–family spillover and problem drinking during midlife. *Journal of Marriage and the Family, 62,* 336–348.

Greenhaus, J. H., & Powell, G. N. 2006. When work and family are allies: A theory of work–family enrichment. *Academy of Management Review, 31,* 72–92.

Hammer, L., Allen, E., & Grigsby, T. (1997). Work–family conflict in dual-earner couples: Within-individual and crossover effects of work and family. *Journal of Vocational Behavior, 50,* 185–203.

Hammer, L. B., Cullen, J. C., Neal, M. B., Shafiro, M. M., & Sinclair, R. R. (2005a). The Effects of Work–family Fit on Depression: A Longitudinal Study. *Journal of Occupational Health Psychology, 10,* 138–154.

Hanson, G., Hammer, L. B., & Colton, C. (2006). Development and validation of a multidimensional scale of work–family positive spillover. *Journal of Occupational Health Psychology, 11,* 249–265.

Hill, E. J., Allen, S., Jacob, J., Bair, A. F., Bikhazi, S. L., Van Langeveld, A., Martinengo, G., Parker, T. T., & Walker, E. (2007). Work–family facilitation: Expanding theoretical understanding through qualitative exploration. *Advances in Developing Human Resources, 9,* 507–526.

Ilies, R., Wilson, K. S., & Wagner, D. T. (2009). The spillover of job satisfaction onto employees' family lives: the facilitating role of work–family integration. *Academy of Management Journal, 52,* 87–102.

Ingersoll-Dayton, B., Neal, M. B., & Hammer, L. B. (2001). Aging parents helping adult children: The experience of the sandwiched generation. *Family Relations: Interdisciplinary Journal of Applied Family Studies, 50,* 263–271.

Kahn, R. L., Wolfe, D. M., Quinn, R., Snoek, J. D., & Rosenthal, R. A. (1964). *Organizational Stress.* New York: Wiley.

Katz, D. & Kahn, R. (1978). *The social psychology of organizations* (2nd ed.). New York: John Wiley & Sons.

Kinnunen, U., Feldt, T., Geurts, S., & Pulkkinen, L. (2006). Types of work–family interface: Well-being correlates of negative and positive spillover between work and family. *Scandinavian Journal of Psychology, 47,* 149–62.

Kirchmeyer, C. (1992). Perceptions of nonwork-to-work spillover: Challenging the common view of conflict-ridden relationships. *Basic and Applied Social Psychology, 13,* 231–249.

Kirchmeyer, C. (1993). Nonwork-to-work spillover: A more balanced view of the experiences and coping of professional women and men. *Sex Roles, 28,* 531–552.

Kossek. E. E., & Ozeki, C. (1998). Work–family conflict, policies, and the job–life satisfaction relationship: A review and directions for organizational behavior/human resources research. *Journal of Applied Psychology, 83,* 139–149.

Marks, S. R. (1977). Multiple roles and role strain: Some notes on human energy, time, and commitment. *American Sociological Review, 42,* 921–936.

Pavalko, E. K., & Smith, B. (1999). The rhythm of work: Health effects of women's work dynamics. *Social Forces, 77,* 1141–1162.

Pietromonaco, P. R., Manis, J., & Frohardt-Lane, K. (1986). Psychological consequences of multiple social roles. *Psychology of Women Quarterly, 10,* 373–382.

Piotrkowski, C. S. (1979). Work and the family system: A naturalistic study of working class and lower-middle-class families. New York: The Free Press.

Powell, G. N., & Greenhaus, J. H. (2010). Sex, gender, and the work–family interface: exploring negative and positive interdependencies. *The Academy of Management Journal, 53.*

Repetti, R. L., Matthews, K. A., & Waldron, I. (1989). Employment and women's health: Effects of paid employment on women's mental and physical health. *American Psychologist, 44,* 1394–1401.

Ruderman, M. N., Ohlott, P. J., Panzer, K., & King, S. N. (2002). Benefits of multiple roles for managerial women. *Academy of Management Journal, 45,* 369–386.

Schaufeli, W. B., & Bakker, A. B. (2004). Job demands, job resources and their relationship with burnout and engagement: A multi-sample study. *Journal of Organizational Behavior, 25,* 293–315.

Seligman, M. E. P. (1998). *Learned optimism: How to change your mind and your life* (2nd ed.). New York: Pocket Books.

Seligman, M., & Csikszentmihalyi, M. (2000). Positive psychology: An introduction. *American Psychologist, 55,* 5–14.

Sieber, S. D. (1974). Toward a theory of role accumulation. *American Sociological Review, 39,* 467–478.

Staines, G. L. (1980). Spillover versus compensation: A review of the literature on the relationship between work and non-work. *Human Relations, 33,* 111–129.

Staw, B. M., Sutton, R. I., & Pelled, L. H. (1994) Employee positive emotion and favorable outcomes at the workplace. *Organization Science, 5,* 51–71.

Stevens, D, Minnotte, K. L., Mannon, S. E., & Kiger, G. (2007). Examining the 'neglected side of the work–family interface': Antecedents of positive and negative family-to-work spillover. *Journal of Family Issues 28,* 242–262.

Stoddard, M., & Madsen, S. R. (2007). Toward an understanding of the link between work–family enrichment and individual health. *Journal of Behavioral and Applied Management, 9,* 2–15.

Thoits, P. A. (1983). Multiple identities and psychological well-being: A reformulation and test of the social isolation hypothesis. *American Sociological Review, 48,* 147–187.

Thompson, J. A., & Bunderson, J. S. (2001). Work–nonwork conflict and the phenomenology of time. *Work & Occupations, 28,* 17–39.

Tiedje, L., Wortman, C., Downey, G., Emmons, C., Biernat, M., & Lang, E. (1990). Women with multiple roles: Role compatibility perceptions, satisfaction, and mental health. *Journal of Marriage and the Family, 52,* 63–72.

Van Steenbergen, E. F., Ellemers, N., & Mooijaart, A. (2007). How work and family can facilitate each other: Distinct types of work–family facilitation and outcomes for women and men. *Journal of Occupational Health Psychology, 12,* 279–300.

Voydanoff, P. (2007). *Work, family, and community: Exploring interconnections*. Mahwah, NJ: Lawrence Erlbaum Associates.

Wayne, J. H., Musisca, N., & Fleeson, W. (2004). Considering the role of personality in the work–family experience: Relationships of the big five to work–family conflict and facilitation. *Journal of Vocational Behavior, 64*, 108–130.

Wayne, A. Randell, J., & Stevens, J. (2006). The role of identity and work–family support in work–family enrichment and its work-related consequences. *Journal of Vocational Behavior 69*, 445–461.

Wayne, J. H., Grzywacz, J. G., Carlson, D. S., & Kacmar, K. M. (2007). Work–family facilitation: A theoretical explanation and model of primary antecedents and consequences. *Human Resource Management, 17*, 63–76.

Werbel, J., & Walter, M. H. (2002). Changing views of work and family roles: A symbiotic perspective. *Human Resource Management Review, 12*, 293–298.

Westman, M., Etzion, D., & Danon, E. (2001). Job insecurity and crossover of burnout in married couples. *Journal of Organizational Behavior, 22*, 467–481.

Williams, A., Franche, R., Ibrahim, S., Mustard, C. A., & Layton, F. R. (2006). Examining the relationship between work–family spillover and sleep quality. *Journal of Occupational Health Psychology 11*, 27–37.

Yogev, S. (1981). Do professional women have egalitarian marital relationships? *Journal of Marriage and the Family, 43*, 865–871.

Zimmerman, K, Hammer, L.B., Kossek, E.E. (2009). Operationalizing the antecedents of work–family positive spillover: A longitudinal study. Unpublished Dissertation.

15

The Impact of Psychological Flexibility and Acceptance and Commitment Therapy (ACT) on Health and Productivity at Work

Frank W. Bond
Goldsmiths, University of London, U.K.

Paul E. Flaxman
City University, London, U.K.

Marc J. P. M. van Veldhoven and Michal Biron
Tilburg University, The Netherlands

Redesigning work and management processes in order to reduce workers' exposure to sources of stress has long been advocated by occupational health psychologists (e.g., Cox et al., 2000). Furthermore, outcome research has demonstrated that work redesign interventions that enhance characteristics such as worker control, role clarity, workplace communication, and social support can improve both the mental health and productivity of employees (e.g., Bond & Bunce, 2001; Bond, Flaxman & Bunce, 2008; Parker, Wall, & Cordery, 2001). Despite these successes, it also seems important to address the psychological styles, or approaches, workers bring to stressful work situations. First, some sources of stress may not be completely avoidable (e.g., immovable deadlines). Second, workers' efforts to modify stressful situations may themselves be inhibited by poor psychological coping strategies (e.g., use of avoidance strategies). Finally, work-related stress does not occur in a vacuum, and psychological styles that increase stress reactions at home (e.g., being overcontrolling and inflexible) may also result in feeling stress at work. Consistent with this line of thought, researchers investigating stress at work have found that psychological styles, such as negative affectivity and an external locus of control are reliable predictors of occupational stress (e.g., Jex, 1998).

Research by Bond and Bunce (2003) confirms the significance of these two individual characteristics in predicting stress, but it also highlights the even greater importance of another psychological style, which is beginning to receive more attention in the work-related stress literature, *psychological flexibility* (or *flexibility*); this is the ability to fully contact the present moment and the thoughts and feelings it contains without needless defense or avoidance, and, depending upon what the situation affords, persisting in or changing behavior in the pursuit of goals and values (Hayes, Luoma, Bond, Lillis, & Masuda, 2006).

Psychological Flexibility and Acceptance and Commitment Therapy (ACT)

Psychological flexibility is the theory of psychological health proposed by Acceptance and Commitment Therapy (ACT; Hayes, Strosahl, & Wilson, 1999). ACT (spoken as the word *act* and not by its constituent letters, a-c-t) is based upon Relational Frame Theory (RFT; Hayes, Barnes-Holmes, & Roche, 2001), which is a comprehensive, behavior-analytic account of language and cognition. Both ACT and RFT maintain that psychological health is largely determined by how people's language and cognition interact with contingencies of reinforcement to help or hinder their ability to pursue long-term values and goals (Hayes et al., 2006). ACT and RFT hypothesize that, depending upon the values-related opportunities afforded in a given situation, people need to be flexible as regards whether they base their actions more on their cognitions or current contingencies. For reasons specified by RFT (Hayes et al., 2001), most people, and especially those who experience psychological disorders, tend overly to base their actions on their internal events (thoughts and feelings) rather than on environmental contingencies. Moreover, these people tend to act in a way that they believe will minimize or avoid unwanted internal events (e.g., anxiety). As researchers such as Wegner and colleagues (see, e.g., Wenzlaff & Wegner, 2000) have shown, such experiential avoidance, itself, can enhance one's distress; in addition, people who base their actions on avoiding unwanted internal events are more likely to act in ways that are inconsistent with what their current context can provide, relative to their values and goals (Hayes et al., 2006).

Psychological flexibility at work

Psychological flexibility, and its promotion through ACT, has primarily been discussed in terms of mental health (see Hayes & Strosahl, 2004); however, the implication that flexibility may help people to be sensitive to, and contact, contingencies of reinforcement that bear on chosen values makes its usefulness to the work setting clear. If people value doing well at work (even if it is just to get paid), greater psychological flexibility increases their sensitivity to performance-related contingencies of reinforcement in their work environment (Bond, Hayes, & Barnes-Holmes, 2006). This is because people who are more flexible are not expending their limited attentional resources trying to change, control, or otherwise avoid their internal events; as a result, they are better able to notice and respond effectively to those performance-related contingencies that exist in their current environment. Put more succinctly, this context-sensitivity hypothesis states that, in the context of work, flexibility allows people to learn how to do their job more successfully and to have better mental health (in particular, through greater contact with values-centred contingencies of positive

reinforcement) (Bond et al., 2006). As we now discuss, ACT postulates six core processes that, together, promote psychological flexibility; and, as we discuss below, ACT,
when used in the workplace, attempts to enhance these processes.

Six core processes of psychological flexibility

Psychological flexibility is established through the following six processes that can
be seen in Figure 15.1. Importantly for flexibility's relevance to the work environment, each of these processes is considered a positive psychological skill and not
merely as a strategy for preventing and alleviating psychopathology.

Acceptance
Acceptance is a psychological stance that seeks to counteract experiential avoidance,
and its tendency, noted above, to compound psychological suffering (e.g., Wenzlaff &
Wegner, 2000). Acceptance involves the active willingness to experience internal

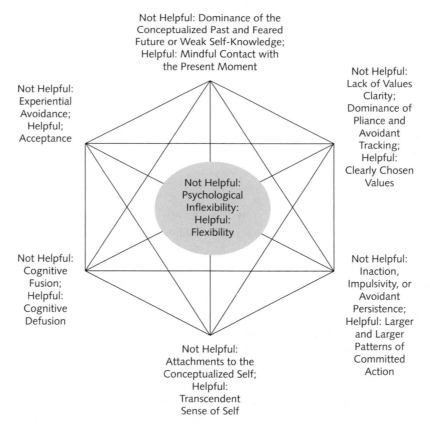

Figure 15.1   The ACT/RFT Model of Psychological Flexibility and Inflexibility

events (e.g., thoughts, feelings, and physiological sensations) without attempting to change their frequency or form, especially when doing so interferes with people working towards their values and goals. For example, anxious workers are taught to feel anxiety, as a feeling, fully and without defense; people with chronic back pain are taught skills that help them to stop struggling with their pain and take steps towards their goals and values.

Acceptance does not mean tolerating or resigning oneself to unwanted internal experiences, such as psychological distress; nor does it mean that one has to like or approve of the experience. Indeed, people can judge or evaluate an experience negatively, but psychologically accepting people would not then base their actions and behaviors (e.g., mental or physical avoidance) upon those evaluations.

Cognitive defusion

Cognitive defusion techniques attempt to change the way that people interact with, or relate to, their internal events. Cognitive defusion occurs when people focus on the process of thinking, rather than the content of their thinking. For example, people concentrate on the sound, pattern, rhythm, temporal frequency, and the individual letters or words that constitute their thinking, rather than on what all of those components can come together to mean or imply. When people are cognitively defused, they have more "psychological space" to decide whether, in a given situation, their values and goals are best served by basing their actions on their thoughts (e.g., fear or uncertainty), or the contingencies that exist in their current context.

Being in the present moment

Cognitive fusion does not merely lead to avoidance and inflexibility (e.g., by creating a repetitive tendency to avoid or overanalyze fearful thoughts, when they occur); it also causes us to lose contact with the present moment: in terms of flexible contact with the immediate physical and social environment, as well as contact with our own psychological reactions. Being in the present moment allows people to make nonjudgmental contact with psychological and environmental events as they occur; they can experience the world more directly, which allows their behavior to be more flexible, and thus their actions become more consistent with the values and goals that they hold. This is accomplished by allowing workability (discussed below) to exert more control over behavior, in addition to acceptance and defusion; that is, by using language more as a tool to note and describe events than as a means simply to predict and judge them.

Self as context

"Self as context" refers to how we perceive our thoughts and other internal events. It is the act of distinguishing the content and process of self-knowledge from the context or perspective of self-knowledge. Through this act, people can observe that they have thoughts, and that those thoughts can change. Importantly, because people can notice that their thoughts change, they can also observe that *they* are not the changing thoughts that they notice: they themselves are something more stable than those internal experiences and, as a result, they are more free to let go of those experiences (those thoughts and beliefs about themselves), when they prove to be unworkable in their lives. As perhaps can be seen, the stability that self as context provides can facilitate defusion and acceptance.

Values

In ACT, values are defined as chosen qualities of action patterns (e.g., being a good manager) that people can work toward, but that they cannot arrive at once and for all (Hayes et al., 2004) (i.e., people have to work constantly at being a good manager or they cease to be one). To the extent that people act according to *their* chosen values, they are living an effective life, *for them*. Thus, in accordance with the functional contextual philosophy of science that underlies both ACT and RFT (Hayes, 1993), judgments regarding personal workability and effectiveness need to be made against a priori statements of values.

Committed action

Finally, ACT encourages the development of larger and larger patterns of effective action linked to chosen values. Unlike values, which are constantly instantiated but never achieved as an object, concrete goals that are values-consistent can be achieved, and ACT almost always encourages people to take action to achieve short, medium, and long-term goals that are linked to their values. Defusion, acceptance, self as context, and being in the present moment facilitate the achievement of people's goals, because working towards them can frequently lead to contact with psychological barriers (e.g., anxiety and sadness) through which these "mindfulness" processes can help people to move.

Interrelations among the six processes

Figure 15.1. highlights the interrelations amongst the six processes that constitute psychological flexibility. Importantly, the four "mindfulness" processes (i.e., defusion, acceptance, being in the present moment, and self as context) are not ends in themselves. Rather, they help people to see situations more clearly and to be more flexible in acting in accordance with their values. Thus, living a valued life provides the raison d'être for defusing, accepting, and contacting the present moment as a conscious person. All of these processes are mutually facilitative; in that they, together, promote psychological flexibility. As a result, and as we now discuss, an important goal of ACT is not only to promote acceptance and defusion and, hence, contact with the present moment as a conscious person; but, it is also to have individuals, and indeed organizations, clarify and specify their values. When people do not behave according to their values, they risk denying themselves contact with positive reinforcers that foster good mental health, and effective action in a given context, such as work. Reinforcement deprivation often results when people avoid difficult psychological experiences, and the values-consistent actions that occasion them (Wilson & Blackledge, 1999).

Overview of Acceptance and Commitment Training

To further illustrate the nature of ACT and psychological flexibility, we now outline some of the strategies we have used as part of a three-session ACT program which has been developed for delivery at the worksite. Over the past 10 years or so, two of us (FB and PF) have been implementing and validating this program in organizations across the United Kingdom. We have labelled this approach *Acceptance and Commitment Training* (rather than therapy) to reflect the fact that we are delivering ACT to groups of employees outside of the therapeutic consulting room (Flaxman & Bond, in press). We usually deliver this training to small groups of between four and ten employees, although we have also used the same protocol to guide one-to-one coaching sessions. In principle, ACT could also be effective with larger groups (e.g., 20 or so), although the format for such groups is likely to be more didactic and less interactive. In general, our experience tells us that smaller ACT groups provide a much richer experience both for the participants and trainer.

When administering ACT in the workplace, we typically employ a "two-plus-one" delivery method (Barkham & Shapiro, 1990) which involves two training sessions in consecutive weeks, followed by a third "booster" session between one and three months later. Each session lasts for between two-and-a-half and three hours. Our data suggest that leaving a gap between sessions two and three allows participants to practice ACT techniques, and it helps to maintain mental health improvements for at least six months (Bond & Bunce, 2000; Flaxman & Bond, 2006).

Because of space limitations, we do not, in this chapter, describe every aspect of our worksite ACT program (see Bond & Hayes, 2002; Bond, 2004, and; Flaxman & Bond, 2006 for greater detail on this program). Rather, we illustrate a few of the techniques and exercises that we have used to cultivate the six interrelated processes that produce psychological flexibility. We have found it useful to conceptualize acceptance, defusion, contact with the present moment, and self-as-context as forming a higher order set of *mindfulness and acceptance* skills; while self-as-context, contact with the present moment, values, and committed action constitute a broad set of *values-based action* skills (Hayes, 2004). The inclusion of self-as-context and contact with present moment in both skill sets reflects the interrelatedness of ACT's mindfulness and values (or behavioral) components (Hayes, Strosahl, Bunting, Twohig, & Wilson, 2004).

Introducing ACT in the Workplace

At the outset of our worksite ACT intervention, we typically provide participants with an overview of the two sets of skills, which we refer to as *mindfulness* and *values-based action*. We highlight mindfulness as a skill for the "internal" world (inside the skin) and describe values-based action as a skill for the "external" world of observable behavior. We explain that the training involves a wide range of exercises and techniques, all of which are designed to help participants develop or enhance these two related psychological skills which, together, promote psychological flexibility.

Throughout the training, the various values and mindfulness exercises are interspersed with group discussions of ACT-consistent principles (see Bond, 2004; Flaxman & Bond, 2006). For example, during the initial stages, we introduce the notion that humans can often become overly wrapped up in the world inside the skin, and we encourage participants to share any related experiences. Here is an extract from this type of discussion between the trainer and two participants:

TRAINER: So, would anyone like to share their own experiences of that happening (*i.e., becoming wrapped up in the internal world*)

PARTICIPANT 1:   It makes me think about when I drive home from work. When I've had a hectic day or someone has upset me at work, I can become completely absorbed in that while driving. I sometimes arrive home without even realizing how I got there!

TRAINER: Thanks Sue—that's a great example of the human mind in action. We can sometimes get so lost in our "mindstuff" that we are not really there at all. In those moments, the automatic part of us is about all that's left in charge of driving while we are off with our thoughts. Does anyone else have an example they would like to share?

PARTICIPANT 2:   Well, I'm a terrible worrier! I'll worry about anything and everything. Like Sue said, I find that I get lost worrying about all sorts of stuff, and sometimes don't know how long I've been doing that for.

TRAINER: And let me ask you this Jane: When your mind is worrying, how *real* do those worries seem to you?

PARTICIPANT 2:   Well… they feel very real. I'm convinced that the stuff I'm worrying about is happening or is going to happen.

TRAINER: It's strange isn't it? Worry is another great example of how our minds work. When we are worrying, it can seem as if we are actually in the situation that we are worrying about. Does that make sense? Of course, we may not be in the actual situation at all, just *having thoughts* about it.

This brief extract illustrates some interesting features of ACT. Essentially, this initial discussion is about *cognitive fusion*—the trainer is highlighting a psychological context in which thoughts are experienced as indistinguishable from the events or situations which they symbolically represent (Hayes et al., 1999; Luoma, Hayes, & Walser, 2007). The trainer's use of language here is designed to promote defusion. For example, notice how the trainer discusses "the mind" almost as if it were a separate entity. Notice also that the trainer uses phrases such as *having thoughts*. This form of "defused" language is modelled and reinforced throughout ACT interventions; it is designed in part to promote contact with the healthy psychological space that exists between thoughts and the person having the thoughts (Hayes et al., 2004).

Promoting acceptance

As noted earlier, acceptance is cultivated in ACT to counteract the problematic context of experiential avoidance. Various techniques are employed to increase one's willingness to experience even the most difficult thoughts, emotions, and sensations, so that the presence of such private events has less impact on well-being, and exerts less control over behavior.

When implementing acceptance strategies, we usually describe the process as one of expanding awareness to "make room" even for undesirable internal events, and to begin seeing such events for what they actually are (e.g., thoughts and feelings). We often employ a "physicalizing" exercise (Hayes et al., 1999), which can help increase acceptance of difficult feelings. For this exercise, participants are asked to think of a current or recent situation that they have found stressful. This doesn't have to be a major life issue, but perhaps a stressful situation being faced at work. As participants think about the situation, they are asked to notice any sensations or feelings that arise. If a sensation or feeling is noticed, the instruction is to imagine it as if it were a physical object set out on the table or floor in front of them. The trainer asks a series of questions such as, "If this feeling or bodily sensation had shape, what shape would it be?"; "What color does it take on?"; "Does it have any surface texture?"; "What does the feeling look like when you step back from it like this?" At the end of this exercise, participants are asked to welcome the feeling or sensation back inside the skin; this is designed to encourage a nonjudgmental, or accepting, stance towards the feeling or sensation, even if it is undesirable and unwanted. To reiterate, the goal of the exercise is not to reduce or change unpleasant feelings, but to take a psychological step back and to observe the feeling/sensation for what it actually is and not what it may represent or imply.

Promoting cognitive defusion

The cognitive defusion techniques in ACT can be powerful, and we have observed them fundamentally change the way people relate to difficult thoughts and self-conceptualizations. In essence, defusion seeks to reveal the basic properties of thought and language (e.g., as words and sounds), so that the dominance of literal meaning is reduced (Strosahl Hayes, Wilson, & Gifford, 2004).

In our ACT program, we use a well-known defusion technique: the *Milk, Milk, Milk* exercise, originally devised by Titchener in 1916 (as described by Hayes et al., 1999, pp. 154–156). We employ this exercise in the following way. First, participants are asked for any meaning they have in relation to the word "Milk". A range of associations are usually offered in response to this (e.g., "it's white and tastes disgusting"; "cows"; "feeding my baby"; "it goes in my tea", and so on). Participants and trainer then repeat the word "Milk" over and over again for approximately 45 seconds. During this time, the trainer occasionally encourages participants to speed up, slow down, say the word louder, and to really experience the word. At the end of 45 seconds, the trainer asks whether the participants noticed anything while performing this rather strange exercise. More often than not, participants notice that the meaning of the word (e.g., white stuff, cows, feeding babies, etc.) disappears as one begins to experience the word 'Milk' simply as a word or sound. Immediately following the exercise, we write the word 'Milk' on a flip chart or whiteboard, alongside some words that summarize various negative self-conceptualizations. (e.g., "I'm weak", or "I'm stupid"). We then offer the following observation: *At the level of literal meaning*, "Milk" and "Stupid" are very different; however, on another level, *the level of word and sound*, "Milk" and "Stupid" are *not* fundamentally different—they are, after all, both just words/sounds. We go on to explain that it is not necessary to "rise above" literal meaning in this way for very long. Rather, the Milk exercise is simply designed to provide a glimpse of the "illusion" that is naturally woven by the literal meaning of thought and language. Nonetheless, an occasional glimpse of this process is often all it takes to reduce thought believability and undermine the context of cognitive fusion (cf. Masuda, Hayes, Sackett, & Twohig, 2004).

In the trainer–participant extract presented earlier, we highlighted some of the other ACT language conventions that promote defusion. For example, instead of using common phrases, such as "I'm anxious" or "I'm stressed", ACT participants are encouraged to adopt the following language practices: "*I'm having the feeling of … anxiety*"; or "*I'm having the thought that I'm stressed*" (Hayes et al., 1999). Participants often instantly recognize how such labeling offers a more defused and descriptive (i.e., less evaluative) way of relating to private events. This technique has additional benefits: it can help participants to practice labeling private events as they unfold in present moment awareness (e.g., now I'm having this thought; now I'm having this memory; now I'm having this feeling; now I'm having this bodily sensation); it also highlights the fundamental (yet often overlooked) distinction that exists between difficult private events, and the person who is having those experiences (Hayes et al., 2004).

Increasing contact with the present moment

To some extent, all of ACT's strategies seek to increase people's ability to contact present-moment experience. This involves cultivating an expanded (and nonjudgmental) awareness of the *process* of thinking and feeling as it is unfolds in the here and now, as well as a heightened awareness of one's external environment. To increase contact with present-moment experience, ACT encourages participants to build *mindfulness* into daily life. Accordingly, a significant proportion of our worksite ACT program is dedicated to imparting mindfulness skills. When introducing mindfulness, we typically describe some of its core features:

- Mindfulness practice involves expanding our awareness to pay attention to here-and-now experience.
- Mindfulness takes practice, similar to learning a musical instrument; in this realm, practice *makes permanent*.
- Mindfulness is not a relaxation exercise, and it is not designed to change or remove difficult thoughts or emotions; instead, mindfulness provides us with a different perspective on our internal world.

- Mind wandering during mindfulness practice is perfectly normal (in fact, becoming aware of mind wandering is part of the practice).

We usually initiate mindfulness practice with a fairly straightforward mindfulness of breathing exercise, which takes approximately 10 minutes. During this time, participants are asked simply to become aware of their breathing. The trainer occasionally encourages participants to notice when they have drifted off with particular thoughts, and to gently escort awareness back to the breath. Participants are instructed not to push thoughts away, but to let thoughts come and go in the background, whilst paying attention to one's breathing as it happens in the here and now. Following this mindfulness exercise (and indeed all subsequent mindfulness exercises), the trainer asks participants to share their experiences. These discussions are not intended to intellectualize the nature of mindfulness, but rather to establish if participants are getting the "experiential gist" of the skill. Over the three sessions of our ACT program, we might introduce nine or so different mindfulness exercises, and we will usually begin the second and third sessions with a brief mindfulness technique. We also provide participants with mindfulness CDs or MP3 files so that they can practice outside of the training sessions.

Contacting the self-as-context

One of the core aims of ACT is to help people contact a stable sense of self that is distinct from (and therefore not threatened by) negative thoughts, memories, emotions, sensations and so on. In ACT, this somewhat transcendent sense of self is often referred to as the 'observing self', and is accessed through various defusion and mindfulness exercises (e.g., Hayes, 2004; Hayes et al., 1999). In our ACT program, we implement self-as-context interventions as part of the mindfulness practice. For instance, we make the observation that there are essentially two processes operating during mindfulness practice—first there is "The Mind", constantly doing what minds are designed to do (i.e., chattering, predicting, imagining, planning, worrying, comparing, judging, criticizing, and so on); and then there is "The Observer" (or Awareness): this is the perspective from which we observe our thoughts, feelings, and sensations. We also use a cloud and sky metaphor to illuminate this process (from Hayes et al., 1999, p.187), in which clouds and weather are the "verbal chatter" of the mind, behind which lies blue sky; we do not have to remove the clouds to know that there is blue sky; whenever we look we will see that it is there.

We would typically guide participants through a brief observer experiential exercise, to encourage experiential contact with the self-as-context (we adapted the observer exercise from Hayes (1999, pp. 192–196); and more recently Harris (2008, pp.176–177). The exercise asks us to notice thoughts, emotions, and sensations as they unfold in the here and now, and become aware that part of us is able to stand back and to *observe* these internal events. Participants are encouraged to experience their thoughts, feelings, and sensations as constantly changing, while the observing self is a constant—always there, noticing these changes.

Clarifying values

Values are discussed in every session of our ACT program, and we regularly seek to illustrate how mindfulness and values skills are mutually related. Time is set aside during the training to administer a *values assessment* exercise, designed to help participants clarify behavioural values and associated goals. Specifically, participants are presented with ten core areas of life (e.g., family relations, work/career, recreation/ leisure, physical health, and so on) (adapted from Hayes, et al., 1999, pp. 224–225). Participants are asked to write down their "chosen life directions" (i.e., values) in each area of life that they rate as personally important. To facilitate this process, the trainer introduces various questions, such as "Imagine you are now 80 years old and looking back, what footprints would you like to see behind you in this area of life"; "What do you want to be about in this area of your life"; and, "If you have goals in this area of your life, in which direction are they taking you?" The trainer illustrates the difference between values and goals—an important distinction in ACT interventions. As noted above, a value is defined as a general chosen life direction that is never achieved, while goals are described as specific and obtainable outcomes that help people to move in the direction of their values. In addition, participants are asked to consider any "internal barriers" (e.g., difficult or unhelpful thoughts, memories, moods, or emotions) that have the potential to interfere with pursuing their valued directions. It is important to raise awareness of specific internal barriers, as these typically provide the richest material around which to practice and develop mindfulness and acceptance skills.

The values component in ACT can also be powerful, and participants occasionally become upset while completing such exercises. Participants are asked to rate how consistently they have recently been pursuing valued life directions, and to recognize that a lack of progress can be painful. For example, one participant who found the values assessment particularly difficult explained to the group that she had become increasingly irritable and curt towards her spouse, and yet she found that one of her most important values was "to be a loving, supportive partner." Such moments are grist for the mill in ACT interventions; they illustrate how internal states can control our behavior to such an extent that we may find ourselves mindlessly pursuing life directions that we would not ultimately choose for ourselves. As the training unfolds, participants are encouraged to begin utilizing their deeply held values as a prominent guide to daily behavior, while using mindfulness skills to make room for the difficult thoughts, emotions, moods, or urges that will inevitably arise.

Increasing commitment to values-based action

By encouraging participants to generate increasingly detailed value, goal, and action plans, we are seeking to increase commitment to values-consistent living. From an ACT perspective, commitment is manifested through the process of engaging in life-enhancing action even when doing so elicits difficult psychological content (Hayes et al., 1999). We particularly focus on commitment in the final session of our ACT program. We distribute diaries and rating forms that are designed to encourage participants to self-monitor their values-based behavior on a weekly basis. We typically end the final session by asking each of our participants to stand before the group and make a public commitment to values-based action (this is referred to as "Taking a Stand"; Strosahl et al., 2004). The underlying rationale is that people are more likely to follow through with valued behavioral commitments if they have been publicly expressed. Also, the process of publicly stating a personal value may itself elicit difficult internal reactions (e.g., anxiety or embarrassment), therefore providing a further opportunity for practicing mindfulness, acceptance, and defusion (Orsillo Roemer, Lerner, & Tull, 2004).

Research on Psychological Flexibility and ACT in the Workplace

This worksite ACT program, and the theory of psychological flexibility underpinning it, has been developing for the past decade. However, research in these areas, as they relate to occupational health psychology, has not, until recently, been very widespread. Fortunately, though, this seems to be changing as scholars and practitioners are looking increasingly at how psychological flexibility and ACT can inform both employee well-being and organizational performance. Over the past decade, several aspects of ACT, in relation to organizational behavior and occupational health psychology, have received theoretical and empirical attention. First, there has been a series of studies on psychological flexibly and ACT in the context of stress at work, and there is now growing research evidence indicating the utility of this construct and intervention in relation to the workplace. Second, there are several topics, such as organizational change and development, rehabilitation after injury or ill-health, and emotional labor, which are beginning to receive more empirical attention. We now briefly review the research evidence in these wide-ranging areas.

Psychological flexibility and ACT in stress management interventions

As noted above, studies in stress management generally seek to identify characteristics of the work environment (e.g., lack of job control) as well as other, individual characteristics (e.g., negative affectivity) that are likely to induce or exacerbate stress and thus impair employee health and performance (Hurrell & Murphy, 1992). To alleviate these stress-related outcomes and promote occupational well-being, work reorganization interventions (aimed at identifying and changing inefficient workplace practices) may be required. At the same time, interventions aimed at providing employees with better tools by which to cope with occupational stressors may also be needed. In this respect, Bond (2004) strongly advocates stress management approaches that *combine* interventions targeted at the work environment with interventions targeted at the person.

Bond and Bunce (2000) were the first to test the utility of promoting psychological flexibility, through an ACT stress management intervention, as a means for reducing mental ill-health at work. Using a randomized, controlled experiment, these researchers found that the ACT program just described improved employees' ($n = 30$) general mental health, depression, and innovation potential relative to a control group ($n = 30$). Importantly, they found that this ACT program produced these improvements, because it enhanced employees' psychological flexibility.

In a subsequent study, these same authors started to examine the utility of combining organizational and personal approaches to reducing stress management, this time in UK customer service centers (Bond & Bunce, 2003). Here, it was expected that psychological flexibility would moderate the well-established positive relationship between job control on the one hand and well-being and productivity on the other (Karasek & Theorell, 1990). Using a two-wave, full-panel design, the authors found that the beneficial effects of having more job control (i.e., better job performance and mental health) were indeed enhanced amongst employees who had higher levels of psychological flexibility; because, as the context-sensitivity hypothesis maintains, employees with greater flexibility did not expend as much cognitive effort in trying to avoid or control their internal events. They had, therefore, more attentional resources to notice the degree to which they had control in a given situation, and, through trial and error learning, they were better able to discover how they could most effectively use this control in order to do their work more efficiently or at least in a way that was less stressful to them. Importantly, results indicated that performance and mental health did not predict psychological flexibility over the one-year period in which the study was conducted. This suggests that psychological flexibility affects subsequent mental health and job performance, not the reverse.

In a recent study, Bond, Flaxman, and Bunce (2008) replicated and extended these findings, demonstrating how psychological flexibility moderates the effects of a control-enhancing work re-organization intervention among customer service employees in a UK bank. In particular, they found that, in comparison to a control group, the intervention improved people's mental health and decreased their absence levels, at a 14 month follow-up; and, these improvements were significantly greater for those employees who had higher levels of psychological flexibility; finally, these researchers found that these improvements were mediated by an increase in employees' perceptions of job control, which were greater amongst those who had greater flexibility (i.e., a mediated moderation effect).

In addition to this series of studies from Goldsmiths, University of London, research from other universities have also successfully employed psychological flexibility-based interventions to increase well-being and performance. For example, Berceli and Napoli (2006) found that these interventions helped professional caregivers such as social workers, police, and physicians learn effective self-directed techniques to maintain equanimity in the face of danger and human suffering, thereby reducing their incidence of secondary or vicarious trauma. In another study, an ACT-based intervention was found to be effective in preventing the development of burnout among workers in a palliative care unit in a Spanish hospital (Ruiz,

Rios, & Martin, 2008). The effect was particularly evident in terms of reducing feel-ings of depersonalization and increasing feelings of personal accomplishment. In the USA, Schwetschenau (2008) examined the effectiveness of an ACT-based inter-vention for stress at work. Using a randomized controlled trial, she found significant reductions in psychological distress, but not on several other outcomes. Finally, and outside of the traditional workplace, Gardner and Moore (2004) report several case studies of athletes who are facing problems in making progress in their respective sport, and report that ACT-based strategies were helpful in moving these athletes forward. This seems to be a promising line of work, considering that under a high-performance paradigm, many professionals in modern organizations can more and more be regarded as a kind of athlete in their job, striving for near continuous peak performance (Boxall & Purcell, 2008).

In sum, evidence regarding the usefulness of psychological flexibility and ACT in work settings is gradually accumulating, and it provides support for the hypothesis that psychological flexibility is very much associated with both mental-health-related outcomes (e.g., depression, burnout, job satisfaction, general well-being) and performance-related outcomes (e.g., computer input errors, absence rates, learning a new computer program), with a healthy average effect size of $r = .42$ (see Hayes et al., 2006 for a meta-analysis). Importantly, research also shows that these effects are evident even after controlling for one or more individual characteristics, such as emotional intelligence, negative affectivity, and each of the "Big Five" factors of personality (see Bond et al., 2006 for a review).

Psychological flexibility, ACT, and organizational behavior

Some initial, yet promising, results suggest that psychological flexibility might improve organizational development (OD) outcomes. OD refers to a set of planned-change interventions aimed at improving organizational effectiveness (French & Bell, 1999), and the features of psychological flexibility—i.e., identifying valued directions towards which to move (commitment), and being willing to experience the psychological events that could function as barriers along the way (psychological acceptance)—could be useful in enhancing OD outcomes (Stewart, Barnes-Holmes, Barnes-Holmes, Bond, & Hayes, 2006). For example, almost every drug-counseling organization would have the policy/mission/value that all of its counselors have nonprejudicial attitudes towards their clients. Hayes et al. (2004) showed that an ACT group intervention (1-day workshop) reduced the stigma and prejudice of drug abuse counsellors towards their patients at post-intervention and at a 3-month follow-up. Instead of directly attempting to change (i.e., reduce or suppress) stigma-tizing thoughts (a process known to produce paradoxical effects; e.g., Smart & Wegner, 1999), the ACT intervention reduced the impact of negative thoughts that counselors retained about their patients (e.g., the believability of prejudicial thoughts), even if the form or frequency of those thoughts changed only slowly or not at all. Similar findings were reported in another study by Masuda et al. (2007), who compared education and ACT-based interventions (a 150-minute workshop) for reducing counsellors' stigmatizing attitudes toward their clients with psychological disorders. While the former was designed to replace stigmatizing and biased thoughts with new, informed ones, the latter was designed to undermine avoidance of difficult thoughts, and this latter approach was found to be more helpful in reducing mental health stigma.

Psychological flexibility may also help improve leadership and management skills. ACT-inspired interventions can teach managers to distinguish between external and internal barriers to accomplishing their values-based goals. Organizational behavior research suggests effective strategies for overcoming *external* barriers (e.g., see Rummler & Brache, 1995) to organizational success. ACT-based interventions, on the other hand, can train managers to use various acceptance and defusion exercises, in order to move through *internal* barriers that may get in the way of pursuing their (units') values and goals. Herbst and Houmanfar (2009), for example, suggest that interventions targeted at the processes underlying values formation in organizations may be an important focus for OD, and a key process they identify in this context is "values clarification", which, as described above, is a standard part of any ACT-based approach.

A second new area for applying psychological flexibility and ACT in the workplace is that of rehabilitation in relation to injury or (chronic) ill-health. Many employees who are rehabilitating from such conditions face chronic fatigue and/or pain (Franssen et al., 2004). In such a context, enhancing psychological flexibility may play a role in managing successful rehabilitation (Donaldson, 2003), although empirical evidence is very limited. Nevertheless, one experiment that compared an ACT program with treatment as usual (e.g., the use of pain relieving drugs) found the former to be more successful in reducing the number of sick leave days and the use of medical treatment resources among public health sector workers who showed chronic stress/pain (at post and 6-month follow-up) (Dahl, Wilson, & Nilsson, 2004).

A third new arena for applying psychological flexibility and ACT principles centres on customer-facing work. In the work psychology literature, there has been an increasing interest in emotional labour, or emotion regulation, targeted at meeting organizationally or professionally specified behavioral displays (Grandey, 2000). As people-oriented service work has become so ubiquitous, insights into emotional labour have become very important. So far, only approaches of emotion regulation have been investigated that are either targeted at role-playing in the face of emotions triggered by the job (surface acting), or targeted at trying to actually feel the emotions that the organization prescribes (deep acting). Biron and van Veldhoven (submitted) suggest that psychological flexibility might be an alternative approach. When service employees are better able to accept emotions and stay committed to valued goals, in line with organizational performance demands, better service as well as enhanced well-being during service encounters can be expected. Survey and diary data collected among 168 Dutch service workers have confirmed these hypotheses.

These three areas of organizational behavior and occupational health psychology that psychological flexibility may be able to inform are not exhaustive; indeed, Stewart et al. (2006) have suggested other areas, such as teamwork and leadership, which future research may wish to explore. A key aim of this chapter has been to highlight the extant theory, practice, and research that have applied psychological flexibility and ACT to the work environment, in order not only to inform but to inspire others to extend this work and test the boundaries of usefulness this construct, and its application, have to occupational health psychology and organizational behavior.

References

Barkham, M., & Shapiro, D.A. (1990). Brief psychotherapeutic interventions for job-related distress: a pilot study of prescriptive and exploratory therapy. *Counselling Psychology Quarterly, 3*, 133–147.

Berceli, D., & Napoli, M. (2006). A proposal for a mindfulness-based trauma prevention program for social work professionals. *Complementary Health Practice Review, 11*, 153–165.

Biron, M., & van Veldhoven, M. (2009) *Alternative emotion regulation strategies and emotional exhaustion: Main and interaction effects.* Manuscript submitted for publication.

Bond, F. W. (2004). Acceptance and Commitment Therapy for stress. In S. C. Hayes & K. D. Strosahl (Eds.), *A practical guide to Acceptance and Commitment Therapy* (pp. 275–293). New York: Springer-Verlag.

Bond, F. W., & Bunce, D. (2000). Mediators of change in emotion-focused and problem-focused worksite stress management interventions. *Journal of Occupational Health Psychology, 5*, 156–163.

Bond, F. W. & Bunce, D. (2001). Job control mediates change in a work reorganization intervention for stress reduction. *Journal of Occupational Health Psychology, 6*, 290–302.

Bond, F. W., & Bunce, D. (2003). The role of acceptance and job control in mental health, job satisfaction, and work performance. *Journal of Applied Psychology, 88*, 1057–1067.

Bond, F. W., Flaxman, P. E., & Bunce, D. (2008). The influence of psychological flexibility on work redesign: Mediated moderation of a work reorganization intervention. *Journal of Applied Psychology, 93*, 645–654.

Bond, F. W., & Hayes, S. C. (2002). ACT at work. In F. W. Bond & W. Dryden (Eds.), *Handbook of brief cognitive behaviour therapy*. Chichester, U.K.: Wiley.

Bond, F. W., Hayes, S. C., & Barnes-Holmes, D. (2006). Psychological flexibility, ACT, and organizational behaviour. *Journal of Organizational Behavior Management, 26*, 25–54.

Boxall, P., & Purcell, J. (2008), *Strategy and human resource management*, New York, Palgrave Macmillan.

Cox, T., Griffiths, A., Barlowe, C., Randall, R., Thomson, L., & Rial González, E. (2000). *Organizational interventions for work stress: A risk management approach*. Norwich:, UK: Health and Safety Executive/Her Majesty's Stationery Office.

Dahl, J., Wilson, K.G., & Nilsson, A. (2004). Acceptance and Commitment Therapy and the treatment of persons at risk for long-term disability resulting from stress and pain symptoms: A preliminary randomized trial. *Behavior Therapy, 35*, 785–801.

Donaldson, E. (2003). Psychological acceptance, and why every OH/HR practitioner should know about it. *Occupational Health Review, 101*, 31–33.

Flaxman, P. E., & Bond, F. W. (2006, March). *Worksite stress management interventions: Identifying the mechanisms of change.* Paper presented at the Sixth APA International Conference on Occupational Stress and Health, Miami, FL.

Flaxman, P. E., & Bond, F. W. (in press).

Franssen, P. M., Bültmann, U., Kant, I. J., & van Amelsvoort, L. G. (2003). The association between chronic diseases and fatigue in the working population. *Journal of Psychosomatic Research, 54*(4), 339–344.

French, W., & Bell, C. (1999). *Organisation development.* London: Prentice-Hall.

Gardner, F. L., & Moore, Z. E. (2004). A mindfulness-acceptance-commitment based approach to athletic performance enhancement. *Journal of Behavior Therapy, 35,* 707–723.

Grandey, A. A. (2003). When "the show must go on": Surface acting and deep acting as determinants of emotional exhaustion and peer-rated service delivery. *Academy of Management Journal, 46,* 86–96.

Harris, R. (2008). *The happiness trap.* London: Constable & Robinson.

Hayes, S. C. (1993). Analytic goals and the varieties of scientific contextualism. In S. C. Hayes, L. J. Hayes, H. W. Reese, & T. R. Sarbin (Eds.), *Varieties of scientific contextualism* (pp. 11–27). Reno, NV: Context Press.

Hayes, S. C. (2004). Acceptance and commitment therapy and the new behaviour therapies: Mindfulness, acceptance, and relationship. In S. C. Hayes, V. M. Follette, & M. M. Linehan (Eds.), *Mindfulness and acceptance: Expanding the cognitive-behavioural tradition.* New York: Guilford Press.

Hayes, S. C., Barnes-Holmes, D., & Roche, B. (Eds.). (2001). *Relational frame theory: A post-Skinnerian account of human language and cognition.* New York: Plenum Press.

Hayes, S. C., Bissett, R. T., Roget, N., Padilla, M., Kohlenberg, B. S., Fisher, G., Masuda, A., Pistoreleo, J., Rye, A. K., Berry, K., & Niccolls, R. (2004). The impact of acceptance and commitment training on stigmatizing attitudes and professional burnout of substance abuse counsellors. *Behavior Therapy, 35,* 821–836.

Hayes, S. C., Luoma, J. B., Bond, F. W., Masuda, A., & Lillis, J. (2006). Acceptance and commitment therapy: Model, processes and outcomes. *Behaviour Research and Therapy, 44,* 1–25.

Hayes, S. C. & Strosahl, K. D. (2004). *A practical guide to Acceptance and Commitment Therapy.* New York: Springer-Verlag.

Hayes, S. C., Strosahl, K. D., Bunting, K., Twohig, M., & Wilson, K. (2004). What is acceptance and commitment therapy? In S. C. Hayes & K. D. Strosahl (Eds.), *A practical guide to acceptance and commitment therapy.* New York: Springer.

Hayes, S. C., Strosahl, K., & Wilson, K. G. (1999). *Acceptance and commitment therapy: An experiential approach to behaviour change.* New York: Guilford Press.

Herbst, S.A., & Houmanfar, R. (2009). Psychological approaches to values in organizations and organizational behaviour management. *Journal of Organizational Behavior Management, 29,* 47–68.

Hurrell, J. J., & Murphy, L. R. (1992). An overview of occupational stress and health. In W. M. Rom (Ed.), *Environment and occupational medicine* (2nd ed., pp. 675–684). Boston: Little, Brown.

Jex, S. M. (1998). *Stress and job performance.* London: Sage.

Karasek, R., & Theorell, T. (1990). *Healthy work: Stress, productivity, and the reconstruction of working life.* New York: Basic Books.

Luoma, J. B., Hayes, S. C., & Walser, R. D. (2007). *Learning ACT: An acceptance & commitment therapy skills training manual for therapists.* Oakland, CA: New Harbinger & Reno, NV: Context Press.

Masuda, A., Hayes, S. C., Fletcher, L. B., Seignourel, P. J., Bunting, K., Herbst, S. A., Twohig, M. P., & Lillis, J. (2007). The impact of acceptance and commitment therapy versus education on stigma toward people with psychological disorders. *Behaviour Research and Therapy, 45*, 2764–2772.

Masuda, A., Hayes, S. C., Sackett, C. F., & Twohig, M. P. (2004). Cognitive defusion and self-relevant negative thoughts: Examining the impact of a ninety-year-old technique. *Behaviour Research and Therapy, 42*, 477–485.

Orsillo, S. M., Roemer, L., Lerner, J. B., & Tull, M. T. (2004). Acceptance, mindfulness, and cognitive-behavioural therapy: Comparisons, contrasts, and application to anxiety. In S. C. Hayes, V. M. Follette, & M. M. Linehan (Eds.), *Mindfulness and acceptance: Expanding the cognitive-behavioural tradition*. New York: Guilford Press.

Parker, S. K., Wall, T. D., & Cordery, J. L. (2001). Future work design research and practice: Towards an elaborated model of work design. *Journal of Occupational and Organizational Psychology, 74*, 413–440.

Ruiz, C. O., Rios, F. L., & Martin, S. G. (2008). Psychological intervention for professional burnout in the Palliative Care Unit at Gregorio Maranon University Hospital. *Medicina Preventiva, 15*(2), 93–97.

Rummler, G. A., & Brache, A. P. (1995). *Improving performance: Managing the white space on the organization chart* (2nd ed.). San Francisco: Jossey-Bass.

Schwetschenau, H. M. (2008). The effectiveness of an acceptance and commitment intervention for work stress. Unpublished doctoral dissertation, Green State University.

Smart, L., & Wegner, D. M. (1999). Covering up what can't be seen: Concealable stigma and mental control. *Journal of Personality and Social Psychology, 77*, 474–486.

Stewart, I., Barnes-Holmes, D., Barnes-Holmes, Y., Bond, F. W., & Hayes, S. C. (2006). Relational frame theory and industrial/organizational psychology. *Journal of Organizational Behavior Management, 26*, 55–90.

Strosahl, K. D., Hayes, S. C., Wilson, K. G., & Gifford, E. V. (2004). An ACT primer: Core therapy processes, intervention strategies, and therapist competencies. In S. C. Hayes & K. D. Strosahl (Eds.), *A practical guide to acceptance and commitment therapy*. New York: Springer.

Wenzlaff, E. M., & Wegner, D. M. (2000). Thought suppression. *Annual Review of Psychology, 51*, 59–91.

Wilson, K. G., & Blackledge, J. T. (1999). Recent developments in the behavioral analysis of language: Making sense of clinical phenomena. In M. J. Dougher (Ed.), *Clinical behavior analysis* (pp. 27–46). Reno, NV: Context Press.

16

Corporate Social Responsibility and Psychosocial Risk Management

Stavroula Leka and Aditya Jain
University of Nottingham, U.K.

Gerard Zwetsloot
TNO Work & Employment, The Netherlands

Organizations may "externalize" problems, i.e., hold external factors responsible for health or environmental issues. Increasingly, the consequences to society of externalization are no longer regarded as normal or acceptable. Organizations are now expected to solve the problems they cause by acting responsibly and by "inclusive thinking and acting," i.e., by taking the consequences of their business activities for society and specific stakeholders into account in their decisions. They are also expected to be active in the solution of global, local, or regional societal problems. Companies are increasingly eager to demonstrate that their business practices are responsible, as they come to discover that many consumers, as well as business customers, may prefer to do business with responsible enterprises.

The increase of psychosocial risks in society offers an example of a societal development to which organizations can directly contribute to reducing the societal problem by managing psychosocial risks at their workplaces properly, thereby preventing the shift of problems to society, workers, and their families. Furthermore, good psychosocial risk management is clearly linked to good business. It may lead to a more productive workforce in terms of less absence, more positive engagement, and greater mental flexibility. In this chapter, the link between corporate social responsibility (CSR) and psychosocial risk management will be explored through the presentation of key findings from a European project that focused on the development of a European framework for psychosocial risk management at the workplace level (PRIMA-EF).

What Is Corporate Social Responsibility?

With increasing globalization and greater environmental and social awareness, the concept of organizations' responsibilities extending beyond purely legal or profit-related aspects has gained impetus. In order to succeed, business now has to be seen to be acting responsibly towards people, planet, and profit (the so-called '3Ps')

(European Commission, 2001). According to the European Agency for Safety and Health at Work (EU-OSHA, 2002), CSR is an inspiring, challenging, and strategically important development that is becoming an increasingly significant priority for companies of all sizes and types.

Early accounts of CSR referred to it as social responsibility; however, in more recent times the CSR concept has transitioned to include alternative themes such as stakeholder theory, business ethics theory, corporate social performance, and corporate citizenship (Carroll, 1999). Over the decades, numerous definitions of CSR have been proposed. In 1980, Thomas M. Jones defined the construct as:

> the notion that corporations have an obligation to constituent groups in society other than stockholders and beyond that prescribed by law and union contract. Two facets of this definition are critical. First, the obligation must be voluntarily adopted, not influenced by the coercive forces of law or union contract. Second, the obligation is a broad one, extending beyond the traditional duty to shareholders to other societal groups such as customers, employees, suppliers, and neighboring communities (Jones, 1980, pp. 59–60, cited in Carroll, 1999).

The European Commission (2001) defined CSR as "a concept whereby companies integrate social and environmental concerns in their business operations and their interactions with their stakeholders on a voluntary basis". The European Multistakeholder Forum on CSR (2004) further extended the understanding of CSR by concluding that it is the voluntary integration of environmental and social considerations into business operations, over and above legal requirements and contractual obligations, that commitment of management and dialogue with stakeholders is essential, and that, when operating in developing countries and/or situations of weak governance, companies need to take into account the different contexts and challenges, including poverty, conflicts, environment, and health issues.

The World Business Council for Sustainable Development (WBCSD, 2000) pointed out differences in the meaning of CSR between countries that included environmental concerns and local community empowerment. This conflict and overlap of meanings has led to research being fractured and lacking a critical agenda. A single, universally accepted definition of CSR would be helpful (Blowfield & Frynas, 2005; Kok, van der Wiele, McKenna, & Brown, 2001) but remains unlikely; however, there are ways of seeing this lack of definition as a benefit to the area. The various definitions do have a commonality of themes in the context of various stakeholders, ethics, employee issues, environment, governance, and policy. The concept, it is argued, needs to be retained as an overarching umbrella term (Blowfield & Frynas, 2005). Companies can "cherry pick" the areas in which they wish to move forward without the constraints of an overly tight definition (Cowe, 2003). Being generic, it is argued that it can be applicable from multinational to small and medium-sized enterprises (SMEs); but a counter argument is that the use of the term "corporate" implies that size is a prerequisite (Schoenberger-Orgad & McKie, 2005).

In recent years efforts have been made by business networks to increase awareness of the CSR concept and promote best practice. CSR Europe is the leading European business network for corporate social responsibility. It was founded in 1995 by senior European business leaders in response to an appeal by the European Commission President Jacques Delors (CSR Europe, 2000). CSR Europe is a platform for connecting companies to share best practice on CSR, innovating new projects between business and stakeholders and shaping the modern day business and political agenda on sustainability and competitiveness. Another such network is Enterprise for Health (EfH) which was set up in 2000 jointly by the Bertelsmann Stiftung Foundation and the Federal Association of Company Health Insurance Funds (Bundesverband der Betriebskrankenkassen) in Germany to promote the exchange of information and experience among committed enterprises and to publicize examples of the success of a corporate culture based on partnership. EfH is a network of international enterprises which devotes itself to the development of a corporate culture based on partnership and a modern company health policy. The key objective of the network is to process the available information related to CSR and employee health and to provide it in a systematic and practice-oriented manner.

Relevance of Corporate Social Responsibility

Proponents of CSR claim that it is in the enlightened self-interest of business to undertake various forms of CSR. The forms of business benefit that might accrue would include enhanced reputation and greater employee loyalty and retention (Moir, 2001). The word "voluntary", which characterizes the commitment of enterprises to CSR practices, covers a large number of possible situations that bear witness to the variety of motives leading enterprises to commit to the path of socially responsible practices. First, CSR may have a positive effect in distinguishing an enterprise's products, which may give it an advantage in its market. It also represents a way of preventing environmental or social risks that may seriously undermine a brand's reputation. CSR can also be a positive factor in attracting and retaining a workforce sensitive to this ethical dimension and willing to put a lot into an enterprise whose socially responsible commitments it shares (Segal, Sobczak, & Triomphe, 2003).

Other studies undertaken to assess the motives of management to engage in CSR practices and adopt CSR policies and codes in multinational corporations (MNCs) suggest two main sources of motivation. First, management may see advantages in reaching an agreed code in terms of the additional legitimacy for a policy that employee representatives' consent or approval can bring (Marginson, 2006). Further, legitimacy comes from linking CSR policies and codes to multilateral instruments such as ILO Conventions, the principles of the UN's Global Compact, and the OECD's Guidelines on MNCs (Hammer, 2005). The second source of motivation is the capacity of trade unions and nongovernmental organizations to bring international pressure to bear on management over a company's practices and those of its suppliers.

The ILO (2007) reported it highly plausible that whether or not a multinational organization sees a need to have a CSR code is shaped by characteristics of the sector, such as how visible companies are in the eyes of consumers, the extent to which they trade on a brand name, and the extent to which their supply networks encompass operations in developing nations. Essentially, according to Moon (2007), "business performs ... to defined standards ... [which is] a key factor in the increasingly institutionalized nature of CSR."

CSR focuses on the effects of organizational strategy on the social, environmental, and economic impact of organizations' activities, as well as achieving an appropriate balance between these three impacts. As such, CSR is considered a leading principle in the development of innovative business practice (Zwetsloot, 2003). CSR evolved from the 1990s approach of developing management systems, which were often based on standards and guidelines such as ISO 9000 (quality management), ISO 14001 (environmental management), SA 8000 (social accountability), and OHSAS 18001 (occupational health and safety), and have as their guiding principle "doing things right the first time". However, as far as these systems focus on planning and rational control of activities, they pay little attention to human aspects. To achieve further development of CSR, it is necessary to combine value-based decision-making and the rationales of prevention and management systems (Zwetsloot, 2003).

Corporate Social Responsibility and Occupational Safety And Health

Although CSR has many definitions it is, in essence, based on the integration of economic, social, ethical, and environmental concerns in business operations. Major social concerns include the welfare of key stakeholders in the business, especially employees (Health and Safety Executive, 2005). One important distinction between different types of CSR policies and activities is whether they are "internal" in that they are targeted at management and employees of the firm itself, or "external" in that they are targeted at outside groups such as suppliers, the society, or the environment (Bondy, Matten, & Moon, 2004).

The internal dimension of CSR policies covers socially responsible practices concerning employees, relating to their safety and health, investing in human capital, managing change, and financial control. Recent Occupational Safety and Health (OSH) promotion strategies by the European Commission (EC) and the European Agency for Safety and Health at Work (EU-OSHA) have attempted to link OSH with CSR, establishing a business case of strategic importance for organizations (EC, 2001, 2002; Zwetsloot & Starren, 2004). Health and safety at work is seen as an essential component of CSR and companies are increasingly recognizing that they cannot be good externally, while having poor social performance internally (Zwetsloot & Starren, 2004). CSR is also identified as a critical component for engaging SMEs to move the area of OSH forward (HSE, 2005).

These recent international and national CSR initiatives are complemented by innovative safety and health activities that go beyond traditional OSH issues and have either an implicit or explicit relationship with CSR. An effect of these initiatives is that they change the context of safety and health at work at company level. Zwetsloot and Starren (2004) in a report for the EU-OSHA categorized these initiatives as:

- raising awareness, awards, and ethical initiatives
- exchange of knowledge: best practice, networks, pilot projects, and guidelines
- standardization and certification
- reporting (external) and communication
- innovative partnerships with NGOs, both public and private
- ethical trade initiatives (e.g., "fair trade")
- financial sector involvement/financial incentives.

The nature of the relationship between CSR and OSH varies widely among the initiatives. Some refer explicitly to OSH items while others focus only on new social issues that have no tradition in companies, or on totally voluntary aspects (such as use of unfair labor practices by suppliers in developing countries and/or new member states). Initiatives for promoting CSR are predominantly private and voluntary, while OSH initiatives are often determined by legal regulation and governmental action.

Corporate Social Responsibility and Psychosocial Risk Management

The nature of working life has changed significantly in recent decades. Psychosocial risks, work-related stress, workplace violence, harassment, and bullying are now major occupational health concerns, joining the traditional problems of unemployment and exposure to physical, chemical, and biological hazards (European Social Partners, 2004).

Increasingly, CSR is becoming a *strategic* platform for health and safety management in enterprises. Companies that are perceived to be frontrunners in supporting human, social, and mental resources are often viewed as "employers of choice." They see value in promoting such resources in terms of the sustainability of the company itself, and that of communities and society. Many address such issues not purely as an obligation in law or in order to deal with symptoms of ill health and absence, but through a framework of common (business) sense and social responsibility. In doing so, many of these companies go beyond their legal obligations in relation to the management of psychosocial risks and view the promotion of well-being as part of their usual business practices.

As CSR is strategic and is regarded by many companies and corporate leaders as an important development, it offers opportunities for psychosocial risk management. However, the link of CSR with psychosocial risk management had not been addressed clearly until recently. The remainder of this chapter will present findings from the PRIMA-EF project that analyzed the link between CSR and psychosocial risk management, and the business case underpinning that link. A number of methods were used to explore this association. PRIMA-EF was funded through the European Commission's sixth framework program and aimed at the development of a European framework for psychosocial risk management at the workplace level.

Research Methodology

The methodology was based on the analysis of the existing literature, as well as on quantitative and qualitative research. This included two focus groups and a pilot of key indicators with business networks—these results are presented here. The focus groups explored two thematic areas that included a number of key questions:

- What are the main business impacts of psychosocial risks?
- What is the business case for psychosocial risk management?
- What is the workers' case for psychosocial risk management?
- Who are the internal and external stakeholders and what is the societal impact of psychosocial risks?
- Who are key stakeholders (and, in particular, nontraditional stakeholders that may be important to communicate with, or to involve in psychosocial risk management)?
- What are the main societal impacts of psychosocial risk management?

Two focus groups on CSR were organized during a 2-day stakeholder workshop. The focus groups lasted approximately 1 hr 30 min each. Fifteen stakeholders representing the social partners (trade unions, employer organizations, and governmental organizations), researchers, and academic experts in the area participated in the focus groups. On the basis of the focus group findings and the literature review, 27 indicators for CSR and psychosocial risk management were defined. These were piloted with member organizations of CSR Europe and the Enterprise for Health Network. Responses from 15 companies within these networks were received.

Results

Main business impacts of investing in the management of psychosocial risks

In Table 16.1. the results of the focus groups on health and business benefits of psychosocial risk management are presented.

Workshop participants highlighted the need to develop a clear business case for psychosocial risk management. Participants observed that ,even though all the tripartite partners accepted that CSR was related to psychosocial risk management, the "win–win" situation often discussed by trade unions and employers alike still seemed very distant.

Participants commented that both the business and the employee benefit from reduced sickness absence: for the worker, reduced sickness meant improved earning capacity while for the employer the benefit was reported to be the potential of earning higher profits. The availability of low-cost interventions for psychosocial risk

Table 16.1   Health and Business Benefits of Investing in Psychosocial Risk Management

Type of benefits	Health/Vitality	Business/Economic
Cost reductions	Improved psychosocial health of workers Reduced sickness absence Reduced health insurance costs	Increased productivity Higher job satisfaction Increased work commitment Knowledge retention Lower staff turnover Reduction in training and recruitment costs Reduced employee turnover Reduced early retirement Less confrontation between the organization and their workers and unions
Added values	Added quality-adjusted life years (QALYs) for employees	Better public image Increased long-term stability Higher employee commitment Engagement of different partners/stakeholders Improved employer reputation More commitment by workers to company's aims Better relations with clients

management was highlighted and the advantages of implementing such interventions were discussed; these included reduced sickness, reduced employee turnover, and reduced health insurance costs that benefit not only the organization but also society, as savings in social security could be allocated to other areas. Participants reported that engaging in psychosocial risk management would help to maintain a healthy workforce; such a workforce was expected to have higher job satisfaction and increased work commitment that would lead to further reduction in organizational costs due to knowledge retention, lower staff turnover, and a reduction in training and recruitment costs.

Participants also noted that the benefits of engaging in responsible business practices that incorporated psychosocial risk management would include increased long-term stability for the business, a better public image, and improved employer reputation, which would, in turn, help attract and retain the best employees. Benefits for workers were noted to include better relations with clients, less confrontation with the organization for workers and unions, and increased participation in organizational aims and policies.

Main stakeholders in psychosocial risk management: Beyond traditional stakeholders

Workshop participants discussed the role and involvement of stakeholders in the OSH area whom it may be important to communicate with and/or to involve in psychosocial risk management. In terms of traditional stakeholder groups, these included: trade unions, employer organizations, government agencies, researchers and academics, and OSH services. These traditional stakeholders remain very important in OSH and also more specifically for psychosocial risk management.

The nontraditional stakeholders with a clear interest in the business impact and/ or societal impacts of psychosocial risks identified are listed in Table 16.2. with an explanation of their respective stakes.

Table 16.2   Nontraditional Stakeholders in Psychosocial Risk Management and Their Main Interests

Stakeholders	Main stakes
Social security agencies	Good psychosocial risk management may reduce the burden of psychosocial problems and help to reduce rising costs of psychosocial problems on social security arrangements[1] (for workers compensation, societal costs of mental disabilities and associated unemployment). Social security agencies have a clear stake in prevention.
Health insurers	Good psychosocial risk management may reduce the rise of health care costs for treatment of psychosocial problems.[2] Health insurers have a clear stake in (primary and secondary) prevention.
Families/partners	The psychosocial health of the workers is a very important issue for partners and their families. First, the stress of a traumatized partner will have a strong impact on family life. Second, they are economically dependent on the worker's earning capacity, which can be seriously threatened by exposure to psychosocial risks.
(Mental) health care institutions	The rising prevalence of psychosocial problems is a challenge and burden to health care systems and institutions. Increasing treatment activities may trigger greater interest in prevention.
Customers/clients	In many jobs people work with clients. If workers suffer from psychosocial illnesses, this is likely to affect the way they work and communicate with customers. This is likely to reduce customer satisfaction.
Shareholders	In some industries psychosocial problems lead to high levels of sickness absence. In companies with severe psychosocial problems, it may also be more difficult to attract talent. As a result the productivity and competitiveness of the company may be affected, resulting in reduced shareholder value.

Table 16.2 (*Cont'd*)

Stakeholders	*Main stakes*
NGOs	NGOs represent civil society groups. Several civil society groups may have an interest in good psychosocial risk management by companies. This may range from organizations of patients of psychosocial disorders, to local groups requiring socially responsible business practices from companies in their neighborhood.
Communities	See item above.
Business Schools and Universities	Good psychosocial risk management clearly has a link with good business practice. This is important for the education of present and future business leaders. Psychosocial risk management should therefore be integrated in the curricula of business schools and universities.
Employment agencies	Psychosocial disorders are increasingly relevant as a cause of reduced work ability and rising unemployment. In some countries, many long-term unemployed people suffer from mental health problems. Recent literature shows that (re)activation of this target group is more successful when it is combined with work than in the traditional model of treatment and cure before people start working. Consequently, employment agencies have a clear interest in tertiary prevention.
Human resource departments and officers	Within companies, psychosocial issues are relevant for well-being at work, company climate, employee satisfaction, and the retention of existing employees. Though coming from another tradition compared to OSH experts, HRM officers are increasingly involved in the management of psychosocial issues at work.
Media	Psychosocial risk management is a societal issue with growing impact. It is important to many people (workers, their families, etc.). As a result the issue is of increasing importance to the mass media (journals, TV, internet, etc.).
Actors in the judicial system	Psychosocial risks are increasingly having economic implications both for companies and their workers. This is likely to lead to a boost in legal cases, and on liability issues. This may form a burden to parts of the judicial system, but might be a source of potential income to lawyers.
Business consultants	As psychosocial risks are increasingly having business impacts, advising on these issues will probably not remain the exclusive domain of psychologists and occupational health and safety services. Business consultants are likely to develop a growing interest in this area.

[1] Social security arrangements differ widely across the EU. This implies variations in the exact nature of their stakes.

[2] The societal arrangements for the insurance of health care cost differ widely across the EU. As a consequence there are variations in the stakes of the health insurers.

Table 16.3   Health and Business Benefits to Workers of Investing in Psychosocial Risk Management

Type of benefits	Health and well-being of workers	Broader benefits to workers
Fewer problems (and associated costs)	Lower stress Improved health	Better work–life balance Increased work ability and employability
Personal benefits (and added values)	Longer healthier work life Better well-being	Increased self-esteem Increased job security Sense of being valued Better satisfaction Better quality of life

Main societal impacts of psychosocial risks emerging from enterprises

In the previous section the involvement of stakeholders and their stake in psychosocial risk management were clarified. It is also important to assess the impact on workers' health and well-being. While it is important for managers to have a "business case" for psychosocial risk management, it is similarly important to have a "personal case" for workers.

Participants observed that enterprises could do more in regard to the responsible and effective management of contemporary issues such as restructuring, organizational change, and work organization. Worker participation in such processes, skills training, improvement of systems to promote better work–life balance, etc. were discussed. As one participant commented:

> There is a need to change today, in terms of current jobs and even when changing jobs; it is reality and needed, but then it must be managed in a responsible way. If people are informed and are assisted, for example, in finding new jobs, or helped with developing new skills, if it is managed in a responsible way then there is a possibility that then they may manage the change more effectively.

Participants also discussed the advantages of linking psychosocial risk management and CSR in relation to workers' health and work–life balance (see Table 16.3.).

Participants reported that engaging in responsible business practices that incorporated psychosocial risk management would likely lead to low levels of work-related stress and related problems among employees and thereby contribute to creating a healthier work life for them, and one in which they enjoyed high work ability and employability. Other related benefits for employees were reported to include more secure jobs, as the risk of absence owing to sickness was reduced, thereby reducing the fear of lost wages. Also, effective changes in work organization, such as flexible schedules, were expected to help improve work–life balance for employees. Employees were also expected to experience better well-being and lead happier lives owing to improved physical and mental health.

Indicators for CSR and psychosocial risk management

The indicators developed are meant to give a strategic overview of the development of psychosocial risk management, using potential synergies with CSR at the enterprise level. Findings indicate that, by and large, all respondents found all the indicators relevant. Sixteen of the 27 indicators that were developed and piloted were found useful for benchmarking at the enterprise level from business network participants (see Table 16.4.).

Table 16.4   CSR Indicators Considered Relevant and Useful for Benchmarking at Enterprise Level

Area	Reasons for indicators in this area	Indicators
Integration into the *systems and structures of business operations*	Both psychosocial risk management and CSR need to be integrated into the companies' business processes. Integration and implementation in existing management systems and structures are key in this respect.	The enterprise has management information on psychosocial risk management (as part of normal business control or a management system in place). The enterprise has an explicit policy to address (prevent, reduce, control) psychosocial risks (and comply with legal obligations). The system for managing psychosocial risks is also relevant and used in cases of reorganization and restructuring. The enterprise has a code of conduct for psychosocial issues. The enterprise has a code of conduct for violence, harassment and bullying. The enterprise has systems for raising harassment, bullying or other psychosocial risk issues confidentially. Company guidance or guidelines on the prevention of psychosocial risks and the promotion of mental health are available.

Table 16.4   (*Cont'd*)

Area	Reasons for indicators in this area	Indicators
Integration into the *company culture*	Both psychosocial risk management and CSR need to be integrated into the companies' business processes. Besides systems and structures, it is a matter of (company) values and culture and "how things are done around here".	Leadership is trained and developed to prioritize psychosocial issues and address them openly as a preventive mechanism. Notification of incidents (e.g. aggression and harassment) is encouraged (it is rewarded, and does not lead to blame). There is active open internal and external communication on psychosocial problems and preventive actions (transparency).
Integration into *learning and development of the organization*	Both CSR and psychosocial risk management are not time limited projects, but rather represent ongoing journeys, where learning adaptation and continuous improvement are key.	All incidents of violence and harassment are recorded and analyzed, and the lessons learned are communicated. The enterprise has a system in place to evaluate interventions on psychosocial risks. Individual workers get feedback on problems notified and solutions proposed or implemented.
Integration into *dialogue with stakeholders*	Stakeholder involvement is key in CSR; it is also useful beyond the social partners that are part of the OHS/psychosocial risk management tradition. External stakeholders as identified in this chapter all have a stake in psychosocial risk management and may help enterprises in one way or another to further develop it.	The enterprise has an internal reporting system in place on psychosocial problems, which is linked to internal planning and control cycle and to external reporting (e.g. in CSR report). The enterprise has identified its main stakeholders in psychosocial issues (e.g. government, social partners, (social) insurance agencies, NGOs, etc.) and has regular dialogue with them.
Explicitly *addressing ethical aspects and dilemmas*	Ethical issues and ethical behavior are vital in CSR as well as psychosocial risk management. Explicitly addressing ethical dilemmas is important for developing ethical awareness and behavior both at individual and company level.	People are trained to use conflicts at work in a positive way (to overcome problems and turn them into productive experiences).

Some participants suggested that the indicators must include the critical aspect of the level of implemented actions. Further, it was considered important that a company had policies, codes of conduct, and guidelines to address psychosocial issues. It was also suggested that differences between small and large enterprises should be considered. A participant advised that a database ought to be created to assist with benchmarking. Building such a database would allow the reliability and robustness of the indicators to be tested. Some respondents also expressed the need for clearer definitions in the form of standards. Whether the organization includes psychosocial risk management indicators within the regular employee attitude survey routine was suggested as a potential indicator, as was active open and external communication of the results of employee attitude surveys.

Discussion

The findings from the focus groups highlighted a number of important issues in relation to the link between psychosocial risk management and CSR. While there was unanimous agreement that CSR and responsible business practices were an important issue in relation to psychosocial risk management, the concept might not be clearly understood in all companies. Lack of clarity might lead to different and/ or unclear practices. These findings are similar to those from previous research by Segal et al. (2003) who, in a study of the link between CSR and working conditions, found that the concept of CSR was still relatively unfamiliar. The findings from the focus groups also indicated that, although companies engage in responsible/good business practices, these are not always encapsulated within the CSR framework, which again confirms previous findings (Leka & Churchill, 2007; Segal et al., 2003). Adopting a single definition of CSR (Blowfield & Frynas, 2005; Kok et al., 2001) and raising awareness of the benefits of engaging in responsible business practices would help improve understanding of the concept. The EU definition of CSR could potentially be accepted as the common definition.

The findings indicated that even though all the tripartite partners accepted that the internal dimension of CSR was related to psychosocial risk management, the "win–win" situation, where employers would voluntarily implement policies to promote workers' health with a view towards the creation of business benefits, often discussed by trade unions and employers alike, still seems very distant. This can potentially be due to variance in the use of the CSR term.

Participants highlighted that in addition to raising awareness of psychosocial issues, a clear business case for psychosocial risk management has to be developed and disseminated to employers.

Findings from the focus groups indicated that participants supported the view that linking psychosocial risk management and CSR had numerous advantages. Engaging in psychosocial risk management was considered to benefit both the business and the employee in terms of reduced sickness absence, reduced employee turnover, reduced health insurance costs, reduced early retirement, increased job satisfaction, and increased work commitment, which would lead to further reductions in organizational costs due to knowledge retention, lower staff turnover, and resulting reductions in training and recruitment costs leading to the much discussed "win–win" situation.

The findings also indicated that engaging in responsible business practices that incorporated psychosocial risk management was considered to contribute to long-term stability for the business, a better public image, and improved employer reputation, which would, in turn, help attract and retain the best employees. In spite of the known and accepted benefits of engaging in psychosocial risk management, many organizations still do not have policies in place to promote such practices; the lack of availability of a common framework for action and unavailability of easy to use tools and standards may contribute to the status quo.

Conclusion

On the basis of the work focusing on CSR and psychosocial risk management conducted through the PRIMA-EF project, a number of opportunities for future activities can be identified. First, it is important for further guidance and standards to be identified and indicators to be formalized and used. These will generate clarity among enterprises and policy makers and facilitate benchmarking. It will then be possible for appropriate actions to be taken to address gaps in practice. These tools should be promoted across experts, practitioners, enterprise networks, government officials, and policy makers and could be also used as an awareness-raising tool. In addition, more effort should be dedicated to raising awareness generally and to involving a wider range of stakeholders, including nontraditional stakeholders. Further research should be conducted into defining the business case for psychosocial risk management, as well as into addressing ethical dilemmas in the psychosocial risk management process. Perhaps the most important challenge, however, lies in instilling a change in perspective so that businesses come to see psychosocial risk management as part of good business practice. A CSR-inspired approach, underpinned by legislation, can prove useful towards this end.

References

Blowfield, M., & Frynas, J. G. (2005). Editorial: Setting new agendas: Critical perspectives on corporate social responsibility in the developing world. *International Affairs, 81*(3), 499–513.

Bondy, K., Matten, D., & Moon, J. (2004). The adoption of voluntary codes of conduct in MNCs: A three country comparative study. *Business & Society Review, 109,* 449–78.

Carroll, A. B. (1999). Corporate social responsibility: Evolution of a definitional concept. *Business & Society, 38*(3), 268–295.

Cowe, R. (2003, October 30). A magnifying glass on businesses' impact. *Financial Times,* 14.

CSR Europe (2000). *Communicating corporate social responsibility.* Brussels: CSR Europe.

EU-OSHA (2002). *Corporate social responsibility and work health*. Conference proceedings— Summary of a seminar organized in Brussels (1 October 2001) by the European Commission and the European Agency for Safety and Health at Work, Forum 3. Bilbao: European Agency for Safety and Health at Work.

European Commission (2001). *Promoting a European framework for CSR,*(green paper). Luxembourg: Office for Official Publications of the European Communities.

European Commission (2002). *Adapting to change in work and society: A new Community strategy on health and safety at work 2002–2006*. Communication from the Commission. COM(2002) 118 final. Brussels: European Commission.

European Multi-stakeholder Forum on CSR (2004). Corporate Social Responsibility – Final results and recommendations. Retrieved from http://ec.europa.eu/enterprise/csr/documents/29062004/EMSF_final_report.pdf

European Social Partners (2004). *Framework agreement on work-related stress*. Brussels: European social partners—ETUC, UNICE (BUSINESSEUROPE), UEAPME and CEEP. Retrieved from http://ec.europa.eu/employment_social/news/2004/oct/stress_agree ment_en.pdf

Hammer, N. (2005). International framework agreements: Global industrial relations between rights and bargaining. *Transfer, 11(4)*, 511–530.

Health and Safety Executive (HSE) (2005). *Promoting health and safety as a key goal of the Corporate Social Responsibility agenda*. Research Report 339. London: HSE.

ILO (2007). *Promotion of the tripartite declaration of principles concerning multinational enterprises and social policy*. Geneva: International Labour Organization.

Jones, T. M. (1980). Corporate Social Responsibility: Revisited, redefined. *California Management Review, 23*, 59–67.

Kok, P., van der Wiele, T. , McKenna, R., & Brown, A. (2001). A CSR audit within a quality management framework. *Journal of Business Ethics, 31*, 285–297.

Leka, S., & Churchill, J. (2007, May). The responsible business agenda: Healthy workers and healthy organisations. Paper presented at the 13th European Congress of Work and Organisational Psychology, Stockholm.

Marginson, P. (2006, March). Transnational agreements in enterprises: The current state of play. Paper for Colloquium on Transnational Collective Negotiations, Europe et Société, Paris.

Moir, L. (2001). What do we mean by corporate social responsibility? Corporate Governance. *International Journal for Effective Board Performance, 1*(2), 16–22.

Moon, J. (2007). *Business and government*. In B. Galligan and W. Roberts (Eds.), *The Oxford companion to Australian politics*, Melbourne: Oxford University Press.

Schoenberger-Orgad, M., & McKie, D. (2005). Sustaining edges: CSR, postmodern play, and SMEs. *Public Relations Review, 31*(4), 578–583.

Segal, J. P., Sobczak, A., & Triomphe, C. E. (2003). *CSR and working conditions*. Dublin: European Foundation for the Improvement of Living and Working Conditions.

World Business Council for Sustainable Development (2000). *Corporate social responsibility*. Retrieved from www.wbcsd.org/web/publications/csr2000.pdf.

Zwetsloot, G. (2003). From management systems to corporate social responsibility. Special issue on Corporate Social Responsibility, *Journal of Business Ethics, 44*, 201–207.

Zwetsloot, G., & Starren, A. (2004). *Corporate social responsibility and safety and health at work*. European Agency for Safety and Health at Work. Luxembourg: Office for Official Publications of the European Communities.

17

Risk Factors, Consequences, and Management of Aggression in Healthcare Environments

Benjamin Brooks
University of Tasmania, Australia

Alice Staniford
PKF Organization Development

Maureen Dollard and Richard J. Wiseman
University of South Australia

Introduction

Internationally, violence is known to be a significant problem in many work environments. In particular, violence against medical staff[1] is an increasing problem in healthcare workplaces, the rate of violent incidents being particularly high in emergency departments and mental health units (Benveniste, Hibbert, & Runciman, 2005; Bowers et. al., 2007).

Healthcare workers are even more likely to be assaulted at work than prison and police officers (International Council of Nurses [ICN], 2007), and also experience more damaging consequences from such incidents than employees in other occupations. Typically, such incidents are underreported within organizational safety management and clinical incident systems. The obvious danger, however, is that the violence becomes "normalized" within the system and tolerated at levels which then significantly increase the emotional demands and stress for these occupational groups (Dollard, LaMontagne, Caulfield, Blewett, & Shaw, 2007). Lack of action could also lead to repeat offenses and escalation of violence. The "epidemiology" or the "who, why, when, and where" of these incidents and injuries is central to controlling the problem. However, there are inconsistencies in the aggregated data associated with aggressive incidents and injuries.

In this chapter we provide a comprehensive review of the international scientific and policy literature on workplace aggression and aggression management in the healthcare sector. Specifically, we examine risk factors, consequences of aggression-related incidents, and injury within the healthcare system. Within this context we also interrogate a workers' compensation claims data set from 2000 to 2004 for public hospitals in one

Australian jurisdiction to explore and elaborate the issues further. We used evidence derived from these sources to build a layered approach to the problem we refer to as the "Culture, Prevention, Protection, and Treatment (CPPT) model". Advice is provided on how to address the cultural environment in which these aggressive incidents occur.

Defining Aggression and Associated Concepts

The behavioral definition of workplace aggression is not straightforward. It occurs on a continuum, ranging from threats (physical and verbal) at one end, to acts resulting in death at the utmost extreme (Wilkinson, 2001). Behaviors may be termed aggressive based on the nature of the behavior itself, and/or its *outcome*. There are also differences in terminology used across the literature. The terms "aggression" and "violence" are often used interchangeably. In addition, whether or not a behavior is classified as aggressive is influenced by many situational and personal variables, for example, attitudes, cultural backgrounds, and operational approaches (Jackson, Clare, & Mannix, 2002).

Given these complexities, the meanings and classifications of aggression ascribed to behavior will vary dependent on location and situation. In a 2005 study, Rumsey and colleagues contended that no single definition applies to all workplaces and situations everywhere (Rumsey, Foley, Harrigan, & Dakin, 2005).

Aggressive or violent acts include *both* physical and nonphysical (e.g., verbal, threatening) behaviors. This is a consideration that some aggression response procedures currently do not account for. For example, NIOSH (2002, p.1) describes workplace violence as "violent acts (including physical assaults and threats of assaults) directed toward persons at work or on duty." It is suggested, however, that an expanded definition describing recognizable features of violent acts is more functional for use in policy. Broad definitions accommodate the full scope of circumstances in which an employee could be assaulted at work or in other situations related to their job (Leather, 2002).

Workplace aggressive behavior may be defined as "incidents perceived or real to individuals, when they are abused, threatened or assaulted in circumstances arising out of, or in the course of, their employment, involving an explicit or implicit challenge to their safety, health and/or wellbeing" (Department of Health Western Australia, 2004, p. 9). According to the U.S. Department of Justice (2004), workplace violence can be classified into four broad categories according to the nature of the perpetrator and the circumstances of the violence. They are:

Type 1. Violent acts by criminals who have no rightful affiliation with the work place, but enter with intent to commit a crime such as theft.
Type 2. Violent acts directed at employees by those who receive services from the organization (e.g., customers, clients, patients, or students).
Type 3. Violence against co-workers, supervisors, or managers by a present or former employee, also known as "horizontal" violence (Rumsey et al., 2005)

Type 4. Violence committed in the workplace by someone who is not employed there, but who has a personal relationship with an employee, e.g., an abusive spouse or domestic partner.

For the purpose of the literature review, Type 2 workplace violence is the focus of investigation, although behavioral definitions and prevention and management strategies for Type 2 may also apply to the other three types. The workers' compensation data considered in this paper includes both Type 2 and Type 3. It is not clear from the data whether Type 4 incidents are also included; however, these are considered to generally be a low percentage of all aggressive incidents in occupational environments.

Literature Search Strategy

To locate the literature used in this review, 25 electronic databases were searched, along with public domain search engines.[2] The search terms used included any or all of the following words or phrases: nurses, doctors, medical staff, health personnel, patients, workplace, hospital, emergency department, ER, psychiatric, mental health, mental health unit, violence, aggression, aggressive incidents, accident, distress, fatigue, job satisfaction, engagement, turnover, retention, risk, incident, accident, safety, quality assurance, quality care, quality indicators, accident prevention, policy, safety system, management, risk management, clinical risk, outcome assessment/methods, hospital/standards, staff supervision, clinical governance, education. Literature was included in the review only if it was

- published in 2001 or later[3]
- written in English
- related to the search terms (see above)
- a review, empirical research paper, report, guideline, policy statement, or case study.

Similarly, literature was included if it explored one or more of the following:

1. preconditions, antecedents, or risk factors for aggressive incidents and their association with staff or patient safety (such as injury, harm, preventable adverse events)
2. best practice principles or strategies for the management of aggression or violence in healthcare settings or other industries
3. consequences of aggressive incidents in the workplace
4. proposes/reviews/outlines existing or future safety systems, policies, programs, or education in relation to managing workplace aggression (beyond the scope of this chapter, but the subject of a further paper by the authors).

Literature related solely to violence directed at staff by another employee or supervisor (including bullying) was not included, although the issue clearly remains a significant one in healthcare and other industries (Dollard et al., 2007). Literature related specifically to incidents where the aggressor had no rightful association with the workplace and where the attack was carried out with the intention of stealing cash or something else of value was also not included (Type 1 workplace violence from US Department of Justice definitions above). The literature was categorized in two summary tables: one for scientific literature, and a second for policy or guideline documents. The tables were used as a quick reference, summary, and record of all papers used to inform the literature review.

Analysis of Workers Compensation Claims Data

This chapter also analyses workers' compensation claims data from an Australian jurisdiction, provided to the lead author in 2007. Between 2000 and 2004 there were 2,141 recorded claims within the Industry Code "Hospitals (Excluding Psychiatric Hospitals), Non-Private Sector". This data set was sorted according to the "Mechanism of Injury" (noting that this category has recently been amended to "Mechanism of Incident") (Australian Safety and Compensation Council, 2008). The mechanism of injury is briefly described as: "the mechanism or process that best describes the circumstances in which the injury/disease occurred" (ibid., p. 10). Filtered from the data-set for further analysis were 293 claims with the following codes:

- '24' Being hit by a person accidentally
- '29' Being assaulted by a person or persons
- '82' Exposure to workplace or occupational violence
- '83' Harassment
- '84' Work pressure
- '86' Other mental stress factors
- '98' Other and multiple mechanisms of injury
- '99' Unspecified mechanisms of injury.

The reason for including this broad list of codes is based on work that demonstrates coding errors exist in this type of data (Brooks, 2007). All claims were reviewed manually, with particular emphasis on the free-text component of the record, which describes the accident in limited detail. Records were excluded if they did not meet the definition of "workplace violence" described in Figure 17.1., below. One hundred and one claims were removed from the data set, leaving 182 claims for analysis. The dataset was then interrogated to provide basic information on a range of demographic and injury-specific issues, and has been integrated throughout the literature review to enhance understanding of the issue.

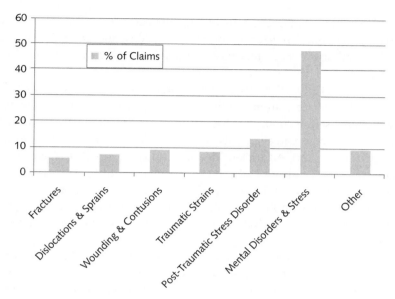

Figure 17.1   Claims by Nature of Affliction for Aggressive Incidents in Public Hospitals of One Australian Jurisdiction, 2000–2004

Consequence of Aggressive Incidents

The consequences of occupational violence are varied and far-reaching. Consequences range in severity on both personal and organizational/industrial levels.

Personal consequences

Incidents involving aggression can result in physical harm or injury and/or psychological and emotional harm to those involved. Overall, the literature shows that physical consequences can range from small injuries (e.g., minor wounds and bruises) to major injuries or even death. Psychological consequences range from shock or short-term distress, to more severe and far-reaching psychological stress that may result in the individual requiring psychological help and/or leaving his or her job (Rew & Ferns, 2005). Evidence indicates that extreme harm is infrequent, yet has recently been on the increase (Cole, 2005; Department of Human Services Victoria, 2005a). Multiple or recurring incidents can result in more severe outcomes (Lam, 2002).

Psychological and emotional harm experienced often appears to be more enduring, yet less obvious to observers, and can affect multiple areas of the employee's life (Rew & Ferns, 2005). An Australian study by Lam (2002) concluded that frequent exposure to aggressive patients is "detrimental" to the mental health of nurses. Forty percent of participants in the study experienced psychological distress after involvement in an aggressive incident, and nearly 10% experienced moderate to severe depression. Long-term psychological consequences may also include trauma-induced disorders such as post-traumatic stress disorder (PTSD) (Hogh & Viitasara, 2005).

As described in Figure 17.1., psychological injury, such as stress and PTSD, were identified as the most common *"Nature of Affliction"*. This category is intended to identify the most serious injury or disease sustained or suffered by the worker. The classification is based on an aggregated version of the International Classification of Diseases (tenth revision)–Australian Modification (ICD-10-AM) (Australian Safety and Compensation Council, 2008). PTSD, mental disorders, and stress represent almost 60% of all injuries in this dataset. The implication is that we should provide a much greater emphasis on the psychological health of workers regularly exposed to aggressive incidents, as it is psychological health that appears most affected by the incidents.

Adverse emotional reactions are also often a consequence of involvement in violent incidents. In 2004, Astrom et. al., conducted a study to investigate the emotional reactions among staff who had experienced violence in residential community care for the elderly. It was found that 97 of 848 staff (11.4%) had been exposed to violence, and the most frequently reported reactions among employees were anger, surprise, and antipathy against the perpetrating patient, as well as insufficiency, powerlessness, insult, and fear. A majority of the incidents were judged as intentionally initiated by the care recipient.

The reactions of employees may vary according to the individual, the nature of the incident, and the extent to which the person is directly or indirectly involved (Department of Consumer and Employment Protection (Western Australia), 2006). In an Australian study by Hegney, Eley, Plank, Buikstra, and Parker (2006), in which nurses were interviewed about their behavioral reactions to workplace violence, it was found that nurses responded to the experience of aggression in a variety of ways. This included taking sick leave or stress leave, using alcohol or drugs, and leaving the profession. All of these reactions can be personally damaging if misused or used for the wrong reasons, and may also affect the quality of care given to patients (Lee, 2006).

Organizational and industrial consequences

In healthcare environments where there are regular and frequent incidents of patient violence, organizational culture and general workplace morale can be adversely affected. Healthcare workers also commonly face a number of industry-specific workplace stressors that may make coping with violent incidents more difficult or stressful. For example, time-critical tasks, heavy workloads, personnel shortages, less predictable client (patient) behavior, and serious or life-threatening consequences of error (Hegney, et al., 2006; Reason, Carthey, & de Leval, 2001). High levels of work-related stress are reported in the sector partly due to the emotional demands arising from dealing with dangerous and violent clients (Dollard et al., 2007). Client-initiated

violence is a common experience particularly for those in emergency service departments, mental health units, drug and alcohol clinics, and in the aged care industry,
and is associated with increased levels of stress (Mayhew & Chappell, 2003b).

For many healthcare staff, and indeed those who do not work in healthcare, violence at work has become accepted as a typical feature of the job (Chang, Hancock,
Johnson, Daly, & Jackson, 2005). In a study by Boyd (2002) investigating emotional
labour in human service industries, it was found that many staff felt customer violence was "part of the job" they had to endure, leading workers to experience low
morale. Low nursing morale has been found to correlate with (among other things)
poor workplace safety and high work stress (Day, Minichiello, & Madison, 2007;
Hegney, et al., 2006).

These unfavourable features of organizational culture can produce broad-ranging
consequences for both individual institutions and the healthcare industry generally.
Consequences may include: an increased cost to the healthcare system, loss of experienced nurses from the workforce, increased staff absence from work, poor efficiency and performance at work, reduced staff numbers leading to increased pressure
on those staff left to cope, higher incidence of patient and family member complaints, litigation, higher likelihood of dissatisfaction felt by patients and staff, security costs, damage to equipment and other property, unfavourable reputation for the
institution and/or healthcare industry, and poor patient ratings of patient care quality (Arnetz & Arnetz, 2002; Chapman & Styles, 2006; Daffern, Mayer, & Martin,
2003; Rew & Ferns, 2005). Another important issue faced by many healthcare institutions is the difficulty of attracting people to the healthcare workforce combined
with the declining number of enrolments in undergraduate nursing programs
(Chang et al., 2005; Jackson & Daly, 2004), and nursing shortfalls (Schubert, 2004).
Between 2000 and 2004 almost 10,000 ($n = 9964$) days of work were lost in public
hospitals of this Australian jurisdiction from RNs, ENs, and nurse managers being
injured through aggressive incidents.

Many of the organizational consequences listed above affect the organization's
fiscal position, for example; insurance claims, legal expenses, property damage, staff
replacement costs, and decreased productivity (American Nurses Association, 2007;
Smith, 2002). As mentioned previously, violent incidents can also result in personal
consequences that require time off from work duties. This ranges from a small
amount of time immediately after the incident, to extended leave which can interrupt
work for an extended period of time (Department of Consumer and Employment
Protection (Western Australia), 2006).

In the United States, the cost of violence at work has been calculated at US$35.4
billion (Di Martino, 2003). In the Australian workers' compensation dataset used in
this chapter the average claim cost (based on claims that were lodged between 2000
and 2004) calculated at the start of 2007 was AUS$ 14,175 or approximately US$
11,660. This is likely to rise slightly given that 18% of claims remained opened (and
therefore payments were likely to rise for those claims). Open claims can be divided
into two categories—those that have remained open (12.6%) and those that have been
closed, then reopened at a later date (5.4%). This suggests that one in twenty claims for

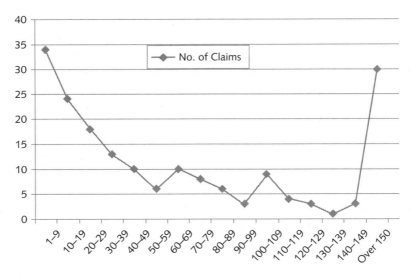

Figure 17.2 Days Compensated for Claims Involving Aggressive Incidents in Public Hospitals of One Australian Jurisdiction, 2000–2004

injuries/illness associated with aggressive incidents will "relapse" within 6 years post-claim. If the number of days compensated (and away from work) can be taken as an extremely crude measure of injury severity, then this also reveals something about the nature of these claims. While the way the categories have been presented in Figure 17.2. amplifies the long or "tail" claims, it demonstrates that 27.5% of claims involving aggressive incidents result in more than 3 months away from work.

Risk Factors, Preconditions, and Antecedents

Increased aggression in healthcare may reflect increased violence in society, making this a very complicated problem to tackle (Australian Patient Safety Foundation [APSF], 2004). However, the development of empirical knowledge about the issue has highlighted the risk factors for patient aggression. This makes it possible to clearly identify which areas should be targets for prevention and intervention.

Importantly, differences have been found between employees' and patients' perceptions of the risk factors that make patient initiated violence more likely. For example, in a study by Duxbury and Whittington (2005), patients and nurses from three in-patient mental healthcare wards were surveyed to examine perspectives on the causes of patient aggression and the way it is managed. It was found that patients perceived environmental conditions and poor communication to be the main antecedents of aggressive behavior, while nurses viewed the patients' mental illnesses to be the main reason for aggression (Duxbury & Whittington, 2005). These differences may be due to the fundamental attribution error; the theory that those being aggressive perceive environmental conditions as causal factors, while those being abused consider it a function of the person being aggressive (Samuels, 2005). Alternatively, it may also be argued that aggressive incidents are in fact preceded by a *combination* of factors; some latent (systemic), and others active (human) (Reason, 2004). Many studies have examined incident rates and gathered information from healthcare staff to show that among healthcare institutions there are a variety of patterns of risk factors or preconditions for patient-initiated violence. Next we discuss risk factors identified in a range of categories comprising the industry, organizational, job-related, and situational factors, and personal characteristics.

The industry

Statistical evidence indicates that employees who experience the largest number of patient initiated aggressive incidents are those in healthcare occupations (U.S. Department of Justice, 2004). Healthcare workers are even more likely to be assaulted at work than prison and police officers (ICN, 2007). Healthcare workers also experience more damaging consequences from such incidents. The prevalence of injury resulting from violence to healthcare workers is more than double the frequency than for employees in other industries (Bureau of Labor Statistics [U.S.], 2005). In fact, verbal and physical abuse is a problem faced by members of the healthcare profession worldwide (AbuAlRub, Khalifa, & Habbib, 2007; ICN, 2007; Lawoko, Soares, & Nolan, 2004).

Organizational factors

The literature is clear that, in addition to the risk posed by merely being a healthcare organization, there are some specific organizational features which may affect the likelihood of patient initiated violence occurring. First, public sector healthcare institutions may be more at risk than private sector institutions. In a study by Hegney and colleagues (2006), it was found that public sector nurses reported a higher percentage of incidents where the source of violence was a patient or a visitor/relative, compared to private sector nurses. This may be because public institutions are perhaps more likely to have inadequate staffing and patient overcrowding, care more often for patients in low socioeconomic categories, and deal with patient substance misuse on a regular basis.

Geographical location is also a risk factor. Remote regional hospitals have been found to be more at risk of violence, particularly at night (APSF, 2004). In a study by Schantz and Meacham (2003), the mean number of experiences of violence was higher among rural than urban practitioners. Rural practitioners also reported significantly higher levels of knowledge of fellow employees working in threatening environments, of others who had experienced violence, and of workers who had been injured due to patient aggression (Schantz & Meacham, 2003). It is also possible that the isolation of rural practitioners may exacerbate the negative psychological consequences of these experiences (Allan, Crocket, Ball, Alston, & Whittenbury, 2007), and that workload (through lack of on-call replacements) increases exposure.

In addition to geographical location, there are types of healthcare units or departments that may be more at risk of aggressive patient incidents. In 2004, an APSF summit identified that units which posed a high risk for patient initiated violence were areas where workers had lower control over events. Settings included ambulances, hospital accident and emergency departments, methadone clinics, psychiatric facilities, and locked dementia wards (APSF, 2004). Interestingly, maternity and paediatric wards were also listed as high-risk areas as most are generally not specifically designed to protect workers against violent patients or their relatives. Aged care facilities, long-term care wards, and acute care wards (Camerino, Estryn-Behar, Conway, van Der Heijden, & Hasselhorn, 2008; Daffernet al., 2003; Hegney, et al., 2006) have also been identified as high-risk locales for patient aggression.

Characteristics of the organizational culture may also influence the occurrence of patient-initiated aggressive incidents. Lack of policies for preventing and managing crises involving volatile patients may be a risk factor for higher severity of consequences (NIOSH, 2002). Additionally, safety climate may be an underlying influence on incident frequency and severity. Hegney and colleagues (2006) found that poor perception of workplace safety was significantly correlated with a high incidence of reported violence. Spector, Coulter, Stockwell, & Matz (2007) found similar outcomes when they adapted the concept of safety climate to violence in developing the concept of perceived violence climate in a study of 200 nurses in a US hospital.

Job-related factors

Particular occupational roles within healthcare are more at risk of exposure to violence than others. Nurses have been found to be at particular risk (Findorff, McGovern, Wall, Gerberich, & Alexander, 2004; ICN, 2007; U.S. Department of Justice, 2004). Nurses are usually the first point of contact for new patients, in their most agitated state. Nurses themselves also often feel that violence is "part of the job" (Boyd, 2002). The normalization of these risks is a reoccurring theme in healthcare environments, and is taken up in the discussion on safety culture and psychosocial safety climate.

Hegney et.al. (2006) indicate that enrolled nurses (ENs) tend to report more frequent incidences of violence than registered nurses (RNs), particularly in aged care settings. Others in healthcare who experience violence on a regular basis include doctors, psychiatrists, psychologists, social workers, mental retardation specialists, substance abuse counsellors, nurses and aides who take care of psychiatric patients, people on emergency medical response teams and those who work in admissions, emergency departments, and crisis or acute care units (U.S. Department of Justice, 2004).

High levels of contact with patients can increase the likelihood of experiences with physical violence among all types of medical staff (Findorff et al., 2004). Perhaps contrastingly, however, it has been found that people working in a permanent part-time capacity, as opposed to casual or permanent full-time, are more likely to experience aggressive incidents (Hegney et al., 2006). Supervision can also reduce the risk of exposure to violence in healthcare. If there is a moderate or high level of supervisor support, risk of violent incidents is less (Findorff et al., 2004).

The Australian jurisdiction's public hospital workers' compensation data may counteract some of these findings. As indicated in Figure 17.3., RNs represent almost 50% of the injuries in the period between 2000 and 2004, with no other single occupational group accounting for more than 10% of the injuries, and all groups except for clerks, receptionists and secretaries accounting for less than 5%. Medical practitioners were not excluded, but were not represented in the data set. Medical practitioners are clearly not immune from exposure to aggression. Possible explanations for their absence from the claims data include being less likely to report injuries, higher perceived and/or actual resilience to psychological injury, or having better access to support resources if an assault occurs. As mentioned above, it is also likely that nursing staff spend a significantly higher proportion of time in contact with patients and their families and therefore have a significantly higher exposure to aggressive incidents.

Situational factors

In general, violent incidents occur when workers are performing their routine tasks (U.S. Department of Justice, 2004). High-risk duties may include handling, carrying, or having access to items of value (e.g., drugs or money); caring for people who are distressed, anxious, in pain, or incarcerated; transporting patients; lifting objects onto high places; caring for people who have unreasonable perceptions of what the organization can provide; carrying out procedures which are unpleasant or painful; and working alone (Mayhew & Chappel, 2001; NIOSH, 2002).

Features of the environmental space may also influence risk of aggressive incidents. Such features include areas with inadequate security; overcrowded waiting rooms and smoking areas; uncomfortable temperature (especially heat); inadequate lighting in corridors, rooms, parking lots, and other areas; high numbers of beds in each room; a ward/unit layout in which beds are in close proximity; lack of privacy; and excessive noise (both common noises such as radios or people shouting, and unexpected noise such as squeaking doors, door bells, or other patients making noise late at night) (Daffern et al., 2003; HCC, 2005; NIOSH, 2002). Additionally, off-site visits to client homes can also put healthcare workers at more risk, as can emergencies where staff must work in car parks or ambulance bays, particularly in high-crime areas (Mayhew & Chappel, 2001a).

There may also be time-related risk factors. There are particular times of the week at which aggressive incidents have been found to be more frequent. In a study by Bowers and colleagues (2007), the number of patient-initiated violent incidents was found to

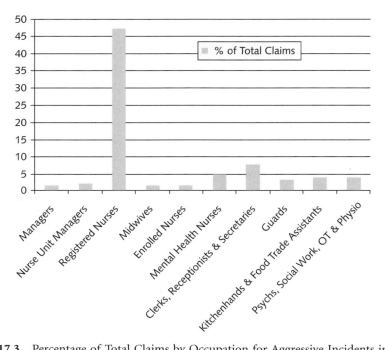

Figure 17.3   Percentage of Total Claims by Occupation for Aggressive Incidents in Public Hospitals of One Australian Jurisdiction, 2000–2004

be lower on weekends and at midweek. Additionally, there were more incidents reported on the days before and after ward rounds but fewer on ward-round days.

Time of day may also influence the occurrence of patient-initiated aggressive incidents; however the literature is conflicting on this issue. Some authors have proposed that night time presents a higher risk of violence than other times of day (NIOSH, 2002; Mayhew & Chappel, 2001; Rumsey et al., 2005; Schantz & Meacham, 2003). However, a psychiatric hospital study in Victoria found that there was an approximately even rate of incidents reported between the hours of 9:00 a.m. and 11:00 p.m. and that no aggression occurred between midnight and 5:00 a.m. This may not be generalizable to other types of institutions (Daffern et al., 2003). Other times found to predict a higher occurrence of patient violence are during mealtimes and visiting hours (NIOSH, 2002).

As shown in Figure 17.4., this Australian public hospital claims data shows a spike in aggressive incidents between the hours of 6:00 a.m. and 10:00 a.m., with injuries tapering off from that point and reaching their lowest levels between 10:00 p.m. and 6:00 a.m. The data should be viewed cautiously as some injury time-values may have been arbitrarily assigned for the purposes of the claim form.

Other situational triggers of aggressive incidents include times when there is understaffing and associated long waits for service; limited security support (e.g., security staff are busy elsewhere); unrestricted movement of the public; inadequate

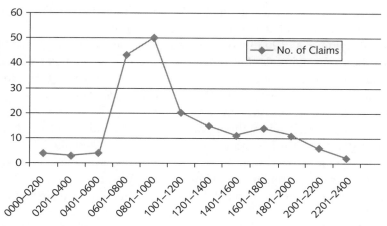

Figure 17.4 Reported Time of Injury for Claims Involving Aggressive Incidents in Public Hospitals of One Australian Jurisdiction, 2000–2004

communication between staff or between staff and patients; lack of teamwork; uncertainty concerning patients' diagnoses/treatment; general confusion over responsibilities; demanding client mix; overcrowding; patients misunderstanding medical staff intentions; difficult journeys to hospital or clinic; and theft of personal belongings among patients or by outsiders (ACSQHC, 2003; Benveniste et al., 2008; HCC, 2005; NIOSH, 2002; Rew & Ferns, 2005).

Certain violence control strategies may also increase the risk of further aggressive incidents occurring. It has been found that in psychiatric hospitals, the use of isolation to control aggressive or potentially aggressive patients may contribute to more frequent aggression and injury to staff (Daffern et al., 2003). This is because staff are physically assaulted more frequently during restraint than by direct assault. Restrictions such as denial of freedom or denial of services can affect the way patients and staff interact, and this change may induce a higher tendency for aggression in both parties (Duxbury & Whittington, 2005).

Personal characteristics

Characteristics of perpetrators
Due to space limitations the review of personal characteristics has been truncated. The reader is directed to the references identified within the section below for further information. Characteristics that have the potential to increase the risk of aggressive incidents include:

- comorbidities (e.g., renal problems and psychoses associated with drug dependence that dictate a reduced security-level for a patient at certain stages of treatment)
- personal circumstances (e.g., pain, substance addictions), demographic factors, and behavioral history, poor coping skills and social skills, lack of self-confidence

and self-esteem (Rew & Ferns, 2005). People with low self-confidence may also be more easily intimidated by other service users (HCC, 2005)

- medical conditions including organic brain disorders (e.g., Parkinson's disease, dementia), schizophrenia and other psychotic illnesses, bipolar disorder, and personality disorders (e.g., antisocial personality disorder) (Department of Human Services [Victoria], 2005; Oster, Bernbaum, & Patten, 2001)
- low score on the Global Assessment of Functioning (GAF) scale used to rate the social, occupational and psychological functioning of adults (Oster et al., 2001). (Noting that situational agitators are also an influence: Nijman, 2002)
- patients regaining consciousness postoperatively, suffering hypoxia or with acute brain trauma (Department of Human Services [Victoria], 2005)
- perceived stigmatization by mental health patients due to their mental illness (Lawako et al., 2004)
- frustration with relationships external to the care environment (e.g., family or relationship problems, criminal issues) (HCC, 2005)
- alcohol abuse and recreational drug use. These are key contributors to violence in hospital emergency departments (APSF, 2004)
- nonsmoking patients who may be frustrated by others' smoking behavior (HCC, 2005)
- negative or uncomfortable side effects, difficulties with treatment compliance, and changes to medication regimes (HCC, 2005)
- prolonged or intense pain (Rew & Ferns, 2005)
- low socio-economic background or those who feel they are marginalized in society have been considered a risk factor (Chappel & Mayhew, 2001), although this has been disputed by authors such as (Daffern et al., 2003; Oster et al., 2001; Winstanley & Whittington, 2002)
- gender seems an unreliable indicator (see Winstanley & Whittington, 2002; Daffern et al., 2003—but see Oster et al., 2001 for a conflicting view).

Of all categories of risk factor, the best predictor of violence may be a prior record of violent behavior, and/or a history of drug and alcohol abuse on the part of the patient (Department of Human Services [Victoria], 2005; NIOSH, 2002; Oster et al., 2001). Some researchers define two distinct types of perpetrator: those with a violent history who may then be expected to behave aggressively, and those who are violent in certain situations, for example, when frustrated by denial of services or medication (Mayhew & Chappel, 2001a). Control strategies should therefore vary between these two groups.

In addition to patient risk factors, there are several immediate predictors of aggression that may be identified by observing patient behavior. Luck, Jackson, and Usher (2007) used qualitative techniques to study these predictors among patients in an ED department in a large Australian hospital. They described observable behavior indicators for potential violence in patients and patient visitors using the acronym STAMP: Staring and eye contact, Tone and volume of voice, Anxiety, Mumbling, and Pacing. These predictors have been used as a potential violence

assessment framework for medical staff and included in training programs for identifying violence (Luck et al,, 2007; Rew & Ferns, 2005).

Characteristics of staff
There may also be certain classes of individuals more likely to be involved in aggressive incidents as victims. The personal characteristics of staff involved in patient initiated violent incidents have been widely researched. Some of the findings include:

- Patients and visitors felt that some staff attitudes and the way they interact with
  patients triggered violent incidents HCC (2005). This included being patroniz-
  ing to patients, being overly custodial, and behaving impolitely or rudely towards
  patients.
- Findings detailing dihfferences in incidents based on staff gender are mixed.
  Some studies suggest elevated levels of males (Daffern et al., 2003) and this has
  been supported by Lawako et al. (2004). Data collected from the Victorian public
  hospital system counteracts these findings. 83.5% ($n = 152$) claims were made by
  females and 16.5% of claims were made by males.

Of the claims in this data set 55% were made by RNs or accounting clerks, receptionists and secretaries. Based on Australian Census data from 2006, 91.6% of registered nurses in Victoria are female (13,455 of a population of 14,690). For
occupational groups "accounting clerks, receptionists and secretaries", females constituted 94.5% of the population (15,236/16,120) in the 2006 census. Although
females are overrepresented in the number of claims based on proportion of males
to females in the general population, the percentage is roughly consistent with the
ratios of females to males in the main occupational groups. In other words there was
no effect due to gender.

HCC (2005) and the ACSQHC (2003) provide evidence that there may be a higher
risk of violence towards staff who are less experienced and therefore have less developed skills. Temporary staff may also be more at risk (ACSQHC, 2003). In opposi-
tion to this however, it has been found in a study based in the UK with psychiatric
wards that when a group of new and inexperienced staff arrived on the wards there
was *no* associated increase in the occurrence of violent incidents (Bowers et al.,
2007). Perhaps those with longer-term experience in high-stress healthcare environments may be burnt out and have reduced personal resources to respond with empathy and care. However, more research is needed in this area.

The public hospital workers' compensation claims data does not necessarily support the assertion that experience reduces the incidence of aggression. The correlation between age of injured employee and severity of injury (in terms of days away
from work) was $r = 0.05$, suggesting virtually no correlation between age and severity. Although not a definitive indication of expertise, older staff are likely to be more
experienced. As highlighted earlier, RNs account for a much higher percentage of
injuries caused by aggressive incidents, and may also be more experienced than
other nurses (such as ENs).

Modeling and Managing Aggressive Incidents

To fully understand the various sources of influence on the propensity for violence among perpetrators it is important to consider the numerous influences on an individual's behavior and the way they interact. The World Health Organization (WHO, 2004) used an ecological model to illustrate that no single factor can explain why some people or groups are at higher risk of interpersonal violence than others. The model depicts interpersonal violence as the result of an interaction among a range of contributing factors at four different levels: the individual, the relationship, the community, and the societal (WHO, 2004). All of the risk factors discussed above fit into this model.

The model reflects the notion that most perpetrators of violence will have been exposed to a number of different environmental influences, both from their immediate environment (relationships) as well as from the wider community and society they live in. This is also consistent with the concept within safety science of an "organizational accident" wherein active failures (violent events) have a range of latent conditions (influences) (Reason, 2004). Combined with this are personal experiences and internal characteristics that may invite or precipitate violent behavior (WHO, 2004). Leather (2002) supports this view, which he terms a social interactionist perspective on violence. From this perspective, aggressive behavior is viewed as a potential outcome of negative interpersonal interactions rooted in the broader social and organizational context. It is suggested that such an understanding of the nature of personal risk factors for violence allows prevention and management strategies to be more comprehensive.

The model demonstrates that there are a number of risk factors at each of the four levels. Societal factors influence whether violence is encouraged or inhibited. Community contexts in which social relationships occur (such as schools, neighbourhoods, and workplaces) also influence the likelihood of violence. Adoption of attitudes and behavior from personal relationships such as those with family, friends, intimate partners, and peers can also influence aggressive tendencies. Finally, at the individual level, personal history and biological/personality factors influence how individuals behave.

Healthcare institutions, by necessity, have many defences, barriers, and controls designed to shield potential victims from these risk factors (Reason, Carthey, & de Leval, 2001). However, even in a well defended system, there is some chance that an incident will occur. James Reason used the analogy of layers of swiss cheese, to illustrate how holes in an organization's defenses can align to allow a hazard to pass through multiple layers of defense, resulting in losses (e.g., aggressive incidents and their consequences). The more defenses and the greater the comprehensiveness of the system, the less likely it is that the "holes" or defensive gaps and weaknesses, occur together in a way that allows an incident to happen (Reason, Carthey, & de Leval, 2001). Some of the holes in defenses are due to the active failures (or errors) of front line staff, for example, forgetting to respond to a patient's request (Reason, 2004). Other holes are caused by latent organizational factors or error producing conditions (pathogens) in the workplace, for example, reducing the number of staff in the ED on weekends, or a poorly designed piece of equipment or procedure (Reason, 2004).

From this perspective, safety management become a process of finding the holes in defenses, and building stronger and more effective safeguards. These safeguards should be both individual/team defenses *and* systemic defenses (Reason, 2004). These defenses are designed to reduce the occurrence of failures, and better protect the system when inevitable failures occur (Reason et al., 2001). This approach is not new, but perhaps the extent of the necessary layers of defense is important to spell out in the context of managing aggression-related risks in healthcare environments.

From the literature and data explored in this chapter it is possible to take the concept of a layered approach to this issue and identify the various layers both before aggressive incidents occur and those required as responses when incidents do occur. This is represented in our Culture, Prevention, Protection, and Treatment (CPPT) model (see Figure 17.5.).

Space limitations within this volume limit the discussion of the components of the safety management system with respect to violence and aggression. For more detailed discussions about these issues the reader is directed to several key documents (ILO, 2002; Occupational Safety and Health Administration, 2003; Occupational Health and Safety Agency for Healthcare, 2005; Wiskow, 2003). In a comparative analysis of major national guidelines and strategies from the United Kingdom, Australia, Sweden, and the USA, Wiskow (2003) effectively summarizes the necessary safety management approach to manage aggression in the workplace:

> Common sense is the recommendation of a multi-component, organization-wide strategy, based on a systematic risk management approach, including risk assessment, risk reduction and review of the strategy. RCN/UK in difference to the others propose a systematic approach, not only addressing the tasks and roles at all organizational levels but also including a wider view on the organization as an integral part of the community. (p. 31)

More specific information is also available on issues such as training (Grenyer et al., 2004) and integrated Aggression Management Programs (AMPs) that describe the components necessary for such programs and offer critical evaluation of known programs against a range of criteria (Farrell & Cubit, 2005).

Discussion

While it is clear that injury caused by aggressive incidents is a significant problem in healthcare environments, the findings of a comprehensive literature review on the epidemiology or the *who, where, when, and how* of these injuries were sometimes contradicted by the workers' compensation data interrogated in this study.

This data suggests that psychological injury: mental disorders, stress, and PTSD, are by far the most significant injuries caused by aggressive incidents. It further

Level	Aim	Strategy Areas	
SUPPORT STRATEGIES	*CULTURE* Encouraging a societal and organizational climate that underpins the entire program	Public Awareness	Gaining community support through development of a communication and public awareness campaign with a variety of partners such as the police, media, and victim support centres.
		Organizational Culture & Climate	Creating and maintaining an organizational climate that supports the goals of the anti-violence program by using principles of organizational justice in all policy and procedures, and measuring and building psychosocial safety climate, ensuring effective communication and collaboration with employees, and management commitment.
PRIMARY	*PREVENTION* Reducing opportunity for violent incidents to occur	Environment & Equipment Design	Making changes to physical aspects of the environment including layout and design of buildings, and the equipment and furniture within. Referred to as 'Crime prevention through environmental design' (CPTED), this strategy aims to minimise the likelihood and costs of violence.
		Job and Task Design	Altering job designs and staffing patterns to reduce situations where staff at higher risk of violence.
		Staff Training and Education	Strengthening the capacity of individual staff members to prevent/ respond to violence in an educational program covering training in post-incident action, response, prevention, and theory.
SECONDARY	*PROTECTION* Implementing effective response strategies	Emergency Situation Response	Planning and educating staff on response strategies for when violence occurs or is imminent to help manage incidents safely and protect people involved.
TERTIARY	*TREATMENT* Abating the impact following violence and learning from incidents	Incident Reporting	Implementing an effective and well used incident reporting system to provide a means of assessing risk and effectiveness of management strategies, and learning form events.
		Support for Victims	Post-incident follow-ups, debriefing and evaluation to support victims and help them to cope after they have been involved in an incident.

Figure 17.5 CPPT Model of Intervention Layers for the Prevention and Management of Aggression

suggests that registered nurses are by far the largest occupational group injured through aggressive incidents, and that almost 85% of injuries are to women, as might be expected given their dominant representation in the industry as registered nurses. Comparing data available in the literature and current dataset, it is not clear whether there is a peak exposure time during the day for aggressive incidents or whether age or experience alter injury and incident rates. There is clearly more research needed to make definitive statements about these possible risk factors.

What to Do?

We propose a model for the management of risks associated with aggressive incidents, the Culture, Prevention, Protection and Treatment (CPPT) model. It reflects Reason's (1997) Swiss-cheese model of accident causation and addresses the WHO's ecological model of risk factors by recommending a layered approach to risk management. The primary and secondary layers, and the associated risks and consequences have been described earlier. We have not previously discussed cultural issues in any detail. It is to this layer of the model that our attention now turns.

Organizational justice

Organizational justice refers to employees' perceptions of *fairness* in their organization in terms of its systems, procedures, and treatment of personal needs and concerns. Employees value fairness in the outcomes of decisions as well as fairness in the procedures used to reach those outcomes (Krause, 2005).

It is logical to suggest that a just culture is a foundation on which to build cultural elements such as informedness (how much everyone knows about risks, health, and safety) and reporting (how prepared people are to report occupational health and safety issues and how comprehensive those reports are). A just culture refers to the use and acceptance of organizational justice principles (particularly procedural justice) and represents "the way things are done" in an organization. A just culture accepts the inevitability of human error and does not punish honest mistakes, but it does discipline unacceptable behavior.

In this type of environment employees are willing to come forward in the interests of system safety and at the same time understand that unacceptable behaviors warrant disciplinary or enforcement action. Visitors need to be brought into this just culture environment, to acknowledge that there are acceptable and unacceptable patterns of behavior, but also to recognize that they have certain rights and responsibilities. There are at least two sound, competing tools for the investigation of incidents that follow just culture principles (see Outcome Engineering, 2007; Reason 1997). An organization should embed a just culture otherwise attempts to improve knowledge (e.g., through reporting aggressive incidents) are likely to fall short.

Engage the community and address organizational values

The WHO model clearly identifies that violent behavior does not only emerge because of the acute stress created in healthcare environments, and the literature demonstrates that certain individuals are more likely to act aggressively. Public awareness of the standards of behavior required in hospitals must be known before people find themselves in stressful situations where aggressive actions may result. Mass media public awareness campaigns and targeted campaigns through police, victim support centres, and other community centres should be an on-going part of the latent defense against these incidents.

We have also mentioned the possibility that people in healthcare facilities accept elevated levels of aggression. So called normalization can sometimes be a function of gender (e.g., male or macho interpretation of resilience to aggression), workload (reporting incidents of a low severity takes time that we don't have), or post-event rationalization (clients must be forgiven because they are under significant pressure, are injured, or sick). The professional imperative to care for the sick and infirm also cannot be discounted as a major driver in the acceptance of risk. For a number of risks—fatigue is another good example—the trade-off between occupational health and safety and clinical risk often finds the healthcare employee on the wrong side of the ledger. This is not a criticism of organizations or individuals, but a reflection of the challenge associated with addressing issues that go to the very core of why people choose this vocation and what function these organizations serve in our society.

Measure and manage the psychosocial safety climate (PSC)

The claims data has highlighted the dominance of psychological injury with respect to aggressive incidents. It is logical to then suggest that healthcare organizations need to address psychosocial safety climate. Psychosocial safety relates to *freedom* from psychological and social risk or harm. Psychosocial safety climate (PSC) is defined as policies, practices, and procedures for the protection of worker psychological health and safety (Dollard, 2007). We see low PSC as *the* preeminent psychosocial risk factor at work, preceding a range of psychosocial risk factors (see Dollard & Bakker, in press), including aggression. We argue that in order to reduce psychological and social harm, PSC should be targeted. Increasing PSC would be a useful strategy to prevent aggression from occurring in the first place, to overcome the culture of acceptance and normalization, and to ensure that policies and practices are in place to assist workers once assaulted.

Building PSC is described in detail elsewhere in this volume (see the chapter by Dollard and Karasek). Specifically here it relates to building policies, practices, and procedures to prevent aggression and should include the following principles: (1) senior management show support for aggression prevention through involvement and commitment; (2) participation and consultation in occupational health and safety issues related to aggression occurs with employees, unions, and occupational health and safety representatives; (3) the prevention of aggression involves all layers of the organization; (4) contributions aimed at resolving aggression concerns in the organization are listened to; (5) workers are encouraged to report and are prepared to report; (6) there is good communication about risks, health, and safety; (7) action is taken to discipline unacceptable aggressive behavior—but does not publish honest mistakes; (8) the public is fully informed about the high PSC standards in relation to aggressive behavior in the healthcare setting, including their own rights and responsibilities; and (9) comprehensive reporting and monitoring systems are developed to identify and control antecedents.

Conclusions

In conclusion, there is still more to be learnt about the risk factors associated with aggression-related incidents and injuries in healthcare environments. There are inconsistencies in the epidemiological data that, if resolved, will offer a better indication of where to focus preventive and injury management activity. It is important to recognize that claims data are lag indicators and represent the consequences, rather than the source of the problem. Ideally, evidence-based interventions for workplace aggression require the identification of factors that precede the aggression and which are amenable to change. An example of such a lead indicator is PSC. It will be important to determine whether factors such as age, experience, gender, occupation, and time of day are indeed risk factors worthy of further consideration and control. Further research is required to test the relationship between organizational justice, PSC, and the incidence of aggression and subsequent psychological injury.

Any sound approach to workplace health and safety issues addresses both proximate and distal causes, building defenses at all levels. The latent defenses to these incidents should include public awareness campaigns that take the message outside the hospitals and other care facilities to the broader community. The data analysed in this study suggest that cultural programs should devote more time to both preventing incidence and also nurturing the psychological health of employees such that they are resilient to, recover from psychological injury, and do not suffer a relapse. Ultimately, programs to address aggression-related injury are likely to meet resistance in the form of risk normalization and risk acceptance. Such programs have the potential to challenge deeply held assumptions about the relationship between the organization, employee, and client and as such require multi-layered approaches to maximise the likelihood of success. We conceived the Culture, Prevention, Protection and Treatment (CPPT) model as a useful way to conceptualise such an approach.

Notes

1. Includes doctors, nurses, midwives, managers, surgeons, anaesthetists, physicians, allied health professionals, and other medical professionals.

2. Academic Search Elite, Academic Search Premier, AGIS Plus Text, Australia/New Zealand Reference Centre, Australian Industrial Relations Database (IREL), Australian Public Affairs – Full Text (APA-FT), CINAHL, Clinical Reference Systems, EJS E-Journals, ERIC, Health Business Fulltext Elite, Health Source – Consumer Edition, Health Source: Nursing/Academic Edition, Humanities & Social Sciences Collection, MasterFILE Elite, MasterFILE Premier, MEDLINE, Pre-MEDLINE, Pre-CINAHL, Professional Development Collection, PsychARTICLES, PsychINFO, Psychology and Behavioral Sciences Collection, Rural and Remote Health Database (RURAL), WORKLIT. In addition to the academic databases listed, internet search engines 'Google Scholar' and 'Google' were also used.
3. Exception is made when a theory or concept originating from before 2001 is referred to.

References

AbuAlRub, R. F., Khalifa, M. F., & Habbib, M. B. (2007). Workplace violence among Iraqi hospital nurses. *Journal of Nursing Scholarship, 39*(3), 281–288.

Agency for Healthcare Research and Quality. (2003). *Patient safety indicators, version 2.1.* Rockville, MD: Agency for Healthcare Research and Quality.

Allan, J., Crocket, J., Ball., P., Alston, M., & Whittenbury, K. (2007). 'It's all part of the package' in rural allied health work: A pilot study of rewards and barriers in rural pharmacy and social work. *The Internet Journal of Allied Health Sciences and Practice, 5*(3), 1–11.

American Nurses Association. (2007). *Workplace violence.* Retrieved from www.nursingworld.org/MainMenuCategories/ANAPoliticalPower/State/StateLegislativeAgenda/WorkplaceViolence.aspx

Arnetz, J. R., & Arnetz, B. B. (2001). Violence towards health care staff and possible effects on the quality of patient care. *Social Science & Medicine, 52,* 417–427

Astrom, S., Karlsson, S., Sandvide, A., Bucht, G., Eisemanne, A., Norberg, A., & Saveman, B. (2004). Staff's experience of and the management of violent incidents in elderly care. *Scandinavian Journal of Caring Sciences, 18,* 410–416.

Australian Commission for Safety and Quality in Health Care. (2003). ...

Australian Patient Safety Foundation. (2004). *Summit May 2004: Aggression and violence in the health care workplace.* Retrieved from www.patientsafetyint.com/events.aspx?ID=13

Australian Safety and Compensation Council (2008). *Type of occurrence classification system,* third ed. Canberra: Australian Safety and Compensation Council.

Benveniste, K. A., Hibbert, P. D., & Runciman, W. B. (2005). Violence in health care: the contribution of the Australian Patient Safety Foundation to incident monitoring and analysis. *Medical Journal of Australia, 183*(7), 348–351.

Bowers, L., Jeffery, D., Simpson, A., Daly, C., Warren, J., & Nijman, H. (2007). Junior staffing changes and the temporal ecology of adverse incidents in acute psychiatric wards. *Journal of Advanced Nursing, 57*(2), 153–160.

Boyd, C. (2002). Customer violence and employee health and safety. *Work, Employment and Society, 16*(1), 151–169.

Brooks, B. P. (2007) Shifting the focus of strategic injury prevention: mining free-text workers compensation claims data. *Safety Science, 46*(1), 1–21.

Bureau of Labor Statistics (United States). (2005). *Workplace injuries and illnesses in 2005.* Retrieved from www.pathfndr.com/bls2005.pdf

Camerino, D., Estryn-Behar, M., Conway, P. M., van Der Heijden, B. I. J. M., & Hasselhorn, H. (2008). Work-related factors and violence among nursing staff in the European NEXT study: A longitudinal cohort study. *International Journal of Nursing Studies, 45,* 35–50.

Chang, E. M., Hancock, K. M., Johnson, A., Daly, J., & Jackson, D. (2005). Role stress in nurses: Review of related factors and strategies for moving forward. *Nursing and Health Sciences, 7,* 57–65.

Chapman, R., & Styles, I. (2006). An epidemic of abuse and violence: Nurse on the front line. *Accident and Emergency Nursing, 14,* 245–249.

Cole, A. (2005). *Four in five nurses on mental wards face violence.* Retrieved from www.bmj. com/cgi/content/full/330/7502/1227-a

Daffern, M., Mayer, M. M., & Martin, T. (2003). A preliminary investigation into patterns of aggression in an Australian forensic psychiatric hospital. *The Journal of Forensic Psychiatry & Psychology, 14*(1), 67–84

Day, G., Minichiello, V., & Madison, J. (2007). Nursing morale: Predictive variables among a sample of registered nurses in Australia. *Journal of Nursing Management 15,* 274–284

Department of Consumer and Employment Protection (Western Australia). (2006). Bullying and violence. *Frequently asked questions.* Retrieved from www.safetyline.wa.gov.au/newsite/worksafe/content/topics/violence/violindx0003.html#B2

Department of Health (Western Australia). (2004). *Prevention of workplace aggression and violence.* Retrieved from www.health.wa.gov.au/publications/documents/Prevention_of_Workplace_Aggression.pdf

Department of Human Services (Victoria). (2005). *Occupational violence in nursing: An analysis of the phenomenon of patient aggression and code grey/black events in four Victorian hospitals.* Victorian Government DHS, Melbourne. Retrieved from www.health.vic.gov.au/nursing/downloads/codeblackgrey.pdf

Di Martino, V., (2003). *Relationship of work stress and workplace violence in the health sector.* Geneva: Joint Programme on Workplace Violence in the Health Sector, ILO, WHO, ICN & PSI.

Dollard, M. F. (2007). *Psychosocial safety culture and climate; Definition of a new construct.* Work & Stress Research Group, University of South Australia, Adelaide.

Dollard, M. F., & Bakker, A. B. (in press). Psychosocial Safety Climate as a precursor to conducive work environments, psychological health problems, and employee engagement. *Journal of Occupational and Organizational Psychology.*

Dollard, M. F., LaMontagne, A. D., Caulfield, N., Blewett, V., & Shaw, A. (2007). Job stress in the Australian and international health and community services sector; A review of literature. *International Journal of Stress Management, 14,* 417–445.

Duxbury, J., & Whittington, R. (2005). Causes and management of patient aggression and violence: staff and patient perspectives. *Journal of Advanced Nursing, 50*(5), 469–478.

Farrell, G., & Cubit, K. (2005). Nurses under threat: A comparison of content of 28 aggression management programs. *International Journal of Mental Health Nursing, 14,* 44–53.

Findorff, M. J., McGovern, P. M., Wall, M., Gerberich, S. G., & Alexander, G. (2004). Risk factors for work related violence in a health care organization. *Injury Prevention, 10,* 296–302.

Grenyer, B., Ilkiw-Lavalle, O., Biro, P., Middleby-Clements, J., Comninos, A., & Coleman M. (2004). Safer at work: development and an evaluation of an aggression and violence minimization program. *Australian and New Zealand Journal of Psychiatry, 38,* 804–810.

Health Care Commission (HCC). (2005). *National audit of violence—Final report (2003–2005).* Retrieved from www.healthcarecommission.org.uk/_db/_documents/04017451.pdf

Hegney, D., Eley, R., Plank, A., Buikstra, E., & Parker, V. (2006). Workforce issues in nursing in Queensland: 2001 and 2004. *Journal of Clinical Nursing 15*, 1521–1530.

Hogh, A., & Viitasara, E. (2005). A systematic review of longitudinal studies of nonfatal workplace violence. European Journal of Work and Organizational Psychology, *14(3)*, 291–313.

International Council of Nurses (ICN). (2007). *Fact sheet: Violence a world wide epidemic.* Geneva: ICN. Retrieved from www.icn.ch/matters_violence.htm#top

Jackson, D., Clare, J., & Mannix, J. (2002). Who would want to be a nurse? Violence in the workplace—a factor in recruitment and retention. *Journal of Nursing Management, 10*, 13–20.

Jackson, D., & Daly, J. (2004). Current challenges and issues facing nursing in Australia. *Nursing Science Quarterly, 17*, 352–355.

Krause, T. R. (2005). The safety leadership model, part 3: Understanding organizational culture and safety climate. *Leading With Safety*, Chapter 4, 59–81. Retrieved from www3.interscience.wiley.com/cgi-bin/booktext/112149875/BOOKPDFSTART

Lam, L. T. (2002). Aggression exposure and mental health among nurses. *Australian e-Journal for the Advancement of Mental Health (AeJAMH), 1*(2), 1–12. ISSN: 1446–7984. Retrieved from http://auseinet.flinders.edu.au/journal/vol1iss2/lam.pdf

Lawoko, S., Soares, J. J. F., & Nolan, P. (2004). Violence towards psychiatric staff: a comparison of gender, job and environmental characteristics in England and Sweden. *Work & Stress, 18*(1), 39–55.

Lee, D. T. F. (2006). Violence in the health care workplace. *Hong Kong Medical Journal, 12*(1), 4–5.

Leather, P. (2002). Workplace violence: Scope, definition and global context. In C. Cooper & N. Swanson (Eds.). *Violence in the health sector: State of the art*, 3–18. Geneva: International Labour Organization. Retrieved from www.icn.ch/state.pdf

Luck, L., Jackson, D., & Usher, K. (2007). STAMP: Components of observable behaviour that indicate potential for patient violence in emergency departments. *Journal of Advanced Nursing, 59*(1), 11–19.

Mayhew, C., & Chappel, D. (2001a). *Occupational violence: Types, reporting patterns, and variations between health sectors*, Discussion Paper no. 1. University of New South Wales: Working Paper. Retrieved from www.health.nsw.gov.au/policy/cmh/publications/violence/DiscussionPaper1.pdf

Mayhew, C., & Chappell, D. (2003b). The occupational violence experiences of 400 Australian health workers: An exploratory study. *The Journal of Occupational Health and Safety—Australia and New Zealand, 19*(6), 3–43.

National Institute for Occupational Health (NIOSH). (2002). *Violence: Occupational hazards in hospitals.* DHHS (NIOSH) Pub. No. 2002 101. Retrieved from www.cdc.gov/niosh/2002-101.html

Nijman H. L. I. (2002). A model of aggression in psychiatric hospitals. *Acta Psychiatrica Scandinavica, 106*, 142–143.

Occupational Safety & Health Administration (OSHA). (2003). *Guidelines for preventing workplace violence for health care and social service workers.* Retrieved fromwww.osha.gov/Publications/osha3148.pdf

Occupational Health & Safety Agency for Healthcare (OHSAH). (2005). *Preventing violent and aggressive behaviour in healthcare: A literature review.* Retrieved from www.ohsah.bc.ca/media/130-ID-Workplace_Violence_Literature_Review.pdf

Oster, A., Bernbaum, S., & Patten, S. (2001). Determinants of violence in the psychiatric emergency service. *Canadian Medical Association Journal, 164*(1), 32–33.

Outcome Engineering. (2007). *Just culture: Training for healthcare managers.* Plano, TX: Outcome Engineering.

Reason, J. (1997). *Managing the risks of organizational accidents.* Aldershot, UK: Ashgate.

Reason, J. (2004). Beyond the organisational accident: The need for "error wisdom" on the frontline. *Quality and Safety in Health Care, 13*, 28–33.

Reason, J., Carthey, J., & de Leval, M.R. (2001). Diagnosing "vulnerable system syndrome": An essential prerequisite to effective risk management. *Quality in Health Care, 10*(2), ii21–ii25.

Rew, M., & Ferns, T. (2005). A balanced approach to dealing with violence and aggression at work. *British Journal of Nursing, 14*(4), 27–232.

Rumsey, M., Foley, E., Harrigan, R., & Dakin, S. (2005). *National review of violence in the workplace.* Deakin West, ACT: Royal College of Nursing Australia.

Samuels, S. M. (2005). A social psychological view of morality: Why knowledge of situational influences on behaviour can improve character development practices. *Journal of Moral Education, 34*(1), 73–81.

Schantz, D., & Meacham, M. (2003). Client-initiated violence directed toward staff. *Rural Society, 13*(1), 54–71.

Schubert, M. (2004). Big nursing shortage ahead states warn. *The Age.* Retrieved from www.theage.com.au/articles/2004/06/25/1088144974353.html?oneclick&oneclick=t

Smith, M. H. (2002). Vigilance ensures a safer work environment. *Nursing Management, 33*(11), 18–19.

Spector, P. E., Coulter, M. L., Stockwell, H. G., & Matz, M. W. (2007). Perceived violence climate: A new construct and its relationship to workplace physical violence and verbal aggression, and their potential consequences. *Work & Stress, 21*(2), 117–130.

U.S. Department of Justice, Federal Bureau of Investigation. (2004). Introduction: What is Violence?. *Workplace Violence: Issues in Response*, 11–14.

Wilkinson, C. W. (2001). Violence prevention at work: A business perspective. *American Journal of Preventive Medicine, 20*(2), 155–160.

Winstanley, S., & Whittington, R. (2002). Violence in a general hospital: Comparison of assailant and other assault-related factors on accident and emergency and inpatient wards. *Acta Psychiatrica Scandinavia, 106*(412), 144–147.

Wiskow, C. (2003). *Guidelines on workplace violence in the health sector. Comparison of major known national guidelines and strategies: United Kingdom, Australia, Sweden, USA, (OSHA, and California).* Geneva: Joint Programme on Workplace Violence in the Health Sector, ILO, WHO, ICN & PSI.

World Health Organization (WHO). (2004). *Preventing violence: A guide to implementing the recommendations of the world report on violence and health.* Retrieved from http://whqlibdoc.who.int/publications/2004/9241592079.pdf

Author Index

Subject Index